DIMENSIONS of COMMUNITY HEALTH

DIMENSIONS of COMMUNITY HEALTH

Second Edition

Dean F. Miller

University of Toledo

ωcb
WM. C. BROWN PUBLISHERS
DUBUQUE, IOWA

Book Team

Editor *Chris Rogers*
Developmental Editor *Sue Pulvermacher-Alt*
Designer *Carol S. Joslin*
Production Editor *C. Jeanne Patterson*
Photo Research Editor *Carol M. Smith*
Marketing Manager *Kathy Law Laube*

wcb group

Chairman of the Board *Wm. C. Brown*
President and Chief Executive Officer *Mark C. Falb*

wcb

Wm. C. Brown Publishers, College Division

President *G. Franklin Lewis*
Vice President, Editor-in-Chief *George Wm. Bergquist*
Vice President, Director of Production *Beverly Kolz*
National Sales Manager *Bob McLaughlin*
Director of Marketing *Thomas E. Doran*
Marketing Information Systems Manager *Craig S. Marty*
Executive Editor *John Woods*
Manager of Design *Marilyn A. Phelps*
Production Editorial Manager *Colleen A. Yonda*
Photo Research Manager *Faye M. Schilling*

Library of Congress Catalog Card Number: 87–070905

ISBN 0–697–01341–3

Printed in the United States of America by Wm. C. Brown Publishers
2460 Kerper Boulevard, Dubuque, IA 52001

10 9 8 7 6 5 4 3 2

Contents

13

Schools: Comprehensive Programs for Better Health 275

14

Health Education/Health Promotion: The Forefront of Preventive Health and Wellness 299

Unit Four
Special Target Groups 317

15

Health of Minorities: Socioeconomic Factors Affect Health Status 319

16

Child and Maternal Health: A Measure of a Community's Well-Being 337

This second edition of *Dimensions of Community Health* has been written for the individual with little or no knowledge about community health. This edition provides an overview of the field of community health, and focuses on many important community health problems and issues facing humanity in the latter part of the 1980s and into the 1990s.

This text is most timely since it discusses many significant changes that will have a direct impact on community health. Some of these changes involve the philosophical and financial foundations of community health. For example, during the 1960s and the 1970s much community health programming centered on the role of government funding and regulation. Since the early 1980s this role of government regulatory activity has been reduced in opposition to the role of pro-competition in the health marketplace. These changes have led to many program variations.

The various problems and issues discussed in *Dimensions of Community Health* focus upon three different dimensions: political, social (cultural), and economic. Each dimension is independently discussed in the first portion of the book, but integrated with other facets of community health in the remainder of the text.

The political dimension of community health, especially, has received attention in the early 1980s due to major philosophical changes in thinking, programming, and funding in community health. Certain programs considered important and necessary during the 1970s are now nonexistent or operating at a very low visibility level. A shift from federal programming to state and local responsibility for

community health activities has occurred, placing greater responsibility on state and local health agencies.

The organization of this edition of *Dimensions of Community Health* is presented in four units. The first unit introduces the reader to the various organizational structures of community health: international, national, state, and local. In unit two the various resources of community health are presented. In unit three the reader will be presented with six different areas of community health programming that usually can be found in most localities throughout the country. In unit four, several special target groups are examined for which community health programming is often of concern.

The first unit, The Community, includes presentations concerning the basic concept of "community" and an overview of federal, state and local, and international organization, activities, and programming. The added importance of state and local health department activities with the "New Federalism" of the 1980s is specially highlighted. The reader is also exposed to a broader interpretation of community, with international health problems being emphasized.

Unit two, Resources of Community Health, identifies several important factors related to the provision of health care and to carrying out programs of community health. Dramatic changes are occurring in the provision of health care in the 1980s with many different kinds of impact upon health care facilities and the provision of medical manpower. These factors are discussed in chapter 5. A new chapter on epidemiology is included in this edition.

In any kind of health program planning today the various skills and knowledge of epidemiology are needed. These matters are presented in chapter 6. With any discussion of health care the problems of escalating costs continue to have an affect. In spite of numerous attempts to bring about containment of health care costs, there has been little success. A discussion of health care costs, cost containment approaches, and the development of several alternative approaches to payment of health care costs are presented in chapter 7.

Increasing responsibility for health and social programming in this country is falling to the private sector. Chapter 8 analyzes the private sector and its role in community health. The private sector embodies business and industry, the philanthropic foundations, religious bodies, and also voluntary health organizations.

The third unit, Community Health Programming, presents six different programs that have traditionally been found in most community health organizations. Since the early days of community health in the United States, health programming has included activities to control diseases and to provide a better environmental setting. For this reason, disease control measures are presented in chapter 9 and environmental health in chapter 10. There is an expanded presentation of chronic diseases in this edition. Also, as current as is possible, matters relating to Acquired Immune Deficiency Syndrome (AIDS) are found in the chapter on disease control. The next four chapters present information concerning community nutrition, mental health, school health, and health promotion/education. In each chapter, selected problems and programs germane to the topic are noted. The impacts of political, social, and economic factors are interwoven throughout these chapters. The chapter on mental health also contains information about the homeless.

Increasing interest has developed in recent years in health promotion. This is an important part of the movement from an emphasis on curative medicine to one on health promotion and disease prevention. This important component of community health is analyzed in chapter 14.

In the last unit, Special Target Groups, are extensive discussions relating to special groups of concern in communities throughout the country.

Any student of community health or health worker can not long escape the cultural dimensions of community health. Many community health activities and programs are designed to meet the needs of different cultural populations. All too often low socioeconomic status, or poverty, has a dramatic impact on the health of many minorities. The health status of three minority populations is presented in chapter 15: blacks, Native Americans, and Hispanics. The text also covers the community health concerns of an expanding minority in the United States—refugees who have left their homeland in an attempt to find peace and stability. This influx of refugees in the past few years has introduced a variety of unique community health problems.

A review of the health status of women and infants tells much about the health situation in any specific locality. Chapter 16 presents information on maternal-child health (MCH) issues. Important concepts such as infant mortality, immunization, and contraception are presented. A matter of specific concern in communities across America in the latter part of the 1980s is the epidemic of teenage pregnancies.

At the opposite end of the life cycle from birth and infancy is old age—the senior citizen. This group is the most rapidly increasing demographic population in America today. With this in mind the need for increased thinking about care and life-style of the elderly is presented in chapter 17.

Chapters 18 and 19 present information about substance abuse—drugs, alcohol, tobacco, and occupational health and safety. Many factors that affect everyone are analyzed and discussed.

The last chapter is a new chapter in this edition on the subject of violence and its impact for community health. Initially, child abuse and neglect, spouse abuse, and elder abuse are discussed. Then concerns relating to rape are presented. The chapter ends with material about homocide and suicide.

A short epilogue is included at the end of the book. Hopefully this material will challenge the reader to consider what responsibilities and challenges there are in the field of community health.

To assist the student in the use of this text, *Dimensions of Community Health,* each chapter contains a chapter outline, a summary, discussion questions, suggested current readings, and endnotes. Most chapters also contain a short story, a case study, an inventory, or other "boxed" information that illustrates the actual workings of community health programs and workers. The charts and photographs also elaborate on textual information. Many of these have been added to this edition to assist the reader.

The dynamic, ever changing nature of community health makes it very difficult to maintain total currentness of information. During the period of time that this revision has been taking place, almost daily some news release or journal article either changes, adds to, or increases information about some concept that is presented. The reader will need to keep abreast of developments in the news as this edition serves as a foundation. Community health and health care are ever developing dynamics in the American culture.

Many individuals with whom I have had the opportunity to interact professionally have provided assistance in the development of this book. I appreciate the efforts of all who have answered my questions, sent information when requested, or just had the time to talk with me about the issues found in the book. It has been particularly refreshing to obtain important insights that keep one current as the professor works with students in internships and field experiences. Through these contacts, I have acquired an expanded view of community health and an appreciation of this dynamic, challenging field of activity.

In addition to the many opportunities in this country, my global consciousness has been expanded by working in community health projects in several countries of the world. Hopefully, this consciousness will be extended to the users of *Dimensions of Community Health.*

Thanks are extended to the many reviewers who critically appraised the text: Jacob A. Gayle, Jr., Kent State University; Dawn Graff-Haight, Eastern Montana College; Rick L. Hosler, Wilmington College of Ohio; Janine Cox, University of Kansas; Linda Olasov, Northern Kentucky University; Martha Lynn Bolt, William Rainey Harper College; and Nikki Mead, Loma Linda University. Their evaluations have helped in refining and therefore improving this publication.

At times it seems that those closest to the author, his children and wife, suffer from such a writing project. There are many hours when one is "tied" to the computer writing or in the library researching new information. I appreciate the understanding of my children, Barb and Brian, and of my wife, Karen, for their support in this experience.

D.F.M.

UNIT ONE

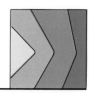

The Community

1

Health: Involvement of Community

Sally had just finished her second week as a public health nurse with the local city health department. Having worked previously in a hospital clinical setting she was not prepared for the broad range of professionals with whom she would interact at the health department. The original concept of public health as being medically oriented is a notion held by many citizens in our communities today. With each new day Sally met new persons whose work responsibilities involved a wide range of interesting activities. All of these encompass what we today know as community health.

She met a young sanitarian whose principal work focused on a rodent control program in a poor inner-city section of the city. Another colleague was conducting a series of awareness classes on the use of seat belts for various population groups. Much to Sally's amazement she learned that the funding for this work came through something called a "block grant."

Her exposure was further expanded one day when she accompanied a nutritionist to a rural community center to work with a group of migrant women. These individuals spoke very poor English. The nutritionist spoke Spanish in explaining various nutritional concepts to these women.

Traditionally, community health programs have principally been directed toward the control of communicable diseases and the improvement of the sanitary conditions of the community. The current scope of community health has broadened considerably. It includes not only these goals but also activities directed at mental health, drug and alcohol control and rehabilitation, improved nutrition, fitness and general wellness, control of chronic diseases such as heart disease and cancer, and a variety of concerns related to the provision of health care. Community health used to be the principal responsibility of the state and/or local department of health. Today numerous programs are conducted in hospitals, in nongovernmental private agencies, in schools, and in a variety of other settings. Since the health of each person has a collective effect upon the health of the community, health and well-being necessitate community involvement.

Historical Perspective

Historically in the United States, the purpose of a public health entity in a community was to prevent communicable diseases, to prevent injury, and to provide an environment free from those organisms and conditions that affected health in a negative way.

The organizations supervising such activities were usually departments of health at the local or state levels that were funded by government monies. These agencies were programmatically directed by legislative mandate and health department regulation, and employed specially skilled personnel such as public health nurses, sanitarians, and physicians.

When communicable diseases were the leading health problems and the principal causes of death, and when the environment contributed greatly to illness and debilitation, the *official health organization* was essential. In fact, in some locations health departments were in operation before statehood was achieved. An evolution in health care and a shift in attention to different health problems have brought about a broadened concept of public health. Though communicable diseases still receive community health emphasis, a different set of problems, one of which is chronic ailments, now results in morbidity and death and so demands attention. Other debilitating conditions have resulted in an expanded community involvement of many agencies, organizations, and programs, all related to the health of the general population.

The roles and responsibilities of a public health agency are no longer clearly delineated, although public health law and sanitary codes are quite specific in identifying many tasks. Previously clear distinctions between the functions of public health departments, hospitals, ambulatory care facilities, and other community health agencies are now somewhat blurred. For example, primary health tasks that were previously conducted by public health departments, voluntary health agencies, schools, and universities are now often performed by hospitals. In fact, one of the newest hospital activities is the development of wellness programs that focus upon a healthier life-style and improved well-being. These community outreach programs may involve fitness measurement and screening followed by prescribed personal exercise and nutrition programs.

Many community agencies, funded by federal or private grant monies, provide a broad range of health care services once fulfilled principally by public health departments. These new programs are not designed by, nor are they responsible to, health departments. In many communities, family planning services, mental health care, maternal and child health activities, and other services are obtainable in settings apart from private medicine and official public health structures.

Local and state health departments are involved both directly and indirectly in medical care functions. For example, they often license various health care institutions, are responsible for issuing credentials for various allied health personnel, and have responsibilities in the administration of Medicare and Medicaid. Some public health departments and public hospitals have combined their resources to provide a full range of health care in both metropolitan and rural areas.

In the early years communicable disease control was often the responsibility of the public health sanitarian. Interest in the relationship between environment and disease causation and control has resulted in a major expansion of community health programming, precipitating concern for a new range of disease problems such as those related to environment, to radiation, and to particular occupations. The Environmental Protection Agency (EPA) and various state environmental health departments provide a wide range of programming activities that focus upon these concepts.

Concept of Community

The concept of community has traditionally been limited to a political or geographical region and its respective subdivisions. In its report, the National Commission on Community Health Services referred to a "community of solution."[1] The Commission suggested that such a community was established ". . . by the boundaries within which a problem can be defined, dealt with, and solved."[2] Each health problem must be considered in light of the population involved. This concept of "community" leads to a new functional definition relating to specifically identified problems. Such a notion may find some health problems very geographically limited, while others take on global dimensions. Yet each, regardless of its magnitude, is of vital importance in attaining the goal of creating a healthy society.

This community concept is illustrated by two health problems. The first example is a common occurrence—an outbreak of a childhood disease in a local section of a metropolitan area. This type of problem is limited geographically, and the local health agency is usually able to solve the problem since the outbreak probably occurred only in a given age group of children within a single school building. The second exemplary health problem, extensive air pollution inversion, necessitates the efforts and services of a number of agencies and political jurisdictions for its resolution. This problem may affect a "community" of several hundred square miles, as is often the case in the Los Angeles area.

As the structure of community health has expanded from the traditional political and geographical entities to the concept of "communities of solution," its scope has broadened. Today, whenever a problem that relates to the health and well-being of people must be resolved, it becomes a concern of community health. Community health closely relates to the provision of health care in the nation since each community health program, activity, organization, and agency, though unique in some manner, contributes to the overall goal of wellness and positive health for all humanity.

Figure 1.1   A vast chasm separates medical technology and health knowledge from effective health care for many.

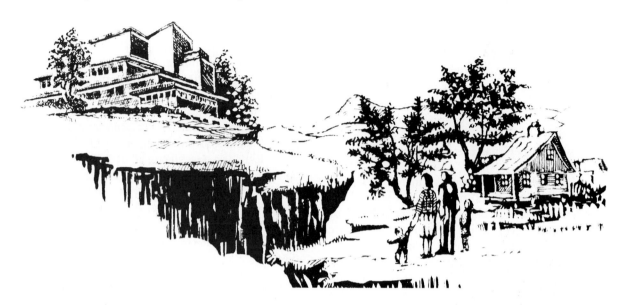

The Great Chasm

Most persons are well aware of the spectacular advances in medical science that have taken place in the twentieth century—new drugs, the control of numerous communicable diseases, body organ transplants, and highly sophisticated technological procedures. The advancement of medical and health knowledge (research and technology) improves the quality of life and has a profound effect upon millions of people throughout the world.

In spite of these developments, the provision of needed health services to multitudes of persons is far from adequate. A vast chasm separates medical technology and knowledge from effective health care for many individuals (figure 1.1). Too often efforts to bridge this chasm have been limited by inaccessible health care, the high cost of obtaining adequate health provisions, and the failure to comprehend the complex system of health and medicine.

Not only is there a notable disparity between the services offered in the United States and in less-developed countries, but even in this country many persons are unable to obtain even minimal health care. Although many reasons can be suggested why this situation exists, the limitations usually belong to one of three categories. These categories relate to the chasm separating medical and health knowledge from the provision of health services and proper effective health care. They are (1) *political considerations,* (2) *economic concerns,* and (3) *sociological* or *cultural ramifications.* Each of these dimensions, though important in and of itself, interacts with others and gives substance to community health.

Health for All by 2000

The importance of projecting long-range goals in the field of health care was highlighted by action taken in 1977 by the World Health Assembly of the World Health Organization. Recognizing the need for mobilizing various aspects of government as well as the health care field, the Assembly called for "Health for All by the Year 2000."

Implied in this declaration is that major program goals that will permit all people throughout the world to lead socially and economically productive lives must be encouraged. It means that new and creative approaches to meeting the health needs of

(a) Total national commitment in the 1960s resulted in the NASA moon expedition in 1969. The same process of goal setting, resource commitment, and national resolve could fulfill the objective of "Health for All by the Year 2000."

(b) Children in the United States and throughout the world will be the major beneficiaries of programs designed to provide "Health for All by the Year 2000."

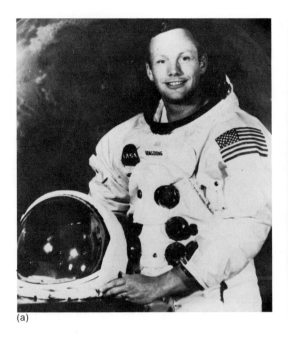

(a)

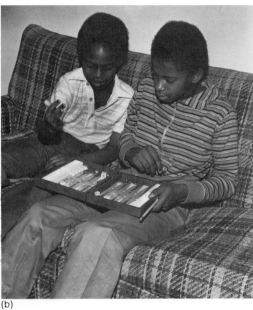

(b)

all people have to be introduced. Emphasis on curative medicine must give way to an emphasis on primary health care and preventive measures. A consideration of social problems relating to hunger, poverty, and overpopulation is needed in addition to traditional efforts at communicable disease control. Two worldwide targets to be achieved by 1990 have been identified by the World Health Organization: (1) the provision of a safe drinking water supply for everyone and (2) the immunization of all children in the world against the major childhood infectious diseases.

Governments must be willing to allocate or reallocate adequate resources for health care needs. Though most governments have been less than supportive of transferring their national resources to the health sectors, some positive measures have occurred. Many governments have reexamined their national health policies and have identified specific health problems needing attention. Reorientation of national health systems toward primary health care

has taken place.[3] Since 1984 various evaluation studies of the progress in implementing "health for all" strategies have also occurred.[4] The need now, however, is for a greater will to provide the needed resources, in terms of both economy and personnel, to achieve "health for all."

Such an international goal is only attainable if individual nations identify goals and establish plans within their countries. "Health for All by the Year 2000" will not be achieved if economic resources, political will, and cultural differences are not addressed by those involved in community health. The chasm separating optimal health care and the present health status of millions in the world must be narrowed if the World Health Assembly goal is to be reached by 2000.

The concept of "health for all," though a creation of the World Health Organization, is applicable to all nations. As an example of how important

National Goals

Populaton Group	Goals	To Fewer Than
Infants (under 1)	35% fewer deaths	9/1,000 live births
Children (1–14)	20% fewer deaths	34/100,000
Adolescents (15–24)	20% fewer deaths	93/100,000
Adults (25–64)	25% fewer deaths	400/100,000
Older Adults (over 65)	20% fewer sick days	30 sick days/year

these factors of national commitment and goal setting are, it must be remembered that in the early 1960s President John F. Kennedy committed the resources and the will of the United States to moon exploration by the end of that decade. Attainment of such a goal seemed out of the question, since no human had even been in space at the beginning of the 1960s. But after extensive economic resources and total government support were applied to the goal, on July 20, 1969, astronaut Neil Armstrong stepped onto the moon, fulfilling the objective set forth by President Kennedy less than a decade before.

National Goals for Health by 1990

If a major commitment is made to the goal of health for all, it is reasonable to suggest that such a goal is attainable. It is hoped that new directions in community health will be charted that will result in "Health for All by the Year 2000" in the United States. This commitment and planning began in 1979. After examining data concerning the leading causes of death and/or morbidity the federal government—through the Surgeon General Report on Health Promotion and Disease Prevention—issued a publication entitled *Healthy People*.[5] Specific risk factors of the leading causes of death were identified, and national goals were then established for five different age groups.

In order to reach these goals extensive professional review and discussion involving individuals and organizations from both the public (governmental) and private sectors took place for the purpose of setting specific, measurable objectives for the nation. These objectives—encompassing such concerns as premature death, diseases, and other disabling conditions—were to be the focus of community health programming for the 1980s.

Fifteen areas were identified that, with planned and appropriate action, would meet these health promotion objectives and so lead to improved health for all Americans. The fifteen health problem areas were: control of hypertension, family planning, pregnancy and infant health, immunization, sexually transmitted diseases, toxic agent control, occupational health and safety, injury control, fluoridation of drinking water supplies, control of infectious diseases, smoking, alcohol, and drug abuse, nutrition, physical fitness, and stress management. These problem areas were grouped into three categories: health services, health protection, and life-style change. In all, two hundred and twenty-six measurable objectives were identified and published.[6] It was felt that if these objectives could be achieved the health status of Americans would be greatly improved.

Two hundred and twenty-six measurable objectives were published by the Department of Health and Human Services in 1980. These objectives were categorized into fifteen different classifications. The national objectives have served as a program guideline in the 1980s.

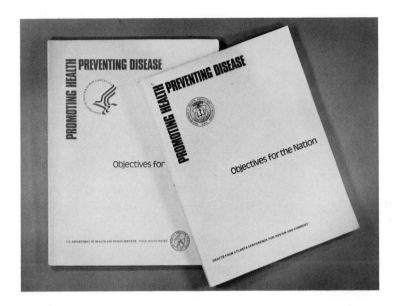

Disease Prevention and Health Promotion Objectives for the Nation

Health services
1. Control of hypertension
2. Family planning
3. Pregnancy and infant health
4. Immunization
5. Sexually transmitted diseases

Health protection
1. Toxic agent control
2. Occupational health and safety
3. Injury control
4. Fluoridation of drinking water supplies
5. Control of infectious diseases

Life-style change
1. Smoking
2. Alcohol and drug abuse
3. Nutrition
4. Physical fitness
5. Stress management

Source: Department of Health, Education, and Welfare (HEW), *Promoting Health, Preventing Disease: Objectives for the Nation* (Washington, D.C.: U.S. Government Printing Office, 1979), p. 4.

Health Objectives for the Nation

Category	Number of Objectives	Responsible Agency
Preventive Services		
High blood pressure	9	National Institutes of Health
Family planning	9	Office of Population Affairs
Pregnancy and infant health	19	Health Resources and Services Administration
Immunization	18	Centers for Disease Control
Sexually transmitted diseases	11	Centers for Disease Control
Health Protection		
Toxic agent control	20	Senior Advisor for Environmental Health
Occupational safety and health	20	Centers for Disease Control
Accident prevention and injury control	17	Centers for Disease Control
Fluoridation and dental health	12	Centers for Disease Control
Surveillance and control of infectious diseases	13	Centers for Disease Control
Health Promotion		
Smoking and health	17	Office on Smoking and Health
Misuse of alcohol and drugs	19	Alcohol, Drug Abuse, and Mental Health Administration
Nutrition	17	Food and Drug Administration
Physical fitness and exercise	11	President's Council on Physical Fitness and Sports
Control of stress and violent behavior	14	Alcohol, Drug Abuse, and Mental Health Administration

―――――

226

Source: Office of Disease Prevention and Health Promotion, U.S. Department of Health and Human Services, *The 1990 Health Objectives for the Nation: A Midcourse Review,* Washington, D.C.: U.S. Government Printing Office, November 1986.

1990 Health Objectives—A Midcourse Review

In 1986 the Department of Health and Human Services published a report of the progress that had been made in the first half of the decade toward the specific health objectives for the nation as identified in 1979. Reports were made for each of the 226 objectives. For each objective the specific objective was identified. The status as of 1985 was noted, followed with a discussion as to the likelihood of reaching the objective by 1990.

The report noted that by mid-decade 13 percent of the objectives had been reached. One-third (34.5 percent) were "on-track," with over one-fourth unlikely of achievement.

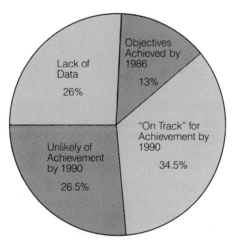

Source: Office of Disease Prevention and Health Promotion, U.S. Department of Health and Human Services, *The 1990 Health Objectives for the Nation: A Midcourse Review,* Washington, D.C.: U.S. Government Printing Office, November 1986.

These "National Health Goals for 1990" have served as major guidelines for state and local health departments, private health agencies, corporations, schools, and other health-related organizations in program development and planning. Many states have established their own state health goals to be achieved by the year 1990.

By the mid-1980s a number of reports and studies had been issued identifying what progress had been achieved.[7] For example, after examining the eleven objectives for sexually transmitted diseases, researchers reported that greater success had been made relative to gonorrhea and syphilis than to chlamydia and herpes virus.[8]

Eleven of the objectives relate to exercise and fitness. Of these, five focus on children and youth. A two-year study of some nine thousand school-age children revealed little progress toward the five objectives relative to the level of fitness for children and youth. In fact, body fat measurement was higher in youth than previously noted and 50 percent did not engage in physical activity.[9] Seventeen objectives to be achieved by 1990 in injury prevention were identified; eight related to health status and nine objectives centered on measures to reduce risk factors, to increase public and professional awareness, and to improve services and surveillance. Some progress had been noted by the mid-1980s; however, it still remained to be seen how many of these objectives could be reached by 1990.[10]

The Office of Disease Prevention and Health Promotion of the Department of Health and Human Services is charged with coordinating and monitoring progress toward attainment of the 1990 national health promotion goals. Specific activities include working with national, state, and local agencies in program development, dissemination of scientific and technical information, and the support of public information on health promotion and disease prevention. The office's activities are also conducted in cooperation with business and industry, and professional and voluntary organizations.

Plans are being implemented to continue review of the progress toward the national goals and to project ahead to the year 2000. New goals with expanded focus on health problems of the 1990s will be developed and released by the start of the last decade of this century.

Health through Prevention

As mentioned earlier, medicine has historically been oriented to *curative* measures. Throughout the United States and most of the industrial world, emphasis in health care has focused upon the treatment and cure of disease. Medical education has prepared the physician to provide service that will cure, resolve, or reduce a maladaptation, and millions of dollars are spent on facilities and equipment to provide such medical care.

In recent years, increasing emphasis is being directed toward the *prevention* of illness and disease and to the promotion of positive health and wellness. The maintenance of a high level of wellness is important to a larger segment of the American population. Individuals who are overweight are concerned about their weight and are looking for ways to reduce. In a society filled with stress-producing situations, the need and desire to find appropriate and effective ways to cope with stress are being examined. Physical fitness activities, such as jogging, bicycling, and participating in active individual sports, are yet other measures being undertaken by millions to contribute to a more positive level of wellness.

Disease prevention is primarily a personal matter. However, there are community dynamics involved in health promotion. Many environmental activities such as pollution control, provision of a pure water supply, and sewage and toxic waste disposal have preventive values for both the individual and for the community. Immunization of children for common childhood diseases also provides a preventive dimension for a community.

The Surgeon General's Report on Health Promotion and Disease Prevention noted that only 4 percent of federal expenditures for health was spent for prevention-related activities. This report pointed out three reasons for the importance of an increased emphasis on disease prevention and health promotion: (1) prevention saves lives; (2) prevention improves the quality of life; and (3) prevention is cost-effective.[11]

An important focus of preventive health care is early intervention. This may involve personal evaluation of one's life-style. It means making decisions concerning factors that contribute to illness or to poor health—nutritional patterns, smoking behavior, stress dynamics, or drinking. In addition to personal life-style, a number of environmental factors affect health. Early intervention in environmental health-hazard recognition and control is equally important in disease prevention.

A basic premise of preventive health care is that it will decrease the incidence, duration, and severity of disease. Theoretically, then, the cost of health care will be reduced and the well-being of people enhanced.

First, though, health promotion strategies must become cost beneficial for individuals, industry, and the community. Some economic incentive must be developed for health care providers to keep people well. With this in mind, hospitals are developing wellness centers or clinics where people in the community receive a variety of preventive services. These services include education, health counseling, screening for hypertension and other chronic disorders, fitness activities, and nutrition awareness.

Health insurance programs have not provided coverage for preventive health services to any great extent. So entrenched is the health insurance payment system in curative medicine that only rarely

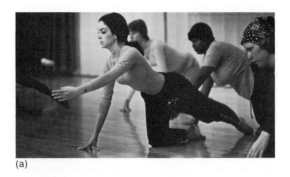

(a)

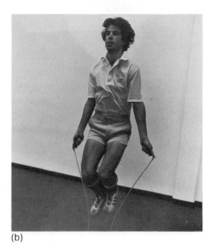

(b)

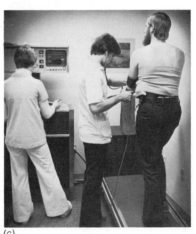

(c)

are routine physical examinations and health counseling services covered by health insurance. Increased interest in group prepaid health programs, known as health maintenance organizations, that provide an emphasis on health preventive measures has occurred in the 1980s. These organizations have economic motivators built into their programs to encourage people to maintain health and wellness.

In several states, efforts have been made to provide special tax funds to promote nonuse or better use of certain health-threatening substances. In one midwestern state, a penny state tax was added to all cigarette sales to finance the development of antismoking education programs in schools and community settings. The more cigarettes that are purchased, the more money that is made available for health promotion activities. With a reduction in cigarette purchases, less monies would be available, but it is hypothesized that the need for such activities would also be reduced. In another state, funds from the state alcohol tax revenues are appropriated for various alcohol programs, including detoxification programs and halfway houses.[12]

Emphasis on prevention creates some interesting dilemmas. Antismoking programs have been somewhat effective. Yet, until recently the federal government and many state legislators have been rather reluctant to pursue antismoking legislation.

This is due in part to the political power of the tobacco-producing industry. For example, during the administration of President Jimmy Carter the Department of Health, Education, and Welfare (HEW) pushed for antismoking legislation. But opposition from the tobacco industry and from the political leadership of the tobacco-growing states resulted in a halt to the HEW's efforts. Since that time measures taken both federally and at the state level to discourage smoking have been met with opposition by the tobacco industry. As a matter of fact, the Department of Agriculture's policy of price supports presently encourages tobacco farming.

Increased emphasis on prevention leads to improved health status. This means less need for curative medicine and the services of the medical care system. The medical profession is then forced to seek revenues for physicians and other health care providers from preventive activities. This has resulted in the development of a variety of health prevention programs by health care provider organizations.

A very important question has been raised concerning preventive health programming. Should prevention be mandated? In the view of many Americans, any preventive health activity is a private matter. A person should have a choice of whether or not to smoke, of what to eat, of whether or not to wear a seat belt when driving an automobile, or of his or her individual drinking patterns. Establishing rules that require certain behavioral patterns, though preventive in nature, is considered by many an infringement of individual rights. A clear example of this is the controversy over the helmet requirement for motorcycle riders. In the early 1970s all but three states had laws mandating that all motorcyclists wear a helmet. But public opposition to these regulations has led most states to rescind this requirement. As a result motorcycle injuries and fatalities have increased, a fact which evidently has had little impact as the issue remains controversial.

Another controversial issue centers on the fluoridation of public drinking water. It is a widely accepted fact that the fluoridation of drinking water will prevent tooth decay. Fluoridation, then, is a common procedure in many communities throughout the United States. But there are many people who are opposed to such a practice, claiming that this is an infringement of their individual rights and is in fact forced medication.

On the other hand, states require children to be immunized prior to enrolling in school. Though an occasional parent may object to this immunization requirement, most comply with little complaint. This issue, however, is somewhat different from the fluoridation and helmet controversies since it relates to the health of the general public. Others can contract communicable diseases from nonimmunized individuals, so immunization is considered by many to not be a matter of individual rights.

Obviously then, in some preventive activities public policy and mandate are viewed as appropriate; in others they are not. When and in which situations preventive health requirements and provisions are an infringement of individual rights is an ongoing debate having no easy resolution.

Another preventive health issue centers around the role of the physician or health clinic. In an interesting California court decision, the supreme court of that state ruled that a physician had an obligation to urge a woman patient to have a Pap smear test.[13] The woman had died from uterine cancer and her family had sued the physician, claiming that the physician was negligent in not insisting that the patient have the Pap test. This ruling, in favor of the family, occurred in spite of the fact that the physician had mentioned to his patient the need for such a test, but did not insist that one be given. The woman did not request the Pap test so the physician did not pursue the issue.

This court decision raises the potential for serious problems for health providers and community health workers as to how much "force" should be exerted to administer preventive measures. Historically, the physician could not insist that tests be taken; the recommendation could only be made. It was the patient who made the final decision. To what degree this court decision in California changes this traditional thinking remains to be seen.

Legislative Mandate to Wear Seat Belts

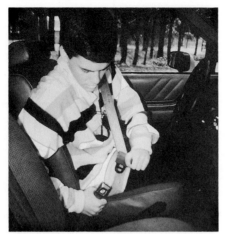

Should state government mandate this young man to wear his seat belt?

By 1987, twenty-six states had passed legislation requiring the wearing of seat belts. The rationale for such legislative action has been that injuries and fatalities are reduced when people involved in accidents are wearing seat belts.

Many individuals, however, are opposed to such requirements. Opposition may center around a feeling that in spite of the data the restraints are not effective in preventing injury and death. More commonly the opposition is centered on a discussion of individual rights.

Does government have the right to tell American citizens what to do while riding in the privacy of their own automobiles? Furthermore, should people be fined for not wearing the belts when they are opposed to such mandates?

Competition or Regulation?

The structure and form of community health programming and of health care provision within a nation is dependent upon that nation's position in an economic and political debate. Some individuals view health as part of the free-market economic system. As such, the health care system operates on the fee-for-service concept with costs determined by the economic principle of supply and demand and by competition in the marketplace. Government involvement in the form of regulatory measures is minimal.

This economic and political view suggests that broad-based geographical planning is not needed. Those health providers—clinics, hospitals, physicians, and pharmacists—that can operate in the competitive economic marketplace will survive. Those who cannot will go out of business. Therefore, overexpansion of hospitals and a surplus of health personnel and equipment do not need to be regulated by government. As in all American private industry, health care costs "find" a level commensurate with the level of the basic national economy. Free-market enterprise principles, it is held, dictate the percent of the gross national product (GNP) spent on health. Highly inflationary governmental controls and regulations do not result and the increases in health care costs, as were seen from the mid-1960s to the 1970s, will be minimized.

Supporters of this marketplace competition concept of health care argue that competition improves the quality of health care. It also makes the consumer more cost conscious. With governmental regulatory programs, there is no incentive to cut costs. If a hospital, through conscious effort, is able to reduce costs to a patient, it does not receive any financial benefit. (See figure 1.2.)

Those supporters also suggest that there should be increased patient cost-sharing measures, more copayments, and greater deductibles in payment for the health care services rendered. It is argued that these measures reduce the demands for minor health care now covered by third-party payment.

Figure 1.2   Philosophical view of health care

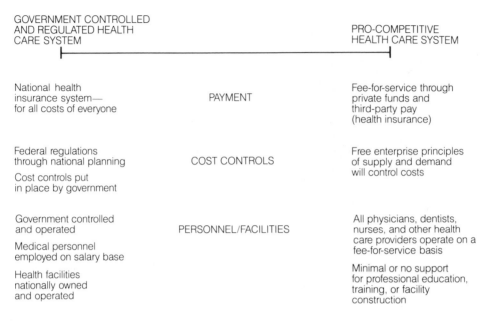

GOVERNMENT CONTROLLED AND REGULATED HEALTH CARE SYSTEM		PRO-COMPETITIVE HEALTH CARE SYSTEM
National health insurance system— for all costs of everyone	PAYMENT	Fee-for-service through private funds and third-party pay (health insurance)
Federal regulations through national planning Cost controls put in place by government	COST CONTROLS	Free enterprise principles of supply and demand will control costs
Government controlled and operated Medical personnel employed on salary base Health facilities nationally owned and operated	PERSONNEL/FACILITIES	All physicians, dentists, nurses, and other health care providers operate on a fee-for-service basis Minimal or no support for professional education, training, or facility construction

Where on the continuum do you place yourself with regard to your philosophical beliefs?

Another competitive measure is to provide employee health insurance options. The worker could then choose the type and amount of coverage, and so dictate personal cost. The employer's cost is the same regardless of the coverage selected, but the employee pays a greater premium for more inclusive coverage. It is believed that with this measure, only the most creative underwriters of health insurance plans would survive and prosper.

Some proponents of this free-enterprise position have suggested that the government withdraw from the health provider business completely with the exception of providing health care for military personnel. Support for community health centers, health facilities for the needy and medically underserved areas, and even some provisions for governmental health care in Public Health Service facilities should be eliminated and provided in the private health care sector. The government then would be removed from the provision of as many direct health care services as possible.

On the opposite end of the political, economic, and philosophical spectrum are those who hold that access to health care services is a *right* and not a privilege. This is based on the assumption that all people, regardless of race, religion, or economic status, have a right to adequate health services and freedom from sickness. When this premise is accepted, provisions must be made available for all to receive the benefits and services they need for healthy lives. As an outgrowth of this belief, the government is forced to play an extensive role in providing these health services.

Supporters of this position suggest that the free-enterprise, open-market system of health care provision fails to meet the needs of many, particularly the economically disadvantaged. There is less accessibility to health care for the poor, the elderly, and those living in medically underserved locations. Price competition often results in health care for only those who can afford to make the payments.

As a result of these concerns, many argue that the government must intervene. The specific intervention measures vary: some nations have a national health care system wherein all health facilities and personnel are controlled and employed by the government; others have national health insurance schemes that provide payment for comprehensive health services at little or no direct cost to the consumer (patient). Though the United States does not have a national health insurance program, the needs of the elderly and the poor are partially met through federally funded insurance and assistance programs.

This approach to health care involves the government in extensive planning and regulatory procedures. Many aspects of health care are regulated, based upon decisions arrived at through a systematic legislative planning process. As a result, health provision independence is often overruled by government direction.

During the 1960s and 1970s the predominant political view in the United States was one of increasing federal support and government regulation of health care services. Numerous federal laws were passed resulting in the widespread regulation of the health scene. Emphasis on curbing environmental pollution, improving industrial health and safety, and reducing the number of automobile accidents resulted in government establishing many mandatory regulatory procedures. Every consumer was affected by government regulations of health and safety matters.

A dramatic reversal of this process came about with the presidential election of Ronald Reagan in 1980. The Reagan administration, with its commitment to a free-market approach in the health field, brought about diverse changes in the budgeting and structure of health care provision.

Those involved in community health and in the provision of health care have had to readjust planning priorities and program directions in order to adapt to these philosophical and political policy changes. Many will accept certain concepts of both the free-enterprise and government-intervention views and find themselves philosophically somewhere between the two positions. This creates a dynamic community health atmosphere that incorporates much more than simple medical answers to health problems.

Your position on this issue will affect your economic and political concepts of the provision of health care. This can be analyzed by using figure 1.2.

Summary

Health and personal well-being are more than an individual matter. Humankind does not live in isolation, unaffected by others. As a result, health must be seen as a dynamic of community.

In the past, collective efforts for communicable disease control, environmental sanitation, and health protection were the domain of public health officials. With expanded programs designed to provide a greater level of wellness, however, community health has evolved into dynamic issues with varying program emphases. The concept of "community of solution" sets a pattern for focusing upon each specific health-related problem in program development and planning.

In bringing needed health care personnel and services to a broader range of citizens, three different—but interrelated—dimensions can be noted: (1) political considerations, (2) economic concerns, and (3) social and cultural ramifications.

The World Health Organization goal of "Health for All by the Year 2000" necessitates a reexamination of traditional community health programming. New and creative approaches are needed if this goal is to be achieved. It means moving away from the curative medical model of solving health problems to a greater emphasis upon disease prevention and health maintenance.

The federal government has identified 226 measurable goals to be achieved by 1990. These goals have been the focus of program planning, implementation, and evaluation by federal, state, and local health agencies, private sector organizations, and professional and voluntary health organizations.

Underlying all community health discussions is your philosophical view of the role of government.

Is health to be managed on the free-enterprise economic system, determined by the law of supply and demand, or is government regulation and control necessary? Your position on this issue determines the extent and types of community health programming, funding, and activities that are supported. Regardless of your view of this issue, the government has and will continue to have some influence on community health.

Discussion Questions

1. What is your understanding of the concept of a "community of solution"?
2. Identify some specific matters in your community that relate to the following dimensions mentioned in this chapter:
   a. political considerations
   b. economic concerns
   c. sociological and cultural ramifications
3. What is meant by the concept of the goal of "Health for All by the Year 2000?"
4. Is it reasonable to expect that the goal of "Health for All" can be achieved in the United States by the year 2000? Explain your answer.
5. What are the National Health Goals for 1990?
6. What are the results of evaluation studies relating to achieving the various health goals by 1990?
7. How does preventive health differ from the concept of curative medicine?
8. How does your understanding of preventive health relate to community health?
9. Do you believe that preventive health programming should be mandated? Why do you take this position?
10. Explain the pro-competitive position of health care provision.
11. Do you support increased federal regulation of the health care industry? Explain your response to this question.
12. What has been the effect of the political philosophy and program implementation of the presidential administration of Ronald Reagan on community health programming?

Suggested Readings

Agich, George J., and Begley, Charles E. "Some Problems With Pro-Competition Reforms." *Social Science Medicine* 21, no. 6 (1985): 623–30.

Caspersen, Carl J.; Christenson, Gregory M.; and Pollard, Robert A. "Status of the 1990 Physical Fitness and Exercise Objectives—Evidence from NHIS 1985." *Public Health Reports* 101, no. 6 (November/December, 1986): 587–92.

Christianson, J. B., and McClure, W. "Competition in the Delivery of Medical Care." *New England Journal of Medicine* 301 (October 11, 1979): 812.

Corbin, Stephen B. "New Opportunities for Enhancing Oral Health: Moving Toward the 1990 Objectives for the Nation." *Public Health Reports* 100, no. 5 (September/October, 1985): 515–24.

Cunningham, Robert M. "Competition and Regulation: We Need Them Both." *Hospitals* 54, no. 19 (October 1, 1980): 63–64.

Fielding, Jonathan E. "Health Promotion—Some Notions in Search of a Constituency." *Journal of the American Medical Association* 67, no. 11 (November, 1977): 1082–85.

Friedman, Emily. "Competition and the Changing Face of Health Care." *Hospitals* 54, no. 14 (July 16, 1980): 64–67.

Friedman, Emily. "Does Market Competition Belong in Health Care?"*Hospitals* 54, no. 13 (July 1, 1980): 47–50.

Hoffman, Richard E. "Tracking 1990 Objectives for Injury Prevention with 1985 NHIS Findings." *Public Health Reports* 101, no. 6 (November/December, 1986): 581–86.

Jones, Jack T., and others. "Workshop on 1990 Injury Prevention Objectives: Progress Review, 1985." *Public Health Reports* 100, no. 6 (November/December, 1985): 612–17.

Jones, Steven. "Hospitals Adopt New Role." *Hospitals* 53, no. 19 (October 1, 1979): 84–86.

Parra, William C., and Cates, Willard. "Progress Toward the 1990 Objectives for Sexually Transmitted Diseases: Good News and Bad." *Public Health Reports* 100, no. 3 (May/June, 1985): 261–69.

Pollard, Michael R. "Competition or Regulation: A Critical Choice for Organized Medicine." *Journal of the American Medical Association* 249, no. 14 (April 8, 1983): 1860–63.

Public Health Service, Office of Disease Prevention and Health Promotion, U.S. Department of Health and Human Services. "Summary of Findings from National Children and Youth Fitness Study." *Journal of Physical Education, Recreation, and Dance* 56, no. 1 (January, 1985—Suppl.): 48 pp.

Quelch, John A. "Marketing Principles and the Future of Preventive Health Care." *Milbank Memorial Fund Quarterly, Health and Society* 58, no. 2 (1980): 310–47.

Endnotes

1. Report of the National Commission on Community Health Services. *Health Is A Community Affair.* Cambridge, Mass.: Harvard University Press, 1967.

2. Ibid., 2.

3. World Health Organization. *The Work of WHO, 1984–1985.* Geneva: WHO, 1986, p. 49.

4. Ibid., p. 50.

5. Surgeon General's Report on Health Promotion and Disease Prevention. *Healthy People.* Washington, D.C.: U.S. Government Printing Office, 1979.

6. Department of Health, Education, and Welfare (HEW). *Promoting Health, Preventing Disease: Objectives for the Nation.* Washington, D.C.: U.S. Government Printing Office, 1979.

7. Roccella, Edward J. "Meeting the 1990 Hypertension Objectives for the Nation—a Progress Report." *Public Health Reports* 100, no. 6 (November/December, 1985): 652–56.

8. Parra, William C., and Cates, Willard. "Progress Toward the 1990 Objectives for Sexually Transmitted Diseases: Good News and Bad." *Public Health Reports* 100, no. 3 (May/June, 1985): 261–69.

9. Public Health Service, Office of Disease Prevention and Health Promotion, U.S. Department of Health and Human Services. "Summary of Findings from National Child and Youth Fitness Study." *Journal of Physical Education, Recreation, and Dance* 56, no. 1 (January 1985—Suppl.): 48 pp.

10. Jones, Jack T., and others. "Workshop on 1990 Injury Prevention Objectives: Progress Review, 1985." *Public Health Reports* 100, no. 6 (November/December, 1985): 612–17.

11. Surgeon General's Report on Health Promotion and Disease Prevention. *Healthy People.* Washington, D.C.: U.S. Government Printing Office, 1979.

12. Fielding, J. E. "Health Promotion—Some Notions in Search of a Constituency." *Journal of the American Medical Association* 67, no. 11 (November, 1977): 1083.

13. *Truman v. Thomas,* 611 P. 2d 902 (1980).

2

Official Health Organization: Federal Government's Role

Official health agencies are those administrative bodies of government involved in programs that are designed to improve the health of people. These are found at the local, state, and national levels of government. These agencies are financially supported by public monies (taxes) and are established for the purpose of implementing health laws, informing the people about health matters, providing various health services, and conducting research.

Federal Involvement in Health Care

The preamble to the United States Constitution states that one of the purposes of the federal government is to "promote the general welfare" of the people. From a broad interpretation of this, the federal government derives its powers to become involved in health-related activities. Yet there is no specific constitutional basis requiring federal control of the nation's health programs.

A number of health activities are supervised by various federal agencies, but most of the responsibility for health belongs to the Department of Health and Human Services (HHS), and in particular, the Public Health Service. There are also health programs that fall under other government departments, though these programs are usually specific to the responsibilities of that department.

The following are examples of specific health concerns of several departments of the federal government.

1. Department of Defense—health of military personnel and their dependents and the operation of several veterans' hospitals throughout the nation

2. Department of Interior—a number of environmental pollution control activities

3. Department of Labor—health concerns of the working person and environmental conditions of the work location

4. Treasury Department—control over the importation of drugs of abuse

Health Services for Governmental Employees

The provision of health services for the general population has historically been a private enterprise concern. The individual physician provided these services on a fee-for-service basis, a concept that has been the cornerstone of medical care provision in this country. Philosophically and constitutionally, health care was outside the realm of government.

At first, the federal government became involved in the health care field on a specialized basis. When health services were needed by governmental employees, the federal government became involved. As early as 1796 the Marine Hospital Service was established to provide health care to sick and disabled American seamen. In 1852, St. Elizabeth's Hospital in Washington, D.C., was established for the purpose of providing health care for federal employees.

The federal government makes provision for the health and medical care of all federal civilian employees. Usually, the health needs of each federal employee are covered by government-paid health insurance. However, the federal government also operates a system of direct medical services for civilian employees. The Federal Bureau of Medical Services Division of Hospitals and Clinics operates the oldest continuous hospital system in the United States, consisting of eight general hospitals and a hospital for patients with Hansen's disease (leprosy). In addition to hospitals, outpatient clinics make available a number of ambulatory services to government employees.

Military hospitals treat military and selected governmental personnel. Any active duty or retired military person, as well as their dependents, may receive treatment at a medical facility administered by the Department of Defense. When, however, these facilities are incapable of treating a particular ailment, the costs incurred by military personnel and their dependents in a civilian hospital are also covered.

The Veterans Administration (VA) operates an extensive network of medical centers and clinics. It is the largest health care system in the United States. Currently, VA medical centers number more than 170, with 226 outpatient clinics, over one hundred nursing homes, and nearly fifty VA satellite clinics. Many different health and rehabilitative services are available in these VA facilities with over 1.2 million patients being seen annually. These facilities are open to any person who has actively served in the military and who has received an honorable discharge with priority being given to individuals who have a problem that is service related. The individual's dependents also qualify for care through the Veterans Administration medical system.

The VA health programs encompass all aspects of medicine. Mental health services are part of the VA system as are physical rehabilitation services. The goal of these services is to return handicapped veterans to their communities as functioning and productive citizens. In addition, ambulatory and dental care are available on an outpatient basis.

The Veterans Administration also sponsors a health professions education program and various research activities. The medical education program provides academic and clinical experiences for students in medicine, dentistry, nursing, pharmacy, social work, and other allied health professions. Research efforts cover a broad range of health problems. Loss of limbs, and spinal cord injury research have been given high priority, but recent programs have focused upon alcoholism and delayed stress disorders in Vietnam-era veterans.

Health Services for the General Population

It was not until after World War II that the government increased its involvement in health care and community health programs for the general population. In 1946, the Hill-Burton Act was passed by Congress. This act provided funds for the building of badly needed hospital facilities in many communities. In the years since the passage of this legislation there have been several thousand government-financed projects for the construction and modernization of various health facilities.

Government funding of actual treatment for illnesses was not an actuality until the 1960s. Prior to that, government involvement in health care was limited to the support of programs for the economically disadvantaged and minority populations. The increase in social welfare programs during the 1960s

resulted in the establishment of numerous plans, projects, and programs, many of which were attempts to make available adequate medical care facilities to citizens who otherwise could not afford or receive such services.

During the 1960s and the early part of the 1970s, Congress passed many social welfare pieces of legislation that involved health programs. The following is a partial list of the federal legislation that was implemented during this period of time.

1. Provisions were made for the establishment of regional planning agencies that would help resolve the problems of water and air pollution, as well as control the building and growth of costly health care facilities.

2. Programs were designed to prevent nonmedical abuse of depressants, stimulants, and hallucinogenic drugs. These programs include research, treatment, rehabilitation, stronger law enforcement, and public education.

3. Support was provided for persons in such professional health training fields as medical schools, nursing programs, and schools of pharmacy, in an effort to reduce the shortage of professional health care personnel.

4. Support was provided for persons enrolled in allied health professional preparation programs in order to strengthen the existing programs and to help eliminate the specialized personnel shortage.

5. Safety and health standards were established for occupational settings.

6. Health services for migrant agricultural workers were introduced.

7. Procedures were established to prevent alcoholism and to treat and rehabilitate alcoholics.

8. Cancer research was funded.

9. Medical libraries received support.

10. Assistance was offered for the establishment of group prepaid health care plans (HMOs).

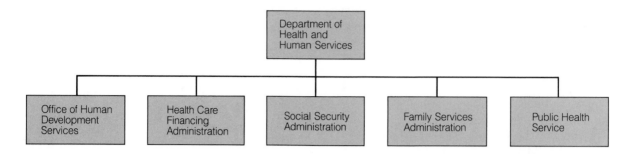

The establishment of Medicare in 1965 inaugurated the first government payments for health services to a certain segment of citizens other than federal government employees. The basic purpose of Medicare has been to make available quality health care for the elderly. Senior citizens who are entitled to Social Security or railroad retirement benefits receive health insurance coverage in the Medicare program.

Another federal medical insurance program established in 1965 was the Medicaid program for low-income individuals. Three population groups were identified for participation in this program: (1) the needy, including all federally aided public assistance recipients—the aged, blind, disabled, or those families with dependent children; (2) the medically needy (as identified in number one) who have the income to meet daily needs but not medical expenses; and (3) children under twenty-one whose parents cannot afford to provide medical care for them.

A major change in philosophy occurred during the first part of the 1980s regarding government involvement in the provision of health care and public health programming. This was primarily the result of the election of a more fiscally conservative Congress and president. Philosophically, the conservative "tide" has advocated less federal government involvement in the field of health. Associated with this philosophical view are the concepts that health care should remain part of the private enterprise system and that the federal budget should be reduced in an effort to control budgetary inflation.

Significant changes have occurred in the structure, function, and programming of federal health programs. Conceptually, federal government involvement in health has been reduced and greater emphasis placed on development and support of programs at the state and local levels of government. This means that federal funds are now provided to the individual states. This funding mechanism is referred to as the New Federalism, or the block-grant program. The state is required to implement and manage the specific programs under this type of programming. A more detailed look at this New Federalism approach to health programming is presented later in this chapter.

Department of Health and Human Services

The Department of Health and Human Services (HHS) was established in May, 1980. Prior to this, federal health administration and programming were part of the Department of Health, Education, and Welfare (HEW), which was organized as a cabinet level department of government in 1952. As the result of expanded legislative mandate, federal programming, and national needs, HEW became the largest department of the federal government. Social legislation passed by Congress during the 1960s and 1970s resulted in such tremendous growth of

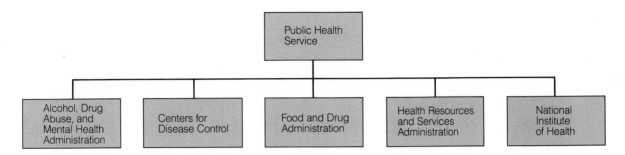

HEW that many felt it should be reorganized. Educators in particular were desirous of the separation of education from HEW. As a result, the Department of Education was organized in 1980 and health concerns were made a part of the new Department of Health and Human Services.

The Department of Health and Human Services is composed of the Office of Human Development Services, Health Care Financing Administration, the Social Security Administration, the Public Health Service, and the Family Services Administration. Each operating division is assigned a special role that contributes to the health of the American public.

The main task of the *Health Care Financing Administration* is to manage the Medicare and Medicaid programs. Medicare provides health insurance coverage for the elderly through the Social Security program. Medicaid is a jointly funded state and federal health insurance program for the economically disadvantaged. Both of these federal health insurance programs were legislated by Congress in the mid-1960s.[1]

The *Office of Human Development Services* provides a broad range of services to special population groups. Services are directed toward the aged, the mentally and physically disabled, the families of the disadvantaged, and other populations with special needs.

The *Social Security Administration* administers the various programs of the Social Security system. Americans pay into this system with payroll deductions. Social Security benefits are paid to an individual at the time of retirement or disability, or to one's dependents in the event of death. The Social Security Administration also administers child support enforcement and refugee assistance programs.

The *Family Services Administration,* formed in 1986, merged the major income assistance programs for families into one administrative unit. The programs included aid to families with dependent children, refugee assistance, the community services block-grant program, and the work incentive and child support enforcement programs.

The *Public Health Service* plays the most direct role in maintaining the health of the nation's general population.

Public Health Service

The Public Health Service is the governmental agency principally responsible for maintaining and protecting the health of the American people. The Public Health Service, headed by the president-appointed Surgeon General, presently consists of five agencies: (1) Centers for Disease Control; (2) Food and Drug Administration; (3) Health Resources and Services Administration; (4) National Institutes of Health; and (5) the Alcohol, Drug Abuse, and Mental Health Administration. This organization, as with most governmental agencies, tends to change with new presidential administrations.

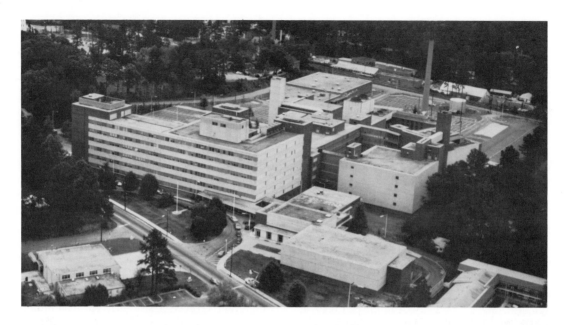

Centers for Disease Control

The Centers for Disease Control (CDC) is the part
of the Public Health Service that has responsibility
for controlling and preventing disease. CDC, head-
quartered in Atlanta, Georgia, was established in
1946 and was known at that time as the Communicable Disease Center. The primary program emphasis at that time was to study and combat various
communicable diseases. The original disease surveillance activities included study of malaria, typhus, smallpox, psittacosis, diphtheria, leprosy, and
plague.[2] As communicable diseases became less of
a health threat in the United States and as other
health problems came into prominence, the program emphasis of the Communicable Disease Center
expanded. This led to the establishment of the Center
for Disease Control in 1970.

Throughout the 1970s prevention of infectious
and chronic diseases became an increasingly important aspect of CDC program activities. This meant
increasing the emphasis upon examining health
problems as they related to environmental hazards.

Prevention of occupational diseases and industrial
safety became important parts of CDC's mission.
The promotion of health and wellness through health
education and health promotion efforts was also emphasized.

In 1980, this expanded focus led to the realign-
ment of CDC, renaming it Centers for Disease Control. Six operational units were established as part
of the newly named agency.

The Center for Infectious Diseases

Efforts to control infectious diseases include investigations of such diseases, diagnosis, surveillance, and
immunization programs. Close working relationships between state and local health departments in
disease prevention programs are established. In addition, CDC works with other nations and with the
World Health Organization to control diseases
throughout the world.

The Center for Environmental Health

Efforts designed to control environmentally related
diseases, particularly through research of environmental matters and their effects on health, are the

The various programs of the Centers for Disease Control include such research activities as (a) electronmicroscopy pathological studies of pesticides in animals, (b) removing fluid from cell cultures in the Maximum Containment Lab, and (c) examining plates with the first environmental isolates of *Legionella pneumophila.*

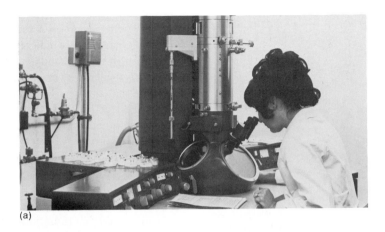

(a)

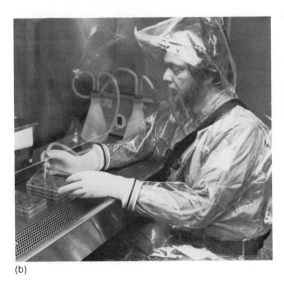

(b)

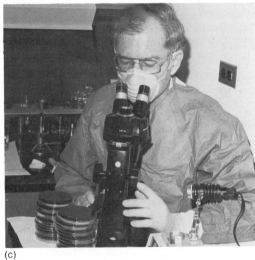

(c)

focus of the Center for Environmental Health. For example, this center conducted extensive investigation into the impact on health made by the Mount St. Helens volcanic eruption in 1980. The center is currently conducting epidemiological studies (dealing with the incidence, distribution, and control of disease in a population) of the effects of low-level radiation on humans.

National Institute for Occupational Safety and Health

Activities designed to encourage a safe and healthful work environment are a primary responsibility of the National Institute for Occupational Safety and Health (NIOSH). Both laboratory research and epidemiological studies are carried out by NIOSH to ascertain the hazard levels of various substances found in the work environment. For example, standards have been established for work-related exposure to a broad range of disease-causing substances.

NIOSH conducts on-site health and safety inspections at the request of both employees and employers, and offers assistance for the prevention and control of occupational health hazards to either group. Most of the authorization for this type of programming comes from the Occupational Safety and Health Act (OSHA). NIOSH also provides medical, technical, and consultative assistance to state and local agencies.

Center for Prevention Services

This agency funds, conducts, and oversees a variety of service programs that have a preventive focus. Several programs specifically identified by the government are the concern of this center: immunizable diseases, sexually transmitted diseases, dental disease, kidney disease, diabetes, and tuberculosis. Special coordination with state and local health departments is designed to provide appropriate services to all citizens.

Center for Health Promotion and Education

Increased awareness that health preventive measures and health promotion are effective in reducing chronic and communicable diseases has resulted in increased activity of the Center for Health Promotion and Education. This activity includes the designing, piloting, evaluating, and dissemination of health education and health promotion programs. These health prevention and risk reduction programs occur in schools, in work environments, in health care facilities, and throughout many community settings.[3]

Center for Professional Development and Training

This center is responsible for the instruction of a variety of health workers. Educational programs, short-term seminars, and workshops are designed to update the professional skills of the nation's health care providers. In addition, health professionals from throughout the world receive training at this center, primarily in disease prevention and control.

Food and Drug Administration

How sure are you that the foods you purchase are safe? When you purchase a prescribed drug, can you be confident that it will be effective in combating the illness you have had for several days? Should health products have labels indicating possible dangers to your health? These and many other questions are seldom considered by most American consumers. We assume that the food we eat is wholesome, that the medicines we purchase are safe and effective, and that health products are labeled accurately.

This assurance of safety is the primary responsibility of the Food and Drug Administration (FDA). The FDA is charged with ensuring that foods are safe and wholesome, that all medicines and medical devices are safe and effective, that cosmetics are harmless, and that radiation emitted from consumer products is not injurious to the health of the consumer. In an effort to make sure that governmental standards are met, FDA personnel inspect factories, warehouses, and stores, collecting samples for testing.

The initial legislative mandate for the Food and Drug Administration occurred in 1906 when Congress passed the Pure Food and Drug Act. In 1938 a much changed Food, Drug, and Cosmetic Act became law. Whereas the previous legislation focused on adulterated and misbranded foods and drugs, the 1938 legislation extended coverage to cosmetics, required predistribution clearance for safety of new drugs, and authorized factory inspections.

For the first time a manufacturer was required to have an effective application for a new drug before it could be introduced for interstate commerce. To obtain the application the manufacturer had to present clear evidence from chemical, pharmacological, and human testing that the drug was safe. However, it was not necessary to prove that the drug was effective. As a result, many new drugs appeared on the market that were safe, but showed no evidence that they could cure diseases for which they were advertised. Not until passage of an amendment (the Kefauver-Harris Amendment) in 1962 did drug manufacturers have to prove to the FDA the effectiveness of the drug before it could be marketed.

Through the years several other amendments to the Federal Food, Drug, and Cosmetic Act have been passed. Such amendments prohibit new food additives from being marketed until proven safe (1958), limit the amount of color additives in foods (1960), outline new procedures for new drug applications (1979), and require that food labeling be honest and informative (1966). Four principal areas within the jurisdiction of the Food and Drug Administration have received major emphasis in recent years: (1) food labeling, (2) food safety, (3) human drugs, and (4) radiological health. Any product that does not meet established federal standards in any of these areas is confiscated. The Food and Drug Administration can remove a product from the marketplace and prosecute either the manufacturer or vendor if it can be shown that the food, drug, or cosmetic is unsafe or contaminated, or if the labeling or advertising can be proven false or misleading.

An important responsibility of the FDA is to make certain that all labeling is truthful, informative, and correctly stated. Consumer interest in the past decade has led to more informative labeling of health products, and especially of food labeling. Food labeling now includes information regarding the specific nutritive ingredients of the food product. For example, federal legislation was passed that required infant formula manufacturers to specify the amount of all nutrients their product contained.

In spite of the fact that many feel it is important to make sure that foods are properly labeled, there are those who have opposed the FDA's increased involvement in these efforts. These groups and individuals suggest that such labeling actions increase the cost of marketing the foods. Others feel that such activities are a government intrusion into the private marketplace.

Food safety is another major concern of the Food and Drug Administration. FDA scientists test foods and food additives to ensure their safety and purity. For instance, food served in interstate carriers, such as planes and trains, must be inspected periodically. Also the FDA ensures that milk has been properly processed and is safe for human consumption.

The Food and Drug Administration certifies the safety and effectiveness of prescription and over-the-counter drugs. Before a drug can be marketed, it must pass certain research standards established by the Food and Drug Administration. It is the responsibility of the drug manufacturer to have all newly manufactured drugs tested and approved. This procedure, from the time of development of the drug until final FDA approval is given and the drug is marketed, often takes several years.

Once a drug is approved by the Food and Drug Administration, it is again tested on a random basis to ensure purity and potency. All insulin and antibiotics marketed for human use, for example, must be certified for purity and effectiveness. In addition, the FDA is responsible for monitoring the proper labeling of prescription drugs.

The FDA is also involved in the protection of consumers from unnecessary exposure to radiation. Of particular concern are such sources of radiation as color television sets and microwave ovens. In addition, the FDA maintains constant surveillance of medical X-ray equipment to ensure the safety of the medical patient. So thorough are the FDA's investigations into possible environmental health hazards, that a recent Food and Drug Administration report warned consumers that some gold jewelry may be contaminated by radioactive materials. The specific dangers associated with wearing this jewelry are dermatitis and, possibly, skin cancer.

Health Resources and Services Administration

The function of the Health Resources and Services Administration is to assist various agencies throughout the nation in improving health resources and in administering the activities of specific organizations that deliver health services. This administration's programs are designed to work with health care providers in an effort to provide excellent health care. The administration makes recommendations for improving access to health care.

The programs administered by this agency fall into one of four bureaus: (1) the Indian Health Service; (2) Bureau of Resources Development; (3) Bureau of Health Professions; and (4) Bureau of Health Care Delivery and Assistance.

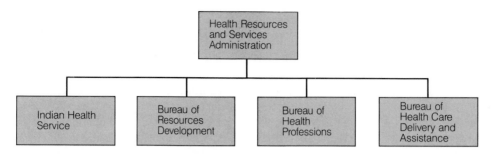

The *Indian Health Service* is the principal federal agency that provides health care to Native Americans living throughout the United States. Health care services are provided in a number of facilities such as health centers, health stations, and satellite field health clinics.[4]

The *Bureau of Resources Development* monitors health facilities that have received federal Hill-Burton funding. This bureau also directs and supports programs of state and local health planning agencies.

The *Bureau of Health Professions* manages a variety of programs designed to enhance the development, distribution, and quality of professional training of health personnel. These activities include the financial support of medical, nursing, and allied health care training, and efforts to improve this training with in-service programs. Since 1980, the federal government has reduced the financial support of such personnel training, and, as a result, the role of this bureau has been somewhat reduced. The recent targets for support from this bureau have been disease prevention, health promotion, bedside nursing and care of the elderly.

The *Bureau of Health Care Delivery and Assistance* conducts several programs designed to meet the needs of people who are not adequately served by the normal private health care system. Some programs are directed at specific health problems and others at certain population groups.

A number of community health centers have provided a wide range of health services in rural and inner-city settings. The centers provide primary health care, mental health services, health education, and other health and social services for the residents of these medically underserved areas.

Since many rural and inner-city localities lacked adequate medical personnel, the National Health Service Corps was established for the purpose of recruiting personnel to serve in such settings. Physicians, nurses, and other health-related personnel are appointed to an underserved locality for a given period of time. Upon completion of this federal service, it is hoped that the health providers will continue serving this same area in a private practice.

Several Bureau programs have focused upon specific health problems. For example, the Genetic Diseases Program provided funds for voluntary genetic testing and counseling programs. Hemophilia diagnosis, treatment, and counseling are supported by grants administered by this agency. Sickle-cell anemia screening and education clinics have also been a program focus, as have hypertension, maternal and child health, Sudden Infant Death Syndrome (SIDS), and family planning.

Two programs are directed at the health problems of certain populations. Over a half million migrants and seasonal farm workers receive medical services through the Office for Migrant Health. The Appalachian Health Program supports comprehensive health services in communities in a number of states. These services may cover home care, preventive health services, dental care, maternal and child health, environmental health, nutrition, and rehabilitation.

The Bureau also provides a number of direct medical services to specific populations. Facilities provide health care for federal employees, inmates of federal prisons, and members of the Coast Guard. In addition, a national program for regional emergency medical services is administered by the Bureau as is the national Hansen's disease program.

The many services offered by the Bureau of Health Care Delivery and Assistance may be reduced in the future. The financial and administrative responsibility for many of these programs will continue to be shifted to the individual states as part of the health block-grant program.

National Institutes of Health

The National Institutes of Health (NIH), one of the largest medical research centers in the world, conducts and supports extensive biomedical research for the benefit of Americans. In addition to this research, conducted in NIH laboratories and in various institutions throughout the nation, the National Institutes of Health trains young researchers and also disseminates research-related information.

The National Institutes of Health began in 1887 in a one-room facility at the Marine Hospital on Staten Island. From that time until 1930 it was known as the Hygienic Laboratory. In 1930 the name was changed to the National Institutes of Health.

From 1953 to 1979, NIH was a part of the Department of Health, Education, and Welfare (HEW). Today NIH is one of the health agencies that make up the Public Health Service of the Department of Health and Human Services.

The National Institutes of Health is organized into eleven research institutes plus a research hospital, the National Library of Medicine, and the Fogarty International Center. Each of these institutes is assigned a specific focus. Research activities are supported and conducted in programs designed to solve the specific health problem.

The research hospital, known as the Clinical Center, houses five hundred beds. It is the world's largest medical research hospital. Admission to this facility is limited to individuals with illnesses and diseases that are Institute study topics and who are referred by their personal physicians.

The National Library of Medicine houses over two-and-a-half million volumes, the world's largest single-subject medical reference center. In addition to housing medical works, the Library publishes numerous periodicals. The other component of NIH, the Fogarty International Center, conducts research into international health concerns and problems. Conferences and seminars involving international collaboration are conducted by this center.

Most of the National Institutes of Health departments are now located outside Washington, D.C., in Bethesda, Maryland. The National Institute of Environmental Health Sciences, however, operates in North Carolina, and several other smaller field stations and facilities are located outside the Bethesda headquarters.

National Institute on Aging

The senior citizen population is rapidly increasing in the United States. As a result, recent years have seen an increased interest in the aging process and in the problems of senior citizens. Research supported by the National Institute on Aging has involved several of these problems.

Research has focused on the interaction of aging and various diseases and disorders associated with aging, such as Alzheimer's disease, osteoporosis, osteoarthritis, injuries caused by falls, and urinary incontinence. Biomedical and psychosocial factors in maintaining health and effective functioning in the middle and later years are another emphasis of research in this institute. The Institute also has responsibility for research concerned with the biological, social, psychological, cultural, and economic factors that affect both the process of growing old and the status and roles of older people in society.

(a) The principal clinical facility for National Institutes of Health studies is the Warren G. Magnuson Clinical Center. This center is a fourteen-story structure containing 540 beds. (b) There are many laboratories throughout the Center where study and research are carried out. Such instruments as the Positron Scanner are used. The scanners can locate minute pieces of tissue in the brain, deeply embedded tumors, and metabolic changes in the body that other noninvasive techniques are unable to detect. (c) About eight thousand patients are admitted annually to this facility, with another 120,000 outpatient visits taking place.

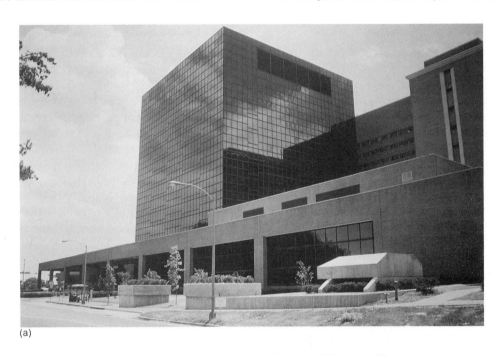

(a)

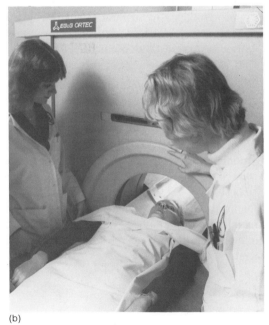

(b)

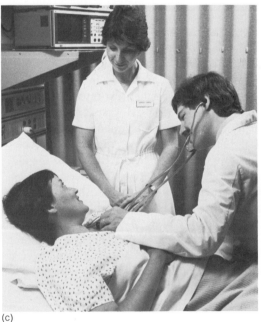

(c)

In 1938, government officials broke ground for the National Institutes of Health in Bethesda, Maryland. These institutes, staffed by scientific personnel, conduct research on a variety of different health problems and diseases.

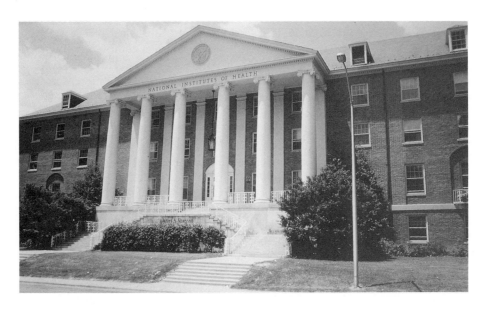

The National Library of Medicine is a part of the National Institutes of Health in Bethesda, Maryland. This is the largest medical reference in the world, containing over 2.5 million items. The medical reference journal, *Index Medicus,* an index to articles in about twenty-five hundred medical journals, is published by the National Library. The Lister Hill National Center for Biomedical Communications and the National Medical Audiovisual Center are a part of the National Library of Medicine.

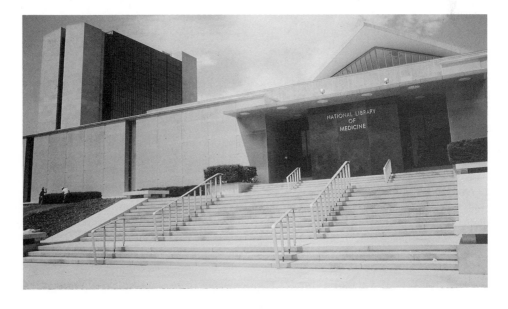

In recent years, among the many research findings in the study of aging was that dioxin, a drug commonly prescribed for patients with chronic heart disease, was ineffective for some elderly patients. Not only was it found to be ineffective in certain people, but it was also found to be toxic if taken in certain amounts.

Another research finding reported by the National Institute on Aging is that the mechanisms for exercise-stimulated muscle building are slowed or turned off in adults. Therefore, exercise results in fat reduction and weight loss in the elderly. An increase in muscle mass is not achieved in these exercisers as it is in younger athletes. This is not to suggest that the senior citizen cannot benefit from exercise, but that muscle growth will not be a major outcome.

The National Institute on Aging has funded research relating to aging and cancer. These research projects have examined the epidemiology of cancer in the elderly with an emphasis on changes in the immune system. In the behavioral sciences, projects have sought the development of effective psychosocial support systems for elderly cancer patients.

National Institute of Allergy and Infectious Diseases

The basic focus of the National Institute of Allergy and Infectious Diseases is to discover why the body's immune system defenses are disrupted and to learn how they can be corrected and prevented. Research efforts at the molecular level expand the knowledge of microorganisms responsible for infectious diseases. Study of immunologic defects, enhancing immunization procedures, and correcting malfunction as in asthma and other allergic disorders are important activities of this institute.

Its research programs are directed at acquiring knowledge that will lead to the treatment and prevention of infectious diseases. This involves research in microbiology looking at isolation, characterization, and biology of disease-causing microorganisms. It also includes the development of successful and safe antimicrobial compounds, particularly for viruses and parasites. The Institute oversees investigations into the nature of infectious diseases. Although these diseases no longer pose the health threat that they did half a century ago, they are still a major cause of acute illnesses in the United States today. Institute scientists are developing and testing new vaccines to combat respiratory infections, particularly influenza. This has been difficult, however, because of the many different microorganisms that cause the illness.

Because allergies are one of the most difficult problems to diagnose and treat, the Institute is conducting research into their cause, pathogenesis (origination and development), prevention, and treatment. Reactions to insect bites, foods, chemicals, and a variety of airborne allergens are being studied by Institute scientists in the hope that some relief for allergic sufferers will be found.

Other research programs have been directed toward the development of new vaccines for pertussis and hepatitis B. The National Institute of Allergy and Infectious Diseases is the principal agency supporting research in parasitology and tropical medicine. This has been accomplished through bilateral projects with other nations as well as through the World Health Organization. Six tropical diseases—filariasis, leishmaniasis, leprosy, malaria, schistosomiasis, and trypanosomiasis—have been the priority diseases of emphasis.

The Institute's research efforts have also increased in the area of sexually transmitted diseases. Attempts have been made to learn more about the biology and physiology of such diseases as herpes, chlamydia, and trichomoniasis. The researchers' efforts are proving effective. A vaccine to protect against gonorrhea has been developed in animal research and is currently being tested in humans. A rapid diagnostic test that allows diagnosis of chlamydial infection within thirty minutes has also been developed.

Along with several other of the National Institutes of Health this institute has placed major emphasis on AIDS in the past few years. Researchers have been working on antiviral drugs, the use of bone marrow transplants, and basic study of the immune system in attempting to help bring about a cure for AIDS.

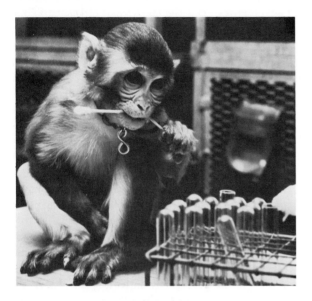

National Institute of Diabetes, and Digestive and Kidney Diseases

This institute focuses its research efforts on a variety of problems related to diabetes and the kidneys.

Research efforts relating to the kidneys are concentrating on developing new methods of preventive therapy, early diagnosis, and more effective treatment. As a result of research work, long-term results of kidney transplants have occurred in recent years. Long-term rehabilitation is now possible.

Kidney stones often present a very painful disorder of the urinary tract. Research has focused on procedures to dissolve these stones and to develop means for medical interventions. By use of a urine sample a procedure has been developed to warn of the possible likelihood of formation of kidney stones.

Improved forms of kidney dialysis therapy continue to be a goal of the Institute. A measure known as continuous ambulatory peritoneal dialysis (CAPD) has been an important research topic in recent years. This procedure, portable and possibly less expensive than other traditional kidney dialysis measures, frees the patient from daily dialysis treatment. Research continues in an effort to make CAPD more efficient and safe.

Diabetes is a metabolic disorder that affects an estimated eleven million Americans. The National Institute of Diabetes, and Digestive and Kidney Diseases conducts a variety of programs attempting to reduce the problems relating to diabetes and to increase early risk identification. Studies of the role of diet and obesity in the development of diabetes among populations at high risk are being undertaken. Interesting research directed at the transplantation of pancreatic tissue for treatment of diabetes has been a new area of work. New procedures for screening the retina of the eye may identify a factor of blood found in patients at risk for vision loss from diabetes.

Not all research is conducted in the NIH laboratories in Bethesda. Researchers at Mayo Clinic in Rochester, Minnesota, are also supported by Institute funds. They have been trying to develop better therapy regimens for diabetics. Their goal is to design a more efficient system of determining individual insulin doses and a better alarm system to warn that the regimen is malfunctioning.

National Institute of Arthritis and Musculoskeletal and Skin Diseases

In 1986 a new institute was created that conducts research in arthritic conditions and human diseases of the skin, bone, and muscle.

Studies of arthritic conditions are concentrated on learning more about the causes of rheumatic diseases, connective tissue diseases, and associated musculoskeletal disorders. Twenty multipurpose arthritis centers have been established throughout the country with research conducted at each center. In addition, medical and community educational programs, and community and health services research programs occur in these centers.

National Cancer Institute

Since cancer is the second leading cause of death in the nation (cardiovascular disease is number one), the importance of the Institute's research into the cause, prevention, diagnosis, and treatment of cancer is obvious.

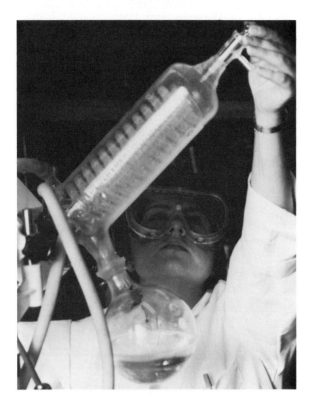

This laboratory technician removes solvent from a rotary evaporator, used to concentrate a chemical solution, while performing an experiment to synthesize an anticancer drug. The National Cancer Institute has been instrumental in the development of several such drugs.

National Cancer Institute grants have promoted cancer prevention, detection, treatment, and rehabilitation activities. Programs about these aspects of cancer have been set up for the education of health professionals and the public. Future directions, however, will emphasize the prevention and screening of cancer, as well as cancer control surveillance activities.

The National Cancer Institute has established the goal of reducing cancer mortality by 50 percent by the year 2000. In order to achieve this goal the National Cancer Institute has established several specific areas for emphasis: reduction in cigarette smoking, dietary changes involving reduction of fat consumption and increase of fiber consumption, increase in breast and cervical examinations, and application of research findings into improved cancer treatment modalities. NCI estimates that achieving a 50 percent reduction would mean saving 250,000 lives a year.[5]

Cancer research takes a variety of directions. Leukemia is one of the least treatable cancers, but recent research has developed an antileukemic therapy program that has had positive results. Some patients have remained disease free for up to four years. The objective of this particular research is to improve the duration of this remission and to prevent a relapse.

Epidemiological research has shown relationships between low incidence of colon cancer among populations with high fiber diets. Other epidemiological studies have established a relationship between use of smokeless tobacco, particularly oral snuff, and excessive rates of oral cancer.

Improvements in cancer patient survival are related to the development of better knowledge of chemotherapy. New drugs that are more effective but less toxic for patients have been developed. For example, the percentage of patients with Hodgkin's disease who are cured with chemotherapy has increased in recent years.

An interesting anticancer research program involves the study of herbal medicine in an effort to discover new anticancer drugs. Thousands of plant samples from throughout the world have been collected and studied. There is great value in such research. Two major cancer drugs used today—vinblastine, used to treat Hodgkin's disease, and vincristine, an effective drug in the treatment of childhood leukemia—come from Madagascar periwinkle. This herb has been used for generations in folk medicine to treat a variety of health problems.[6]

Another new National Cancer Institute program is the diet, nutrition, and cancer program. This program includes research into the relationship between dietary patterns and cancer incidence. This program also helps the cancer patient to cope with dietary problems provoked by the disease.

National Institute of Child Health and Human Development

The program activities of this institute do not focus upon any one disease, but upon a wide variety of health problems related to maternal health, child

Ten Research Areas of the National Institute of Child Health and Human Development

Category	Sample Research Project
1. Pregnancy, birth, and the infant	Genetic and environmental factors related to abnormal pregnancies
2. Congenital abnormalities	Inherited defects with emphasis on Down's syndrome
3. Sudden Infant Death Syndrome	Search for ways to identify infants at risk for Sudden Infant Death Syndrome
4. Nutrition	Dietary management of inborn errors of metabolism
5. Child and adolescent development	Study of the biological bases of behavioral development from infancy through childhood to adolescence
6. Mental retardation	Biological, behavioral, and social variables relating to mental retardation
7. Contraceptive development	Research of safe contraceptives for both men and women
8. Contraceptive evaluation	Research into the long-range safety of currently marketed contraceptives
9. Fertility and infertility	Biological, chemical, and endocrinology as they affect fertility
10. Population dynamics	Population change in terms of fertility, mortality, and migration

Source: Department of Health and Human Services, Public Health Service, National Institutes of Health, *Research Programs of the National Institute of Child Health and Human Development*, NIH Publication No. 83–83, March 1983, Washington, D.C.: U.S. Government Printing Office.

health, and human development. Such concerns as fertility regulation, pregnancy, and labor have been recent emphases of this institute. Prenatal development has also received much attention.

Research designed to reduce abnormalities during pregnancy has been an important emphasis in both the biomedical and the behavioral sciences. The nutritional needs of the pregnant woman, the fetus, and of the newborn infant are determining factors in the early life development of the child.

The more that is known about these nutrition-development relationships, the better the chance of having healthy young children.

A center for population research is also part of this institute. Here programs are conducted to develop better methods for regulating fertility. The development of more effective contraceptive methods is one area of study. Under study are new drugs, devices, and methods, including hormones for male use.

National Institute of Dental Research

The efforts of the National Institute of Dental Research focus upon the control of plaque and prevention of tooth decay. Other oral health programs emphasizing such problems as malocclusion, dental caries, viral diseases of the mouth, mineralization, and periodontal disease are also supported by this institute. These programs have provided a wealth of new information on dental health.

Since the ultimate goal of the National Institute of Dental Research is the elimination of tooth decay as a major health problem, there is interest in identifying a vaccine that would accomplish this goal. The problem with obtaining such a vaccine, though, is that antibody levels decrease after a period of time. It is hoped this problem will soon be resolved and an effective vaccine made available to the public.

Oral health research of the National Institute of Dental Research covers work in fourteen different areas:

Dental caries
Periodontal diseases
Congenital craniofacial malformations
Acquired craniofacial defects
Dentofacial malrelations
Soft tissue disease
Craniofacial pain and sensory-motor
  dysfunction
Salivary glands and secretions
Mineralized tissues and fluoride studies
Pulp biology
Nutrition impact on oral health
Behavior studies
Implants, replants, and transplants
Restorative materials

Source: National Institute of Dental Research, NIH, Bethesda, Md., 20205.

Other research activities involve such areas as salivary glands and secretions, mineralization and fluorides, tooth pulp biology, nutrition, and research related to dental implants, replants, and transplants. Interest has also centered recently on various dental restorative materials.

Canker sores, lesions that form inside the mouth, are yet another facet of dental health in which the Institute is involved. Research now suggests that the tendency to develop these mouth ulcers may be genetic. NIDR-funded projects are investigating this possibility.

National Institute of Environmental Health Sciences

This institute focuses on the chemical, physical, and biological components of the environment that adversely affect health. Researchers are concerned about the effect of long-term exposure to low concentrations of these dangerous components.

Institute scientists, for example, have discovered that anticonvulsant drugs used to manage human epilepsy cause birth defects in animals. Such adverse reactions to the drugs in humans are unknown, but such findings are cause for concern among women of childbearing age who use these drugs.

Every year new synthetic chemicals are introduced in the form of food additives, drugs, cosmetics, insecticides, and herbicides. Many of these chemicals have not been tested to ascertain their adverse effects on humans. Some, previously thought to be safe, have now been shown to cause genetic mutation in animals. This mutation process and other dangerous side effects of synthetic chemicals are yet another concern of the National Institute of Environmental Health.

National Eye Institute

A number of visual problems result in blindness or limited vision for millions of people throughout the world. The National Eye Institute conducts research to learn more about visual disorders and diseases of the eye such as cataract, strabismus, amblyopia, retinal and choroidal diseases. Related research is directed at the rehabilitation of the visually handicapped.

Aplanation tonometry, a technique for measuring pressure within the eye, is used for glaucoma testing at the National Eye Institute. A flat disc is placed on the eye and pressure is exerted until the cornea is flattened. The amount of pressure needed to flatten the cornea is equal to the pressure inside the eye.

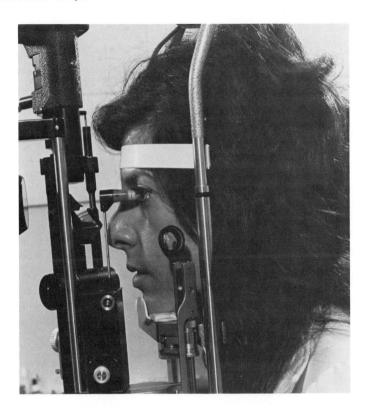

Research programs have made it possible to detect glaucoma in the early stages, to learn more about the cause of cataract in the aged, diabetics, and other population groups, and to study the chemistry of the normal lens as it relates to cataract problems.

The Institute has supported training programs aimed at improving the prevention, diagnosis, and treatment of visual disorders. It has also supported research on the epidemiology, treatment, and cell biology of ocular tumors. The two most frequent ocular tumors are choroidal melanoma and retinoblastoma—conditions that can not only cause loss of sight but may also be fatal. Of particular interest has been the hereditary relationship of retinoblastoma. Close to 40 percent of these cases are hereditary.

National Institute of General Medical Sciences

A broad spectrum of health concerns is included in the research subjects of the National Institute of General Medical Sciences. This institute supports research into genetics, trauma, anesthesiology, pharmacology, and diagnostic radiology.

Researchers at the National Institute of General Medical Sciences are also studying the structure and function of human cells in order to help the medical world better understand the body's response to trauma. Special attention is given to the care and treatment of posttraumatic infections and the rehabilitation of injured individuals. Adjuncts of this attention are the study of pain, and the metabolic and respiratory changes that result from exposure to anesthesia.

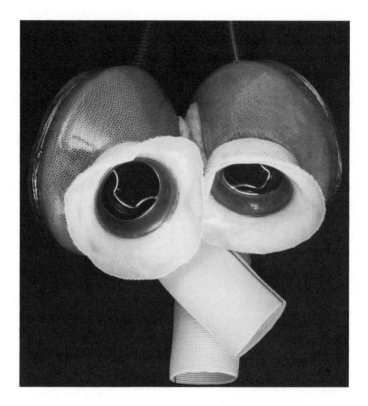

National Heart, Lung, and Blood Institute

Research into heart and lung diseases and circulatory system problems is conducted by this institute. Coronary heart disease, hypertension, congenital heart disease, and pulmonary problems (the Institute is developing a vaccine for Type B hepatitis) are the specific areas of Institute study.

Research, both basic and applied, in identifying the possible causes and prevention of atherosclerosis has been supported by this institute. Such factors as elevated blood lipids, high blood pressure, and cigarette smoking are given special attention. Educational workshops have been sponsored by the Institute to inform professionals and public groups about such problems as sickle-cell anemia and Cooley's anemia.

National Institute of Neurological Diseases and Communicative Disorders and Stroke

This institute conducts research into a wide range of health problems. The causes and early detection of stroke, especially, have received much attention from this institute. For instance, new monitoring devices and techniques have been developed to identify transient ischemic attack (TIA), which is often a forerunner of a major stroke. Studies of tumors of the brain, the spinal cord, and the peripheral nerves have been current research activities. These studies often lead to the development of surgical techniques.

Research in the diagnosis, treatment, and prevention of several communicative disorders has also been conducted. Specific emphasis has been placed upon hearing, language, and speech disorders, including the development of measures to assess hearing loss in infants and young children. Disorders of taste and smell in adults have also been project topics.

Many neurological disorders have been studied. Cerebral palsy, autism, and dyslexia are childhood problems that have been of interest to institute research teams. A wide range of other neurological conditions such as Parkinson's disease, muscular dystrophy, myasthenia gravis, and narcolepsy have also been studied. Research seeking new methods of prevention, diagnosis, and treatment of epilepsy and the development of an antiepileptic drug have taken place.

Other research programs have been directed at studying the cause of headaches, particularly migraine, and seeking effective treatment measures. Biological research with emphasis on the neurology of pain is also an emphasis of this institute.

National Center for Nursing Research

Congress created a new national institute of research in 1986 that supports research related to nursing. Emphasis is directed toward nursing issues and patient care, health promotion and disease prevention. In addition research programs focusing upon nursing interventions, delivery methods, and the ethics of patient care are other important objectives of this new institute.

Alcohol, Drug Abuse, and Mental Health Administration

This federal agency was established to prevent and treat alcohol abuse and alcoholism, drug abuse, and mental and emotional illness. The programs designed to combat these problems most often include research, prevention, training, or the delivery of various treatment services.[7] Much of the agency's work is accomplished with the aid of federal grants.

The New Federalism

The 1980 election of a conservative president (Ronald Reagan) and Congress resulted in a change in political philosophy concerning federal and state government programming. The states now assume responsibility for most programs that had previously been federally legislated and funded. This change stemmed from the desire of the president, Congress, and many citizens to reduce the role of the federal government in the lives of the people of the United States. The Reagan administration termed this reduced role "New Federalism."

A major vehicle to effect these transferrals of responsibility was the 1981 congressional passage of the Omnibus Budget Reconciliation Act. This legislation created a block-grant program for federal funding to consolidate federal support programs.

Congress felt that each state could best determine its own health needs and priorities. Thus, it was argued, the individual states should play the major role in developing and administering the health programs for the citizens of the state. Instead of appropriating money for specific programs, the federal government would deliver funds to each state in the form of block grants. The individual states could then select the specific areas in which these "health" dollars would be of greatest benefit. This has resulted in increased responsibilities, program planning, management, and evaluation being carried out at the state and local health departments.

As a result of the passage of the Omnibus Budget Reconciliation Act most of the existing health programs and services were lumped together under three health block grants: (1) preventive health and health services; (2) alcohol, drug abuse, and mental health; and (3) maternal and child health.

The *preventive health and health services block* includes eight formerly categorical programs:

1. home health
2. rodent control
3. water fluoridation
4. health education/risk reduction
5. health incentive grants

Health Services Categorical Program Funds, 1985

Program	Percent of Total
Community Health Centers	48.8
Family Planning	18.1
Maternal and Child Health Services	9.1
Migrant Health	5.6
Sexually Transmitted Diseases	5.6
Immunizations	5.4
Cancer Control Services	4.9
Mental Health Community Support Program	.8
Mental Health Children and Adolescent Services Assistance Program	.5
Black Lung Clinics	.4
Home Health Services	.4
Pediatric Emergency Medical Services	.3

6. emergency medical services
7. rape crisis centers
8. hypertension

The *alcohol, drug abuse, and mental health block* understandably includes programs concerned with mental health, alcohol abuse, and drug abuse. This has been the largest of the block grants in terms of funds made available.

The *maternal and child care block* involves several programs for maternal and child health care. Adolescent pregnancy services and several childhood-disease research programs are part of this block-grant program. In addition, genetic disease, Sudden Infant Death Syndrome, and hemophilia research are included.

Each block grant has certain regulations stipulating the percentage of money the state can spend on administrative costs, the percentage that can be transferred to other programs, and whether state matching funds are required in order to receive the federal money. For example, the provisions of the alcohol, drug abuse, and mental health block require the states to spend a major portion of these block-grant funds for alcohol and drug abuse programs. At least 35 percent of these funds must go for alcohol abuse programs, 35 percent for drug abuse, and at least 20 percent for prevention programs.[8] The individual states have to match three dollars to every four dollars of federal money received under the maternal/child block-grant program.

To its proponents, the health block-grant concept is a good idea. The idea of allowing states to decide health priorities and to administer these programs at the state level seems meritorious. The New Federalism program has given state health departments more responsibility and greater authority than they have had in the past.

In addition twelve health programs receive categorical support. Nearly half (48.8 percent) of the total amount for categorical health grant funding is to support community health centers.[9] Originally, under provisions of the health block-grant program, funds for community health centers were to be shifted to a primary care block grant. This attempt has not been successfully implemented.

The effectiveness of this concept of community health funding continues to need to be evaluated and reviewed. Those who question the block-grant approach point out that federal services developed primarily because the health needs of certain individual groups were not met in the past by individual states' services. Opponents also argue that politics may affect the distribution of grant monies, with groups wielding less political clout left wanting. Also, economically poor states would not have the matching funds in some instances. This could result in the same situation that originally led to extensive federal intervention and programming in the 1960s and 1970s.

The Legislative Process

The authorization for and appropriation of federal governmental funds for community health programs are most often the result of the legislative process. A basic understanding of this process—how it works and in what ways one can influence it—is useful to those involved in community health.

Legislative proposals come from many sources. Some originate in the executive branch of government (the presidential administration usually submits a number of proposals to the legislative body). Other bills are submitted by the members of Congress; or the idea for a legislative bill may have originated in special interest groups or individuals. The broader the organized support, and the greater the amount of congressional backing for a bill, the better the chances of the bill's ultimate passage.

Once an idea for a legislative proposal is formulated, a member of Congress agrees to author, or coauthor, the bill. The Congressional Research Service of the Library of Congress then researches data regarding the proposal and, working with the staff of the supporting senator or member of Congress, drafts the bill. This Library of Congress service is invaluable in the development of the legislative proposal.

When the proposed bill has been written it is introduced as similar proposals in both the House and the Senate. The bill is then referred to the standing committees which have appropriate jurisdiction over the bill in both the House and the Senate. The standing committees then send the bill to the appropriate subcommittees for action.

In the United States Senate, the Committee on Labor and Human Resources is the standing committee having authorization over most health-related legislation. This committee, for example, has jurisdiction over public health service programs, the Food, Drug, and Cosmetic Act, and mental health legislation.

Another important Senate standing committee that deals with health-related issues is the Committee on Environment and Public Works. This committee works with legislation dealing with air pollution, toxic substances, environmental policy and research, noise, solid waste, and water pollution.

In the House of Representatives, the Committee on Energy and Commerce delegates responsibility for all public health legislation to the Health and Environment Subcommittee. Legislation for hospital construction, mental health and biomedical programs, food and drug matters, and all environmental health legislation comes to this subcommittee.

There are several points in the legislative process where the individual or organized lobby groups can offer input and influence legislation. Prior to the actual writing of the proposal, interested individuals should provide relevant information on the topic. Possibly the most effective time to provide this information is at the subcommittee hearings, because once the bill is reported "out of committee" to the floors of the House and Senate, there is less likelihood of influencing the shape of the proposal.

Many important decisions concerning the proposal occur at the subcommittee level. The subcommittee chairperson is extremely powerful in determining the outcome of a proposal since this individual determines the agenda and decides which legislative proposals will receive a hearing and which will not. If the subcommittee chairperson opposes a piece of legislation, it becomes extremely difficult to get any action. In fact, many legislative proposals never get a hearing but are left to "die" in subcommittee. The key to effective lobbying, then, is to get the support of this individual.

Legislation begins with an idea that leads to a proposal. A series
of activities takes place until the idea becomes a law and is
signed by the president.

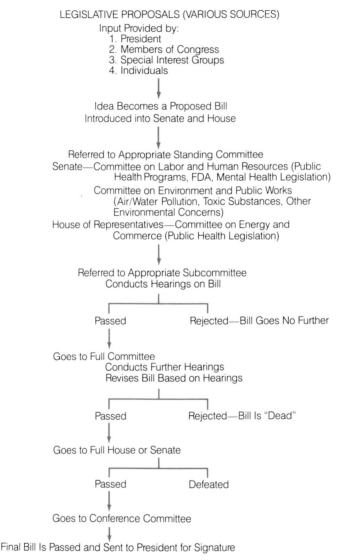

LEGISLATIVE PROPOSALS (VARIOUS SOURCES)
Input Provided by:
1. President
2. Members of Congress
3. Special Interest Groups
4. Individuals

Idea Becomes a Proposed Bill
Introduced into Senate and House

Referred to Appropriate Standing Committee
Senate—Committee on Labor and Human Resources (Public
Health Programs, FDA, Mental Health Legislation)
Committee on Environment and Public Works
(Air/Water Pollution, Toxic Substances, Other
Environmental Concerns)
House of Representatives—Committee on Energy and
Commerce (Public Health Legislation)

Referred to Appropriate Subcommittee
Conducts Hearings on Bill

Passed   Rejected—Bill Goes No Further

Goes to Full Committee
Conducts Further Hearings
Revises Bill Based on Hearings

Passed   Rejected—Bill Is "Dead"

Goes to Full House or Senate

Passed   Defeated

Goes to Conference Committee

Final Bill Is Passed and Sent to President for Signature

Once a subcommittee decides that a legislative proposal will be acted upon, hearings on the proposed legislation are scheduled. It is during the hearing process that interested individuals or groups and lobbyists may be asked to appear either on behalf of or against the proposal. It is vital, then, to make certain prior to the hearing that the appropriate people are invited by the subcommittee to serve as witnesses. Only individuals who can provide effective information and whose testimony is respected by committee members will be called to testify.

When the hearings are concluded, the subcommittee either defeats the proposal or sends it to the full committee. If the proposal passes the subcommittee, it goes through a process known as "markup" before it is sent to full committee. This activity involves going over the proposal, line by line, and marking any changes—additions, deletions, or revisions. Only when this process is completed is the proposal sent to the full committee.

The full committee usually discusses the proposal, makes whatever changes it feels necessary, votes on it, and (if approved by a majority vote) submits the bill to the House or Senate floor. There are instances where a proposal is returned to subcommittee or where the committee votes not to report it to the full congressional body.

Once the proposal has entered the House and Senate, it is debated and oftentimes amended. A vote is than taken and the bill is either passed or defeated.

If the proposal is passed, another step will usually be necessary. Despite the fact that basically similar proposals were introduced into both the House and Senate, by the time the bill is passed on the floor of Congress differences will probably have developed. Before a final piece of legislation can be sent to the president for action, a compromise between the House and Senate versions of the bill must be achieved. A conference committee composed of House and Senate members is appointed by the congressional leadership to arrive at this compromise. Each house of Congress must then vote again to approve the conference committee's action.

When the bill has been signed by the president, it becomes law. However, this action only authorizes a given program or activity. Until funds to support the authorized legislation are appropriated by Congress, nothing will happen.

Several very powerful congressional committees act on appropriation legislation. In the Senate, the Committee on Finance and the Committee on Appropriations are both very strong entities. The Committee on Finance has jurisdiction over all tax and revenue matters. The Committee on Appropriations considers the budget and recommends legislation as it relates to fiscal appropriations.

In the House of Representatives, the Ways and Means Committee and the Appropriations Committee are extremely powerful. Tax and revenue affairs, including Medicare, health costs, and national health insurance legislation, must be channeled through the Ways and Means Committee. All legislation must be approved by the Committee on Appropriations before funds can be authorized for a program. It is not uncommon that a bill authorizing a program is passed but no monies are appropriated to fund the program. This situation "kills" the program.

After the legislative process produces an authorized bill with appropriated funds, implementation regulations must be drawn. The government agency to which the particular law applies must write these regulations. Oftentimes, the writers of the regulations are forced to interpret what was the intent of the congressional legislation, a process that is often very lengthy, time-consuming, and political.

Summary

Official government agencies at the federal level play important roles in community health programming. These agencies are supported financially by public tax monies. Many health programs are administered by the Department of Health and Human Services (HHS). The Public Health Service (within the Department of HHS) is the governmental agency primarily responsible for maintaining and protecting the health of the American citizens. The Surgeon General is the chief officer of the Public Health Service.

The Public Health Service is composed of five different agencies. These agencies are (1) the Centers for Disease Control, (2) the Food and Drug Administration, (3) the Health Resources and Services Administration, (4) the National Institutes of Health, and (5) the Alcohol, Drug Abuse, and Mental Health Administration.

Since the early 1980s, the prevailing political attitude has been to reduce federal programming activity in all areas. Health programs, it is believed, should be the responsibility of state and local governments. As a result, funding for federal programs has been reduced and a renewed and redirected emphasis, in the form of block grants, has led to a broader program concept by state and local health departments.

Federal health programs and the allocation of funds by Congress result from a well-defined legislative process. Legislative proposals are introduced to both the House and the Senate. These proposals are passed to a committee for review and vote. After committee passage, they are brought to the complete congressional body for debate and vote. Throughout this entire process, interested individuals have the opportunity to provide input and testimony so as to influence the legislators' decisions regarding final passage of the proposal.

Discussion Questions

1. In what ways can political changes in government affect a nation's health program?
2. To what groups has the federal government historically provided health care?
3. What types of legislation in the 1960s and 1970s influenced health programming in the United States?
4. Explain some of the types of services provided by the Veterans Administration.
5. What is the basic organizational structure and what are the responsibilities of the Department of Health and Human Services?
6. What is the function of the Public Health Service?
7. Explain some of the program activities of the Centers for Disease Control.
8. Trace the legislative mandate for program activities of the Food and Drug Administration.
9. What role does the Food and Drug Administration play in the approval of prescription drugs?
10. Discuss some of the issues involved in food labeling.
11. How does the Health Resources and Services Administration differ from other agencies of the Public Health Service?
12. Describe some of the research efforts of the National Institutes of Health.
13. Do you believe that there should be an increased or decreased involvement by the federal government in health programming? Explain your answer.
14. What is the significance of the Omnibus Budget Reconciliation Act?
15. What is the health block-grant program?
16. Explain how the different block-grant programs differ from one another.
17. At what point in the legislative process is one likely to be most effective in the lobbying process?
18. How are potential pieces of legislation introduced by legislative bodies?

Suggested Readings

Publications explaining the various federal agencies are available
from the specific agencies. Most governmental documents
are also available from the United States Government Printing
Office, Washington, D.C.

Endnotes

1. An expanded discussion of Medicare and Medicaid is found in chapter 7.

2. Centers for Disease Control, M M W R, *Surveillance Summaries, 1985,* Vol. 34, no. 255, p. 3SS.

3. These activities are discussed in greater detail in chapter 14.

4. A more complete discussion of Native American health problems and the role of the Indian Health Service is found in chapter 15.

5. National Cancer Institute, *Directors Report and Annual Plan FY 1986–1990,* p. 1.

6. *News and Features From NIH* (June, 1981): 12.

7. Specific program activities of the three national institutes of this agency (National Institute on Alcohol Abuse and Alcoholism, National Institute on Drug Abuse, and the National Institute on Mental Health) are discussed in more detail in chapters 12 and 18.

8. Zwick, Daniel I. "Federal Health Services Grants, 1985." *Public Health Reports* 101, no. 5, (September/October, 1986): 500.

9. Ibid., 501.

3

State and Local Health: Expanded Importance in the 1980s

State and local public health departments have always played important roles in the health of American society. In 1940 the American Public Health Association defined public health as having six basic functions: (1) communicable disease control, (2) health education, (3) laboratory services, (4) maternal and child health care, (5) sanitation, and (6) vital statistics.

Historically, the responsibility for the general health and well-being of America's communities has not been federal but rather state and local. Increased federal legislation and budget appropriations, beginning with the "Great Society" legislation in the 1960s, resulted in a reduction of program responsibility for state and local health departments. Federally funded programs either replaced state and local efforts or provided controls that effectively reduced the program identity at the community level. Since the development of the New Federalism concepts of the 1980s, where responsibility for social and health programs were returned to the local communities, state and local health departments have assumed a renewed importance.

State Health Department

Article X of the United States Constitution states that "the powers not delegated to the United States by the Constitution, nor prohibited by it to the States, are reserved to the States respectively, or to the people." Since there is no direct mention of health in the Constitution, under a broad interpretation of the tenth amendment, the responsibility for the health and well-being of the people rests with the individual states. States are expected to develop the various rules, regulations, and laws that are necessary for the positive health status of their citizens.

Each of the fifty states has a state health department, headed by a state health commissioner. The health commissioner is usually a physician who is either selected by the state governor or is appointed by the state board of health.

The policy-making decisions, overall planning, budgeting, program development, and evaluation responsibilities rest with the particular state board of health. Selection to the state board of health is usually by appointment by the governor or by legislative confirmation. Health professionals serve in a majority of the health department board positions, while consumers occupy only a minority of the memberships.[1]

Funding for the operation of the state health departments is obtained from several sources. The major funding comes from state tax revenues. Other major sources of state funding include bonds and fees for license permits, and various types of registrations.

Federal funds are provided for some state health department activities through the block-grant program. This system of federal funding of health programs resulted from the passage of the Omnibus Budget Reconciliation Act in 1981.[2] This legislation provided "block grants" to the individual states for the support of previously federal categorical-grant support programs. This concept of funding through the "block-grant" program gives the state health department greater responsibility in the programming and management of a range of health activities.

Private foundations also support various programs developed and managed by state departments of health. These are usually programs specific to a given activity.

The operational organization and administrative structures of the state health departments are not the same for any two states. In most states, district or regional offices throughout the state provide the direct health department services. For instance, in Texas and Florida there are eleven public health districts, in Minnesota and Illinois there are eight, and in the state of Ohio there are four health department districts. The number of districts or regional offices and the specific services rendered are determined by the needs and geographical distribution of the state's population.

There are many similarities in the various health services provided by the state health departments. Each department's services are provided by physicians, dentists, public health nurses, nutritionists, dietitians, educators, sanitarians, researchers, environmentalists, and other related health professionals. State health departments also employ economists, engineers, attorneys, computer programmers, and a variety of other professional staff members.

Vital statistics are maintained by each state health department. These data are sent to the state health department from the local health departments. Vital records include data concerning births, deaths, marriages, and divorces. These data are useful in providing information about the prevalence and incidence of various diseases, for analyzing trends for program planning, and for research purposes.

The role of environmental sanitarians is important in every state health department. These personnel work to assure a healthful environment in the state. Their tasks include developing standards, conducting regular inspections, regulating licensure and certification, and enforcing sanitary codes and public health laws. They also monitor the health and safety regulations in mobile home parks, in migrant labor camps, and at recreational areas and youth camps. Food and water sanitation is yet another very necessary responsibility of the sanitarian. The state health department must ensure that water supplies and food are safe for human use.

The state health department is also responsible for the prevention and control of communicable diseases. Epidemiology and immunization programs enable the department to successfully accomplish this task. State health departments are becoming more involved in chronic disease control with cancer, hypertension, and diabetes control programs.

Another important state health department facility is the public health laboratory. A state health department public health laboratory provides a number of essential services. In addition to the laboratory testing necessary for the prevention and control of communicable diseases, these laboratories provide specialized services unavailable in many private laboratories to diagnose and treat a broad range of health problems.

Most state health departments have zoonosis control programs. These activities are designed to detect and control animal diseases that can be transmitted to humans. Control of rabies, a disease that can be fatal to humans, is a principal concern. Other zoonotic diseases of concern to state health departments include several types of encephalitis, ornithosis (a poultry disease), and psittacosis (parrot fever).

In many states the state health department administers various hospital, nursing home, and health professional licensing laws. Hospital and nursing home licensing activities assure that these facilities are meeting various state and local codes for providing a safe environment. They also assure that high standards of patient care are occurring. Professional licensing includes such groups as dietitians, audiologists, and medical technicians. In Texas the licensing of athletic trainers is a responsibility of the Texas Department of Health.

The various state health departments are responsible for their individual state Medicaid programs. The administration of the Medicaid program and the establishment of specific regulations are responsibilities of the state health department.

A primary function of most state public health programs is to support the local health department. State-directed health care institutions, with some exceptions, are not direct service providers. A direct service institution that is found in all states is the mental health establishment. Generally, mental health facilities are operated by state departments of mental health. Occasionally hospitals for crippled children and cancer institutions are state operated.

Local Health Department

Actual person-to-person public health services are most often provided at the local level. The local health department is the official governmental agency having legal responsibility for the health and well-being of the citizens within its jurisdiction. This jurisdiction may encompass any of the geographical divisions of a region. Though a wide range of services is offered, the most common services provided by the local health department include immunization, environmental surveillance, tuberculosis control, maternal and child health care, nursing, sexually transmitted disease control, chronic disease programs, home care, family planning, education, and ambulatory care. Over half of the local health departments provide these services.[3]

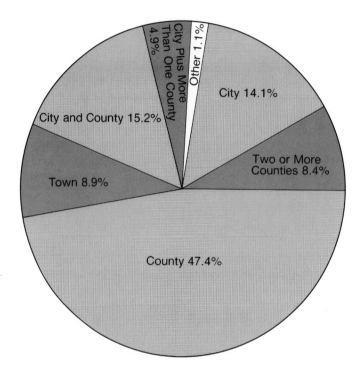

City Plus More Than One County 4.9%

Other 1.1%

City 14.1%

City and County 15.2%

Two or More Counties 8.4%

Town 8.9%

County 47.4%

Some public health clinics have scheduled appointments. However, most health department services are available on a first-come, first-served basis. Fees for these services vary—some services are provided free of charge; others require a small charge. Follow-up visits are not made unless the problem is severe, and preventive-care visits are rare.

The services of the local health department are often targeted at the poor. Because many citizens view the local department of health as a program for public funding of health services for the economically disadvantaged, its acceptance in the community is not widespread. It is important, though, that the local health department be seen as a health care provider for the entire community, not only for a limited sector.

The local health departments were created because of local sanitation and disease control needs. These health departments were originally established to serve limited political and geographical jurisdictions, such as townships, counties, or cities.

These early local public health departments included a physician, a public health nurse, and a sanitary inspector.

Today the county health department is the most common in the United States. Other local health department jurisdictions include city and town departments, units combining city with county, or other multiple jurisdictional arrangements.

Organization and Structure

The organization and structure of most local health departments are patterned after the state health departments. As at the state level, there is a local health commissioner (historically a physician) as well as a board of health. Today one-third of all local health directors and an increasing number of local health officers (administrators) are not members of the medical profession.

There are a number of reasons for this recent development. The shortage of qualified physicians who are interested in public health is one reason.

Economics have also contributed to this change. The salary of a physician serving as the public health commissioner is much greater than that paid a nonmedical person. Most physicians can make a greater income from private medical practice than they can from work in public health. Finally, the nature of the administrative position favors employment of a person who is not medically trained. Many of the skills necessary for administering a public health department involve budgeting, public relations, management, and other business-related skills. The chief administrator of a public health department need not have earned a medical degree if he or she possesses these skills.

However, before the nonmedical health officer is accepted in many jurisdictions, the laws must be modified to permit such officials. In nearly one-half of the states, a nonmedical health officer is not yet permitted by law.[4] But in those states allowing nonmedical public health directors, they have been received very positively by the community. A nonmedical director does need the services of a medical advisor or a medical advisory committee, however, to compensate for the lack of medical training. Medically related decisions are then the responsibility of this individual or committee.

Programming

Local health department activities are determined by state and local laws and other governing codes. Forty-four services that are commonly authorized by state statute have been identified.[5] Included among these are communicable disease control and the keeping of vital statistics. Tuberculosis and venereal disease control and the establishment of quarantine are mandated by 90 percent of the states' health laws.[6]

In order to be most effective, a local health department should serve a population of at least fifty thousand residents. Because larger agencies are more efficient, the trend in recent years has been to merge small health departments into larger units and to consolidate the services of other social services with the public health department. Such mergers have

economic benefits, too. Administrative costs are reduced and funds can be reallocated to better serve the needs of the community.

Today local health department programming must identify the health status and needs of the citizens it serves. Part of this identification process includes an evaluation of the effectiveness in meeting specific needs of current programs. Those areas that are found lacking then become the focus of future planning and programming.

During the 1970s much of the responsibility for health planning was not centered in the local health department. The national health-planning legislation required that local health planning be done by nonprofit private corporations. Thus, local health department planning was basically ignored by this legislation in favor of separate regional health-planning organizations, supported with federal funding. This was extremely frustrating for many local health departments.

Increasingly, health departments are realizing the importance of community (consumer) input into the planning and programming processes. The people of the community must feel that they are participating in the identification and resolution of their specific health needs.

The local health department conducts many of its activities in cooperation with the state health department. This relationship exists in three different organizational structures.[7] One such structure is the *centralized organization* where the state department of health operates the local health unit. All local health department functions, then, are authorized by the state.

A *decentralized organization* occurs when local government operates the health department. The state health department provides only support and consultative services. Thus, there is much more local control in the programmatic decision-making process in these units.

The third structure is *shared organizational control*. Local government operates the health department, which falls under the authority of the state

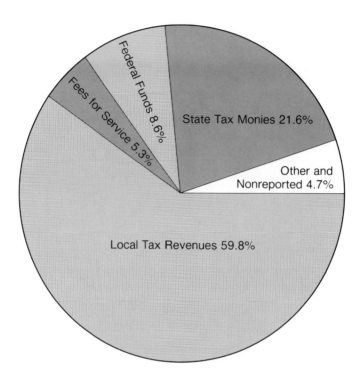

Federal Funds 8.6%

Fees for Service 5.3%

State Tax Monies 21.6%

Other and Nonreported 4.7%

Local Tax Revenues 59.8%

health department. Though developed locally, such aspects as budget planning and programming are submitted to the state for approval.

Budget Problems

More than one-half of the local health department budget comes from local tax revenues. The second greatest source of funding is state monies. In recent years reduction in both state and local tax revenues in some communities, combined with greater demand for health department services, has led to serious program constraints. Many localities have experienced great program cutbacks. This lack of funds has led to a reduction in local health department staffing, which in turn has resulted in the inability to perform seriously needed and at times legislatively mandated services. Usually the first programs eliminated are those with health prevention as a focus such as nutrition services, health education, and visiting nurses' services. Only those programs that are mandated by legislation are retained and these are often operated at a bare minimum.

With the increased demand for funding made by various state and local agencies and organizations, the health department will continue to have to "fight" for a necessary share of the tax dollar. And when the cost of health care increases, so do the operational costs of an effective local health department. If funding is unavailable, it then becomes necessary for the local health department board and staff to make difficult decisions about the programs that can be continued and those that must be eliminated.

Over last weekend, fifteen students living in the north wing of Smith Dormitory became ill with diarrhea, vomiting, and stomach cramps. Some type of food poisoning was thought to be responsible.

Food samples were sent to the state health department for laboratory analysis. It is hoped that this analysis will identify the actual cause of the students' illness.

Public Health Laboratories

The services and information obtained from a health department laboratory are very important to a community health agency. The World Health Organization (WHO) has suggested that any health administrator must have available the information that a health laboratory can provide. In order to achieve maximum efficiency and usefulness, each laboratory must be adapted to the specific needs of the population it serves. Therefore, the functions of a health laboratory vary from one locality to another.

A health laboratory performs numerous services. Lab work is performed by different agencies. Much laboratory work takes place at the Centers for Disease Control in Atlanta, Georgia. Some laboratory services are conducted by the state health department and others by the local health department; and sometimes they are fulfilled under contract with a private laboratory.

Microbiology and serology laboratories are important in any communicable disease control program. The bacteriology laboratory does blood tests and cultures to help diagnose such communciable diseases as syphilis and gonorrhea. In addition microbiological examinations of throat cultures for streptococcal infections, tuberculosis, and parasites are conducted.

The health laboratory also conducts tests for viruses in order to prevent the outbreak of a viral epidemic. For example, animals suspected of having rabies are often examined in a health laboratory. This laboratory service is networked with communicable disease departments so that outbreaks are quickly and efficiently controlled.

Before a new well can be used the water must be tested by the health department and certified as safe for use. Existing water sources, such as private wells, public drinking water, water in parks, camps, and schools, are also tested periodically to ensure safety. These laboratory tests determine the presence of various toxic materials and pesticides as well as the level of bacteria present in the water. If any one of these tests indicates a contaminated water supply, the health department will not certify it for use.

The various sanitary program activities of a health department must be supplemented by a laboratory facility. Water, milk, and various foodstuffs are tested to ensure that they are free of disease-causing organisms. This laboratory testing can also help to identify the specific cause of food poisoning.

Blood samples of newborn infants are analyzed for hereditary and metabolic diseases. Screening for sickle-cell anemia, phenylketonuria, hypothyroidism, galactosemia, and homocystinurea is a regular function of a public health laboratory. Early detection and treatment of these diseases are important in preventing mental retardation and other health problems.

Laboratory testing relating to environmental concerns is another important activity of the health department laboratories. Tests are conducted for such hazards as air pollution contaminants, radioactivity, and various solid waste contaminants. These tests ensure compliance with pollution-control laws.

Many public health laboratories have provided services free of charge. However, because of greater need for laboratory services, it is becoming increasingly necessary to limit public health laboratory work to problems that are clearly of a public health nature. Personal laboratory testing would then be performed by the many private health laboratories throughout our communities.

Community Dental Health

It has been estimated that each person in nearly 95 percent of the population in the United States has at least one dental cavity. Dental caries (tooth decay) and periodontal diseases are the most common causes of tooth loss. Malocclusion, or misalignment of the teeth, is another dental concern that can also lead to tooth loss and cause numerous social and emotional difficulties as well. An estimated two billion dollars a year is spent on dental treatment to combat such problems.[8]

Dental caries are the result of decalcification of the enamel or cementum by bacteria-produced organic acids. Dental caries develop under a bacterial mass on the tooth structure referred to as dental plaque. The principal preventive procedure to protect against both tooth decay and periodontal disease is the removal of this dental plaque through brushing, flossing, and regular visits to the dentist.

The objective of dental health services is the prevention of dental disease of all kinds, as well as the treatment of dental disorders. Most Americans receive this preventive and curative treatment from a dentist in a private practice on a fee-for-service basis. In addition, public dental health services are available through local health department clinics and health dispensaries in many communities. Usually charges for services rendered in these settings vary with the ability to pay.

Fluoridation

Possibly the most effective public health preventive measure against dental caries and related problems is fluoridation. Historically, the dental profession has played a major role in encouraging the fluoridation of public drinking water and other measures designed to result in better dental hygiene.

As early as the 1930s, epidemiological studies indicated that dental caries were reduced in localities having naturally present fluoride in the drinking water. These observations increased the dental interest in the role of fluoride as a preventive to tooth decay. It was not until the 1940s, though, that fluoride was purposefully added, in controlled amounts, to the public drinking water. In 1945 Grand Rapids, Michigan, became one of the first large communities to have fluoride added to its water.[9]

This practice verified the 1930s studies: where fluoride had been added to the community water supply, the amount of tooth decay had decreased significantly. Through the years, a significant body of data has only added weight to the argument that fluoridation of public water is not only safe, but contributes to better dental health. It has been estimated that for every one dollar spent on fluoridation, fifty dollars can be saved on dental treatment.[10]

The American Medical Association Council on Foods and Nutrition, after carefully reviewing the clinical effectiveness of fluoride in public drinking water supplies, concluded that this measure is safe and desirable in the reduction of dental decay. This council also noted that fluoride may be helpful in preventing or alleviating osteoporosis (a condition where the bones become weakened) in the aged.[11] The concept of fluoridation of public drinking water is endorsed by seventy-five national science and health organizations.

As of 1986, 61 percent of the United States population having access to public water supplies received fluoridated water. Eight states had mandatory fluoridation laws. However, only two states, Minnesota and Illinois, required that all public water supplies be fluoridated. The other six states required fluoridation in communities of certain population sizes. The federal goal for the nation is that 95 percent of the population with public water systems will have fluoridation by 1990. This goal will be most difficult to attain.

The recommended concentration of fluoride in the water supply is 0.7 to 1.2 parts of fluoride per million parts of water. Not until rather large amounts of fluoride (eight to twenty mg./day) are ingested for several years have adverse effects been noted.

In spite of the fact that the benefits of fluoridation have been known for many years, many Americans do not have access to fluoridated drinking water because they have individual water systems, a well, or are on a community water system that is deficient in natural fluoride. Another important reason why many people have no access to fluoridated water is the strong opposition to such programs by small but vocal groups.

Antifluoridation

The reasons for the opposition to fluoridation of public drinking water vary from an ignorance of the value of fluoridation in the prevention of tooth decay, to concern over forced medication, to religious beliefs. Often the rejection of fluoridation has been expressed in emotional terms, unsubstantiated by facts.

Opponents have publicized their opinions in a number of approaches. Most commonly, these people take their concern to the voters of the community. Another approach used recently involved local groups attempting to pass statewide legislation to prohibit any community from fluoridating its water supply.[12] In the 1980s nearly two out of every three public referendums on fluoridation of public drinking water were defeated.[13]

Several reasons for opposing fluoridation are listed by these people. Some believe fluoride causes cancer, although the American Cancer Society has found no evidence that this is the case. Others think that fluoridation of the public water supply is a violation of federal clean water statutes. The addition of fluoride to the water supply, they argue, is polluting or contaminating the water by the addition of a foreign substance, which is illegal and an environmental hazard.

Another antifluoridation argument is that this action is an infringement upon the Constitutional guarantee of freedom of choice. Their view is that this addition constitutes forced medication. A citizen has no choice but to drink the fluoridated, or "medicated," water.

Opponents of fluoridation have used AIDS as a reason for opposition. They remind people that a majority of AIDS victims come from urban communities with fluoridation, hence suggesting that fluoridated water fosters AIDS. No medical and/or scientific evidence in any way links fluoridation with AIDS.

Opponents also claim that fluoride can be obtained in other ways, without affecting the community water supply. Fluoride mouth rinses are effective but must be used continually and regularly. Dietary fluoride supplements have been used quite successfully but these, too, must be given on a daily basis from infancy through adulthood. Another approach has been the application of fluoride directly to the teeth, particularly to children's teeth. This procedure usually is necessary twice a year throughout the growing years if it is to be effective.

The dental profession has proven to be fluoridation's greatest advocate. Members have played a major role in support of community fluoridation programs, primarily with programs in preventive dental health care. Public health dentists and dental hygienists continue to educate the general public on good dental health practices, including fluoride treatment, a very important aspect of the public dental health service program.

Health Department Personnel

Of the many personnel employed by state and local health departments two categories of public health personnel have a long tradition of service and importance: (1) the community health nurse and (2) the environmental sanitarian. Every health department has such individuals in its employment. Public (community) health nursing has a long and storied history in its role with state and local health departments. In the early years of public health in the United States public health nurses often played important roles as social reformers.[14] Since those early years the scope of responsibilities of the community health nurse has expanded. The environmental sanitarian has also played an important role in the health of communities since the early days of state and local health departments in this country. Their tasks and opportunities, like those of the community health nurse, have expanded and changed with the passage of time.

The public health nurse serves people of all ages. For youngsters, the nurse (a) administers oral polio vaccine and (b) performs visual testing. (c) The senior citizen is given flu shots by the local public health nurse.

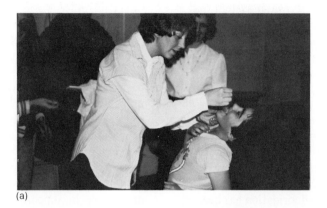

(a)

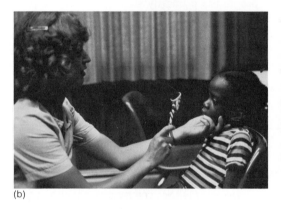

(b)

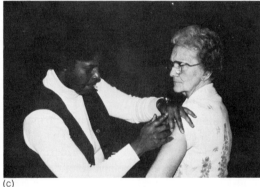

(c)

Community Health Nursing

Possibly the most visible public health person in many communities is the public (community) health nurse. As public health has expanded from a traditional official agency to a broader community-based health service, so the role of the community health nurse has expanded. Community health nursing provides services to a variety of people. These services are offered in industrial settings, in schools, in homes, or through community health screening programs. The community health nurse also performs a variety of services in clinical settings, community mental health centers, with visiting nurses associations, and in nursing homes. Health education and maternal-child health programming are major components of the work of community health nursing today.[15] Most commonly, however, the community health nurse operates in schools, in homes, or in community clinics.

Schools

The community health nurse provides many services in the community schools. The roles and responsibilities in the schools vary, but a common activity of the community health nurse is to conduct various health screening and appraisal activities. Oftentimes, such screening programs as those for vision and hearing are required in many states. Also,

The public health nurse provides many services in the home for patients who are unable to travel to a medical care facility.

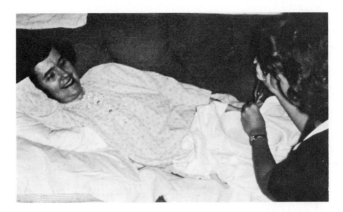

scoliosis evaluation and screening for communicable diseases commonly are conducted in the schools by the community health nurse.

The community health nurse may make periodic visits to the classroom. He or she observes the children and notes those who seem to deviate from normal well-being. The children who appear to have a health-related problem are referred to the appropriate school authorities. Their parents, too, are notified of a potential problem. The nurse's responsibilities also include follow-up of these referrals since no school screening program is effective if the recommended medical care is not obtained.

If the child's parents are not familiar with the appropriate community medical resources for treating the problem, the public health nurse will assist them. This may mean recommending the social services available in the community. The role of the nurse, then, includes not only the education of the parents about appropriate care, but also the actual follow-up treatment for the child.

The community health nurse is often called upon by health education instructors to help in the planning of a health lesson or to serve as a content resource person. Though the community health nurse usually does not teach regularly scheduled health classes, he or she may talk to the children about special topics. Not only are presentations made for the children, but classes for parents on specific health

concerns are given. One very common classroom situation is the presentation on menstruation and feminine growth and development for preteenage girls and their mothers. On occasion the nurse will conduct a class on growth and developmental concerns for boys.

Home Visitation Service

Many community health nurses provide health care services with visits to the home. Historically, such visits investigated cases of chronic and communicable diseases. But today home visitation has expanded so that a very large portion of the nurse's time is now directed toward maternal and child health concerns.

In some communities, health department services are provided to any new mother and her infant. The nurse visits the home and evaluates the health status of the mother and the baby. He or she advises the mother on the care and feeding of the infant and counsels her on an appropriate immunization schedule for the child. The nurse attempts to direct the mother to a medical care service if there is no family physician.

The community health nurse also becomes involved with families having multiple health problems. Most of the people who seek the health department services are the economically disadvantaged. This population group all too often has a

The dairy inspector (a) checks dairy product storage in local dairies, (b) checks the bulk tank to assure that standards are maintained, and (c) examines pasteurizing equipment.

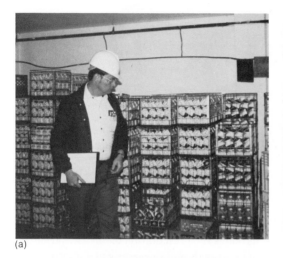
(a)

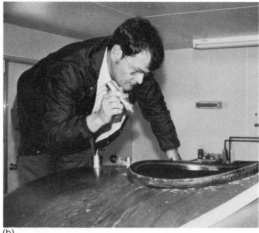
(b)

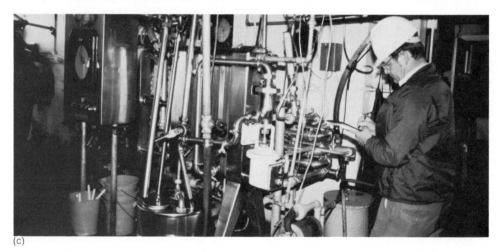
(c)

number of compounded health problems. Their needs are made known to the health department by many sources including direct visitation, school referral, court referral, or referral from a community social service. In all instances, the nurse enters the home and attempts to work with the family as a unit.

Clinics

Most local health departments operate a variety of clinics. It is in one of these clinics that the community health nurse provides a number of basic nursing services. Here the nurse assists the physician in conducting medical examinations, in taking health histories, in maintaining records, and in a host of other services. For example, many people come to the health department clinic for immunizations. Children most frequently require the nurse's services for those inoculations, but many adults (those considering international travel or working in a specific environment) will also seek these immunizations. Another important role played by the public health nurse in the clinical setting is that of patient counselor. This counseling may involve informing the patient of the health condition, helping the patient to cope or adjust to the situation, or recommending additional measures.

The Environmental Sanitarian

Within most state and local health departments are a variety of programs that contribute to the improvement of environmental conditions. These programs include safe water supply, restaurant sanitation, adequate safe housing, swimming pool inspection, milk sanitation, pest and rodent control, and a variety of other activities. These programs are often mandated by state or local laws, codes, and ordinances. These laws, codes, and ordinances are in the public domain and are designed to protect the general public from sickness, disease, and disability. The public health sanitarian is important to the function of an environmental sanitation program.

The public health environmental sanitarian plays an important role in maintaining an environment that is conducive to good health. In the past, this individual was instrumental in the control of communicable diseases. In recent years, as a result of the greater awareness of environmental problems, the responsibilities of the environmental sanitarian have expanded.[16]

Air and water pollution have always been a challenge to the sanitarian. State and federal legislation in both of these areas have transferred power and responsibility to the environmentalist. Today, the environmental sanitarian is concerned—in addition to the problems of air and water pollution, noise abatement, and radiation—with food sanitation, housing, rodent control, and a variety of other environmental conditions and their effects upon individual health and quality of community life.

The sanitarian performs the tasks that are mandated by law at the local, state, and federal levels. These actions may include inspection of food service establishments, of mobile home parks, of public housing centers, or of public schools. A sanitarian may also respond to a complaint and conduct a search to ascertain if a given condition is in violation of the law.

The county health department sanitarian checks the municipal swimming pool for pH level and chlorine residual. Such inspections help to assure a safe swimming area for local residents.

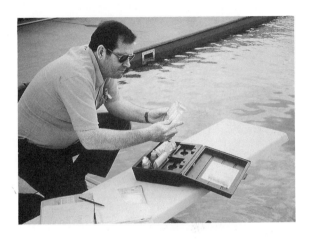

The sanitarian conducts inspections to make sure that public facilities meet appropriate laws and regulations. For example, a food service establishment must be inspected and approved before it can open to public customers. On a periodic basis the sanitarian will conduct additional inspections to assure that the restaurant is still in compliance with appropriate regulations. Where conditions do not meet standards, the sanitarian must inform the owner and then take action to assure correction of the defect or to close down the facility.

Searches occur in response to specific complaints and are not conducted on a regular basis. The sanitarian, upon receiving the complaint, must visit the facility and determine if any violations of laws and regulations exist. If evidence of wrongdoing is noted, the sanitarian files an appropriate report, and correction must be made or a penalty paid.

An inspection can be viewed as a preventive health measure since compliance with certain laws and regulations is checked. On the other hand, a search is more corrective in nature, looking specifically for wrongdoing as reported by another party. Most sanitarians prefer to conduct inspections where they can teach the public about a sanitary environment, rather than searches, where they act as enforcers.

Vending machines that provide coffee, tea, and other drinks must meet certain standards of cleanliness. These are inspected by the local health department sanitarian.

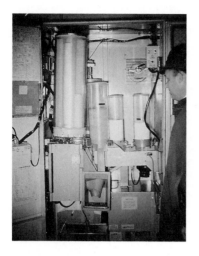

In order to assure that the milk we buy in the local store is safe for human consumption it is important that the farm from which the milk comes meets certain standards of sanitation. It is the task of the local health department sanitarian to periodically inspect dairy farms.

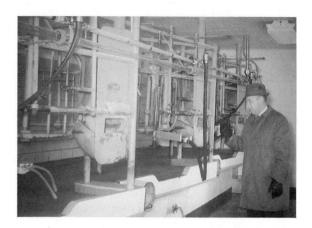

Food Sanitation

The prevention of foodborne disease and illness is the basic objective of public health food sanitation programs. The most widely known cause of food-borne disease outbreak in the United States is salmonella. This usually results from insufficient cooking and improper holding temperatures of the food. The usual signs of food poisoning are vomiting, abdominal cramps, and diarrhea. The public health sanitarian inspects restaurants and other food services to identify unsafe and unclean conditions and to prevent food poisoning and contamination.

Eating at public food establishments has increased dramatically in recent years. Fast-food preparation techniques have resulted in a number of fast-food franchises operating in nearly every city of the country. Because so many people eat out on a regular basis at such establishments, maintaining environments that meet food service codes is of greater importance today than in the past.

The responsibilities of the sanitarian include checking the quality of the food served. Thus, sanitarians are specially trained in food, meat, and milk

sanitation measures. These procedures call for meat and milk inspection. In addition, the sanitarian must certify that the food establishment meets all regulations for the general sanitation of the food preparation and eating areas.

There are several factors that contribute to foodborne diseases. The food itself may be contaminated with microorganisms that cause disease in humans. Often the source of this contamination may be mishandling in the food processing plants or contact with a contaminated employee. For this reason, it is not only important to make sure that food service facilities meet regulations, but that the food processing procedures are sanitary as well.

Inadequate heat processing of food can result in foodborne disease. If foods are not heat processed, toxins are ingested and disease results. Toxins vary in heat stability, but most are destroyed after a few seconds in temperatures reaching 165 degrees F. Bacteria in foods can be killed at lower temperatures if exposed for longer periods of time. Cooking food at too low a temperature or for too short a time will not kill toxins and disease results.

Unhealthy living conditions are manifest in a variety of ways. Poor sanitation and an old structure are an attraction for rodents.

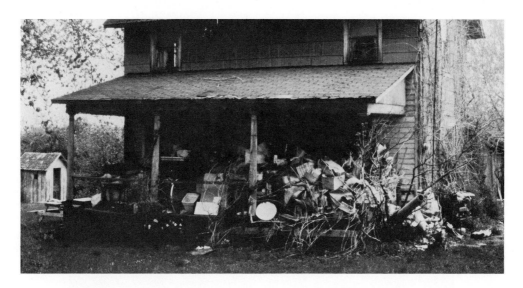

In addition to improper cooking of food, disease can be the result of improper storage of certain foods. Foods that should be refrigerated but are left in warm surroundings are likely to become contaminated and so cause illness.

Disease can be spread with the use of inadequately cleaned cooking equipment. Also the cleanliness of personnel handling food is a contributing factor. There are numerous items that must be inspected to assure that cleanliness and sanitary procedures are maintained.

Some organisms cause food poisoning, or more accurately, intoxication, because the organisms release a toxin on the food that will be eaten. Clostridium perfringens and staphylococcal infections are capable of causing such food intoxication.

Housing

In many cities throughout the United States, there is a shortage of adequate housing, and problems of overcrowding and substandard buildings exist. These problems have grown in recent years as the cost of housing has risen. Lower-income families cannot afford the price of houses, when perhaps a decade ago they could have purchased a home. As a result, these families establish their households in older buildings, apartments, or housing that is only marginally standard.

Most communities have regulations that ensure a safe and healthy living environment. These regulations have to do with water supply, waste removal, and pest control. Usually, local public health departments are responsible for upholding these regulations.

Since housing inspectors usually do not conduct regular inspections and are too few in number in most large cities, housing often becomes substandard or even creates a threat to human well-being. In most instances, the building inspectors approve the construction of new buildings. After this initial approval, they are likely to return only to deal with occupants' complaints or if social workers or public health personnel consider that conditions warrant an inspection.

Inadequate housing has both direct and indirect effects upon the health of people. Unintentional injuries in the home are a cause of many deaths and disabling injuries each year. Over twenty thousand deaths occur each year in the home as the result of

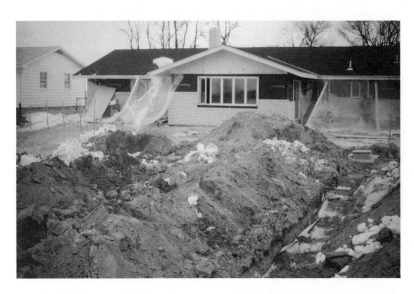

accidents.[17] More than half of these fatalities involve children under five years of age and the elderly over the age of sixty-five. The National Safety Council has estimated that in a recent year, there were more than 3.1 million disabling injuries from home accidents, resulting in a cost of at least fourteen billion dollars.[18] Not all of these accidents occurred in substandard housing, but many times improperly maintained structures were responsible for accidents and related fatalities or injuries.

Inadequate housing is also responsible for the high incidence of lead poisoning among children living in older homes and apartments. Lead poisoning is a problem particularly among preschool children living in old, dilapidated houses where lead-based paint has peeled from walls, floors, doorways, and other parts of the building. The young children chip at the peeling lead-based paint, then eat the pieces that fall off the wall. Lead is a toxic element that causes a number of health problems: anemia, headaches, weakness, and impaired kidney functioning. If untreated, the nervous system may be affected, resulting in blindness, paralysis, and eventually coma and death.

A number of gastrointestinal diseases are caused by poor sanitation, inappropriate water supply, and lack of adequate waste disposal. In many localities, particularly in rural settings, septic systems do not meet required standards. As a result, leaching from the septic system contaminates the water table. In many communities, private contractors remove wastes. Among some poor, rural families it is impossible to pay for such service, so solid waste accumulates and results in problems with insects, rodents, and other disease-causing agents.

In an indirect manner, overcrowding contributes to a lower level of health and well-being. When people are forced to live in an overcrowded housing situation, respiratory diseases are likely to spread. Also, crowding over a long period of time has detrimental effects on the mental health of individuals.

There is a need to establish and support programs that rehabilitate existing housing, both in urban communities and in rural settings. It is important that housing improvement is considered a public health concern because poor, substandard, unsanitary living conditions have a major effect on the health of a community.

Pest Control

Insects and rodents are a public health concern throughout the United States. Flies, especially, constitute a serious public health problem. The household fly feeds upon human waste, garbage, and other filth and debris. It then travels into the home or restaurant and feeds upon food prepared for human consumption. By carrying the pathogens on parts of its body the fly is carrying disease. As a result, many different diseases are spread by domestic flies, including typhoid, cholera, dysentery, hookworm, and pinworm. Mosquitoes, too, are a reservoir of infection and a mode of microorganism transmission. They are particularly a problem in the transmission of malaria, the most widespread disease in the world. Cockroaches also carry various disease organisms.

Pesticides are helpful in controlling insects. Nevertheless, the importance of maintaining a clean, sanitary environment cannot be overlooked. Garbage must be covered and kept where insects cannot invade it.

Possibly the most widespread pest control problem is rodent control. Rats have caused extensive sickness and death throughout the history of humanity. Bubonic plague, or the "black death," is transmitted to humans chiefly by fleas from infected rats. This plague killed millions of people in Europe during the Middle Ages. In India, as many as ten million people died from bubonic plague at the turn of this century. Today the plague is controlled somewhat by medicine and public sanitation.

Another disease caused by fleas that live on rats is typhus. This disease is symptomatically similar to bubonic plague, but is usually less severe.

Several thousand cases of diseases caused by organisms that live on rats are reported in the United States each year. The rat carries fleas and a number of internal parasites that can affect humans.

Because of a weak bladder, the rat urinates often and spoils food and grain. Public health authorities speculate that many cases of indigestion and "flu" in people living in poor inner-city neighborhoods where there is a rodent population are the result of eating food contaminated by rodents.

Rodents are indigenous to the entire United States. But they are particularly populous in urban communities among the lower socioeconomic populations and in cities located on international waterways. There is always the danger that infected rodents are aboard incoming ocean vessels.

Numerous rodent bites are reported each year. Children are the most common victims of rat bites. Most of these bites occur in the home, not out-of-doors. All too often a small child is bitten while asleep in the crib. In such cases, rabies transmission is feared.

The rodent population has increased in recent years because of several circumstances. The natural predators of rodents in the wild are foxes, hawks, and owls. As society has become more urbanized, it has encroached upon the natural habitat of these predators, thus decreasing their population.

Rat poisons have been used widely to control rodents but are only moderately effective. Unfortunately, rodents have developed a resistance and immunity to certain of the more effective rodenticides. It has thus become necessary to develop a more effective poison. The problem with this, however, is that such poisons will kill domestic animals as well as humans.

Improved sanitation and cleanliness have been emphasized as the most positive public health measures in rodent control. Preventive procedures include the cleanup of environments that attract rodents: picking up garbage and other waste materials, covering garbage cans, repairing cracks and holes in walls of buildings, and cleaning areas where rats may be living. If a rodent cannot find a place to burrow and live and cannot obtain food, it will not remain in the area.

Rodent-control programs emphasize prevention, cleanliness, and education. The environment should be as unattractive for rats as is possible. Some communities have mobilized citizens in efforts to clean city lots and old, dilapidated structures, and to mow long grass. As people learn rodent-control procedures and the importance of cleanliness, this public health problem will improve.

Summary

The official health organization at the state and local level is the health department. Each of the fifty states has a state department of health, with many local health departments serving the states' many communities. Funding for these departments comes principally from tax revenues.

State and local health departments provide a range of services, the most common being immunization, environmental surveillance, tuberculosis control, communicable and chronic disease programs, school health services, maternal and child health, and family planning. Legal mandate and budgetary constraint affect the number of services provided. The activities of the local and state health departments are often conducted in cooperation with each other.

Health departments rely on the services of public health laboratories. The functions of a health laboratory vary from one locality to another. Microbiology and serology laboratories are important for communicable disease control activities. Chemical analysis, blood analysis, and various laboratory testing of environmental factors are also part of the health department laboratory activities.

Dental health is more than a personal matter, especially in terms of one issue. Possibly the most effective public health preventive measure against dental caries is the fluoridation of public drinking water. Though a proven measure in reducing the incidence of dental problems, fluoridation of public drinking water has been very controversial. Some people see it as mandated health care, social medicine, or environmental pollution of the drinking water and have fought for its prohibition. These matters have placed the state and local health departments in the middle of a continuing controversy.

Two of the most visible state or local health department personnel are the community health nurse and the sanitarian. The community health nurse provides nursing, education, counseling, and social service skills in a variety of settings. Most commonly, the community health nurse is found working in the health department clinic, in the schools, or in private homes providing home health care.

Health department sanitarians perform a broad range of services. They conduct food and food establishment inspections to ensure that proper sanitation measures are being met and that the food being served is safe for consumption. Other health concerns of the sanitarian involve housing inspections and the control of insects, rodents, and other pests. Rodent-control programs have involved cleaning up waste material, garbage, and other materials that attract rodents. Such problems and related programs are more commonly found in poor, urban neighborhoods.

Discussion Questions

1. Review the annual report of the state health department program in your state and discuss the various programs conducted.
2. Identify the relationships that are important in your local and state health departments.
3. What are the most common services provided by local health departments?
4. Do you believe that the local health department commissioner should be a physician? Defend your answer.
5. What laboratory services are usually found in health departments?
6. Trace the working relationships between the federal health administration, state, and local health departments in relation to laboratory services.
7. Identify several reasons why fluoridation of the public drinking water is beneficial.
8. Discuss some of the reasons given for opposition of fluoridation of public drinking water.

9. How has the dental profession effectively educated the public on dental hygiene?

10. Identify some of the responsibilities of a community health nurse.

11. What does the public health nurse do in the school setting?

12. If you were a public health department sanitarian, what would you look for during food inspections?

13. Explain the difference between a sanitarian's inspection and a sanitarian's search.

14. What procedures for rodent control should a community implement?

Suggested Readings

Materials, data, and assorted information concerning state and local health departments is available from: Association of State and Territorial Health Officials, 1311A Dolley Madison Blvd., Suite 3A, McLean, Virginia 22101

Berkseth, Janet Kempf. "Public Health Nursing for America's Children." *Public Health Nursing* 2, no. 4 (December, 1985): 221-31.

Browne, Sanford M. "A Comparison of Inspection and Search." *Journal of Environmental Health* 44, no. 5 (March/April, 1982): 245-48.

Buhler-Wilkerson, Karen. "Public Health Nursing: In Sickness or in Health?" *American Journal of Public Health* 75, no. 10 (October, 1985): 1155-61.

Cameron, Charles M., and Kobylarz, Anthony. "Nonphysician Directors of Local Health Departments: Results of a National Survey." *Public Health Reports* 95, no. 4 (July/August, 1980): 386-97.

Combs-Orme, Terri. "Effectiveness of Home Visits by Public Health Nurses in Maternal and Child Health: An Empirical Review." *Public Health Reports* 100, no. 5 (September/October, 1985): 490-98.

El-Araf, Amer, and Baca, Thomas E. "The Administration of State and Local Environmental Health Programs: Who is Responsible?" *Journal of Environmental Health* 43, no. 2 (September/October, 1980): 86-100.

Jain, Sagar C. "Role of State and Local Governments in Relation to Personal Health Services." *American Journal of Public Health, Supplement* 71 (January, 1981): 1-95.

Loe, Harold. "The Fluoridation Status of U.S. Public Water Supplies." *Public Health Reports* 101, no. 2 (March/April, 1986): 159-62.

Roberts, Doris E., and Heinrich, Janet. "Public Health Nursing Comes of Age." *American Journal of Public Health* 75, no. 10 (October, 1985): 1162-72.

Vandusen, Karen. "The Challenge of Chronic Physical and Mental Disease to Environmental Sanitarians." *Public Health Reports* 95, no. 3 (May/June, 1980): 223-38.

Endnotes

1. Gossert, Daniel J., and Miller, C. Ardon. "State Boards of Health, Their Members and Commitments." *American Journal of Public Health* 65 (1973).

2. Discussed in chapter 2 under The New Federalism.

3. Miller, C. Ardon, et al. "A Survey of Local Public Health Departments and Their Directors." *American Journal of Public Health* 67, no. 10 (October, 1977): 934.

4. Cameron, Charles M., and Kobylarz, Anthony. "Nonphysician Directors of Local Health Departments: Results of a National Survey." *Public Health Reports* 95, no. 4 (July/August, 1980): 386-97.

5. Miller, et al. "Local Public Health Departments." 932.

6. Ibid., 943.

7. Ibid., 932.

8. *Healthy People: The Surgeon General's Report on Health Promotion and Disease Prevention.* Washington, D.C.: U.S. Government Printing Office, 1979: 116.

9. Arnold, F. A., Jr. "Grand Rapids Fluoridation Study: Results Pertaining to the 11th Year of Fluoridation." *American Journal of Public Health* 47 (1957): 539.

10. Loe, Harold. "The Fluoridation Status of United States Public Water Supplies." *Public Health Reports* 101, no. 2 (March/April, 1986): 157.

11. "Revised Statement on Fluoridation." *Journal of the American Medical Association* 231, no. 11 (March 17, 1985): 1167.

12. Rosenstein, David I., et al. "Fighting the Latest Challenge to Fluoridation in Oregon." *Public Health Reports* 93, no. 1 (January/February, 1978): 69-72.

13. Loe, Harold. "The Fluoridation Status of United States Public Water Supplies." 159.

14. Combs-Orme, Terri. "Effectiveness of Home Visits by Public Health Nurses in Maternal and Child Health: An Empirical Review." *Public Health Reports* 100, no. 5 (September/October, 1985): 490.

15. Ibid., 491.

16. Vandusen, Karen. "The Challenge of Chronic Physical and Mental Disease to Environmental Sanitarians." *Public Health Reports* 95, no. 3 (May/June, 1980): 223–38.

17. National Safety Council. *Accident Facts, 1986.* Chicago, Ill.: National Safety Council: 79.

18. Ibid., 3–4.

4

International Health: Need for Cooperation in Problem Solving

The World Health Assembly, the governing body of the World Health Organization, meets annually at WHO headquarters in Geneva, Switzerland.

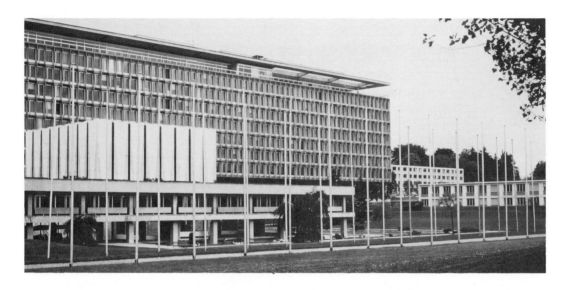

Humanity has rarely made a concerted effort to solve international health problems. Through the years attempts have been made to develop global cooperation in solving the problems of disease, sickness, and starvation. Yet warfare, natural disaster, poverty, and illiteracy continue to thwart these efforts at international cooperation.

In the past, this cooperation may not have been as necessary as it is today. Peoples of the world were isolated from one another by space, time, and culture. Contact between nations and cultural groups within nations was limited so disease was slow to move from place to place. But with the advent of increased mobility and communication, world exploration, industrial development, and growth in population, health problems can no longer be contained by national boundaries or tribal geography. In the latter part of the twentieth century the need for cooperation and improvement of health programs on an international scale is a vital necessity. Quality of life is much more likely to be affected by conditions half the world away than was ever the case before.

International Agencies

World Health Organization

In 1946 an International Health Conference was held in San Francisco. At this conference representatives of sixty-one different governments agreed on the need for an international health organization. As a result, the constitution of the World Health Organization (WHO) was written. It was not until April 1948, however, that ratification of the constitution took place and the World Health Organization was created. It was founded as an agency of the United Nations with central headquarters located in Geneva, Switzerland. Since its founding, this international agency has met with varied degrees of success in improving the quality of health and well-being throughout the world.

The basic objective of WHO is to "help nations to help themselves" in dealing with specific health problems and concerns. One of WHO's earliest contributions to the health professions was the development of a definition for health: "Health is a state of complete physical, mental, and social well-being, and not merely the absence of disease or infirmity."

This definition has received worldwide recognition and acceptance and has served as a foundation for program planning, development, and implementation.

The World Health Organization consists of two official bodies: a governing body and an executive body. (1) The governing body, the World Health Assembly, meets annually to establish policy, program, and budget. A nation does not have to belong to the United Nations in order to belong to the World Health Organization. In 1987 there were 166 member nations—each represented by three official delegates—in the World Health Assembly. However, each nation has only one vote. (2) The executive arm of the World Health Organization is the Executive Board. Representatives of thirty nations, selected on a rotating basis, constitute this board, whose responsibility is to conduct and guide the routine activities initiated by the World Health Assembly.

Six regional offices for WHO have been established. (See table 4.1.) Personnel from these offices supervise and coordinate the actual field work in their respective regions. Specific program focus and emphasis vary from one region to another, depending upon the principal health problems.

The World Health Organization helps nations in planning and providing health services. Projects are conducted for the most part in the developing nations, with professional expertise provided by scientists, educators, engineers, nurses, physicians, dentists, administrators, and other staff personnel. These personnel from developed nations are made available to the developing nations on a short-term, consultant basis. In addition, programs for the education and training of Third World inhabitants are established so that they can eventually assume the duties of the consultants.

Programs tend to be extensive, depending upon the need. Wide-scale activities that the World Health Organization has undertaken include development of an international disease classification system; world communicable disease control; establishment of international standards for foods, drugs, and vaccines; standardization of statistics on disease and

Table 4.1 Regional Offices of the World Health Organization

Area	Office Location
Africa	Brazzaville, Zaire
Americas	Washington, D.C.
Europe	Copenhagen, Denmark
Eastern Mediterranean	Alexandria, Egypt
South East Asia	New Delhi, India
Western Pacific	Manila, Philippines

mortality; health manpower development programs; and development of modern laboratory facilities for comprehensive diagnostic purposes. WHO activities in health manpower development have included the training of health science personnel and specialists; the design, production, and distribution of teaching materials; plus the promotion of health development centers. Other activities include maternal-child health activities and energetic immunization programs.[1]

The sanitation and improvement of water supplies are examples of specific needs that the World Health Organization believes are vitally important objectives in its overall programming. For example, potable water—water that is suitable for drinking—is unavailable for 75 to 80 percent of the citizens living in rural areas of some developing nations. One person out of every four in the world suffers from some type of waterborne disease. As a result, the decade 1980 to 1989 has been designated the International Drinking Water Supply and Sanitation Decade. WHO's objective is for every nation to provide a clean water supply for its inhabitants by 1990.

Since 1948, WHO priorities have been expanded, revised, shifted, and redirected according to changes in the needs of a particular period of time and geographic location. Original WHO priorities included eradication of malaria and tuberculosis and control of venereal disease. Starvation and malnutrition, also serious health problems, have been the focus of various World Health Organization programs, too.

An example of the modification in priorities is the smallpox eradication program. In 1967 the World Health Organization decided to inaugurate a program designed to eradicate smallpox. At that time smallpox was endemic in forty-four nations of the world.[2] Through surveillance, vaccination, and education, this long-feared disease, which had killed millions throughout history, has been eradicated. The last known case of smallpox was diagnosed in a resident in Somalia, East Africa, in 1977.[3] In December 1979 the World Health Organization officially declared the world free from smallpox, and an official certificate of eradication was issued. This program has been without question one of the most successful programs developed by the World Health Organization. It demonstrates that international cooperation and program efforts can solve health problems.

Hanson's disease (leprosy) is another example of a health problem that WHO has worked to eliminate. Assisted by the World Health Organization, a number of nations today have control programs for Hanson's disease. Not only are case finding and treatment important, but research is also conducted in a number of localities.

Not all WHO disease prevention and eradication programs have been successful. In the early 1950s malaria was identified as a "priority disease" for eradication programming. Malaria-control programs (where all buildings were sprayed with DDT) were developed in some ninety-five different countries. The largest program was in India where over 150,000 people were employed in the eradication project. But despite the fact that the program was the largest disease eradication effort in history, in the 1980s malaria continues to be one of the most widespread international diseases. It is still considered to be a very serious problem in many parts of Africa, Asia, and Latin America.

A primary reason for the malaria-control failure was the international ban on DDT because of biological magnification in the food chain. This action required the use of alternative insecticides with shorter residual times and higher costs. Another major reason for the failure of malaria eradication programs has been that the mosquitoes that transmit the microorganism of malaria have become increasingly resistant to insecticides and drugs used to combat the disease. In addition, efforts to educate people to remove standing water, a breeding source for mosquitoes, have not been successful.

The World Health Organization, in conjunction with many nations of the world, continues to study ways to control malaria. It is felt that an effective program must include more than just spraying of DDT. A more comprehensive program is needed that removes standing water sources, implements effective educational efforts, and is a regular aspect of primary health care.

Joint Agency Programs

The World Health Organization has joint programs with other international agencies such as the United Nations Children's Fund (UNICEF)—formerly the United Nations International Children's Emergency Fund, the Food and Agricultural Organization (FAO), and the International Fund for Agricultural Development. In addition to jointly sponsored programs conducted with WHO these agencies conduct a variety of health-related programs having a special focus on activities of a nutritional nature.

UNICEF conducts programs to help children, particularly those in the developing nations. Numerous programs have been implemented to control communicable diseases and to improve nutrition. Funding for this agency results from voluntary contributions from governments and private citizens.

The Food and Agriculture Organization oversees programs designed to relieve hunger and malnutrition throughout the world. Research, school lunch programs, education, and direct services to those in need are vital parts of FAO involvement.

An example of an interagency program is the Onchocerciasis Control Program which has been implemented in eleven countries of West Africa.[4] Onchocerciasis is a debilitating disease that has caused blindness in several million people worldwide. The Onchocerciasis Control Program has brought together the resources of the United Nations Development Program, FAO, the World Bank, and the World Health Organization. Research has been conducted to find effective drugs to counter the filariae in the human body that cause this disease. Various measures have been developed to train field personnel in ways to assist people with onchocerciasis.

Many other agencies and organizations throughout the world have programs designed to meet the health needs of people. Some are government sponsored, such as the United States Agency for International Development (AID). AID provides funds for health and nutrition programs to Third World countries. Other medical- and health-related activities are conducted by nonprofit, volunteer organizations, referred to as nongovernmental organizations (NGOs). NGOs include many religious agencies such as Catholic Relief Services, Compassion International, and World Vision. Other nonprofit groups that are active in many health, nutrition, and population projects include Save the Children, and Helen Keller International. In March 1980 the World Bank announced that funds would be directly available for health projects.[5] The purpose of supporting health projects is to strengthen a nation's primary health care system. It is hoped that such actions will improve access to basic health care, particularly for the poor of the world.

Primary Health Care

Changing concepts have led the World Health Organization and other agencies involved in international health to place more emphasis upon primary health care, not just disease control. Primary health care is now considered a major program objective in the Third World nations.

In 1978, an international conference on primary health care was held in Alma-Ata, USSR. This conference was organized and sponsored by the World Health Organization and the United Nations Children's Fund (UNICEF), and followed worldwide national and regional meetings on primary health care. A major objective of the conference was to promote the concept and development of primary health care in all nations of the world.

The most important outcome of this conference was the Declaration of Alma-Ata. This document has provided significant direction for World Health Organization programming as well as for other international health agencies and organizations, both governmental and voluntary.

The concept of primary health care varies from one location to another. However, there are certain health problems that most agree fall into the category of primary health care. As stated in the recommendations of the Alma-Ata conference, primary health care should include at least:

. . . education concerning prevailing health problems and the methods of identifying, preventing, and controlling them; promotion of food supply and proper nutrition, an adequate supply of safe water, and basic sanitation; maternal and child health care, including family planning; immunization against the major infectious diseases; prevention and control of locally endemic diseases; appropriate treatment of common diseases and injuries; promotion of mental health; and the provision of essential drugs.[6]

Primary health care focuses attention on principal health problems and so must be a part of the health policy planning of any government. The government may have to reevaluate its health priorities, however, in incorporating primary health care into its policy planning. This may mean the development of different types of health personnel and reduced emphasis on curative facilities, particularly in the Third World. Or it may mean integrating the traditional methods of healing with the modern concepts of medicine in many nations.

The Declaration of Alma-Ata has served as an impetus for the World Health Organization, other international agencies, and the governments of the world to set specific, practical goals in their health planning. The Declaration called for all governments to formulate national policies and action plans and to include primary health care as a part of their national health systems. The Declaration called for the cooperation and commitment of governmental bodies in striving for "an acceptable level of health for all people . . . by the year 2000."

Honduras—death rate from diarrheal diseases among children under two years of age fell 40 percent within a year and a half after start of ORT program.

Haiti—at University Hospital death rate of infants with diarrhea was lowered from 35 percent to 14 percent during the first year of ORT program.

Egypt—Diarrhea-related deaths in children under two were reduced by two-thirds from 1980 to 1985 due to the introduction of oral rehydration therapy.

Source: U.S. Agency for International Development, *AID Highlights*, Vol. 3, no. 1, Winter 1986, p. 2.

Whereas Alma-Ata emphasized primary health care, previous international conferences focused upon curative health provisions emphasizing facilities, research, technological development, and increased health care personnel. The emphasis on primary health care should result in lower costs and be much more effective in attaining the long-range goal of improving people's lives.

UNICEF: State of the World's Children

In a statement issued in 1982 UNICEF suggested that developments in social and biological sciences make it possible at very low cost to significantly improve the health of children throughout the world.[7] UNICEF stated that a serious commitment by nations' governments and international health organizations could significantly reduce disability and death among children by as much as one half within a decade. This could be accomplished by conducting programs of simple oral rehydration, universal child immunization, promotion of breast-feeding, and mass distribution and use of simple cardboard weight charts for coping with malnutrition.

Oral Rehydration Therapy (ORT)

The world's largest killer of children throughout the Third World is diarrhea. The World Health Organization estimates that five million children a year die from diarrhea. As recently as fifteen years ago the standard treatment for dehydration was intravenous infusion of fluids. This was not only costly but necessitated the presence of trained medical personnel and sterile equipment. However, a procedure of rehydrating patients by oral administration of a solution of water, sugar, and salts has now become widely used. This procedure, known as ORT, is inexpensive, can be prepared by the patient's parents, and has been shown to be very successful. Through the use of oral rehydration therapy many children have been saved from death.

Universal Child Immunization

Millions of children die each year throughout the world from common childhood diseases for which protection is available in the form of immunization. Measles, diphtheria, tetanus, whooping cough, polio, and tuberculosis account for about one-third of all childhood deaths. Two million children a year die from measles.[8] The development of more heat-stable, effective, and inexpensive vaccines has made it possible to immunize children in the remotest of Third World nations. For agencies conducting child survival programs immunization must be a top priority.

Breast-feeding

Children who are breast-fed are healthier and obtain all the necessary nutrients needed for early childhood growth and development. Breast milk alone is adequate until most infants are four to six

Simple, cardboard growth charts can be helpful to the mother in identifying deviations from normal health related to proper growth and development. This chart and instructional information have been used by thousands of village health workers throughout the world.

A typical **ROAD TO HEALTH CHART SHOWING A CHILD'S PROGRESS:**

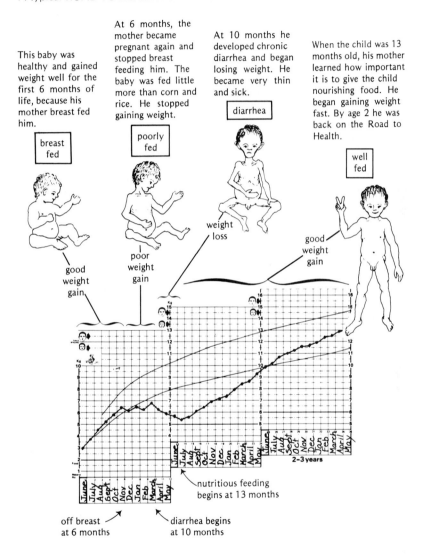

This baby was healthy and gained weight well for the first 6 months of life, because his mother breast fed him.

At 6 months, the mother became pregnant again and stopped breast feeding him. The baby was fed little more than corn and rice. He stopped gaining weight.

At 10 months he developed chronic diarrhea and began losing weight. He became very thin and sick.

When the child was 13 months old, his mother learned how important it is to give the child nourishing food. He began gaining weight fast. By age 2 he was back on the Road to Health.

Road to Health charts are important. They help mothers know when their children need more nutritious food and special attention. They help health workers better understand the needs of the child and his family. They also let the mother know when she is doing a good job.

Source: Werner, David. Where There Is No Doctor, *1985, p. 304.*
Permission for use provided by the Hesperian Foundation, P.O. Box 1692, Palo Alto, Calif. 94302.

The China Medical College in Taichung, Taiwan, R.O.C., includes education for both traditional Chinese doctors and modern medicine. This medical college provides a setting for the integration of both medical care systems.

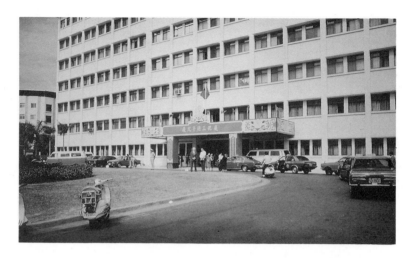

months of age, yet mothers in many Third World nations are choosing to stop breast-feeding and use bottle-feeding.[9] At the time of weaning the child is at high risk for infection, diarrheal diseases, and malnutrition. This is the result of such factors as: illiteracy, in which mothers are unable to read the instructions on the infant formula labels; the use of impure, polluted water resulting in diluted formula; and basic economic poverty. It is important that women be educated regarding the advantages of breast-feeding and the disadvantages of switching to the use of infant formula and bottle-feeding.

Malnutrition

Millions of children worldwide suffer from malnutrition. Protein and vitamin A deficiencies are often present, but malnutrition may not be noticed by mothers until the problem has become serious and life threatening. With the use of rather simple, inexpensive cardboard growth charts mothers can be taught to enter a monthly weight of the child. Over a period of time they can see abnormal changes in growth and can be taught to seek help when these abnormal growth patterns develop.

Health Care Needs

The lack of medical care in many countries is related to inadequate health care facilities and work force. In most Third World nations whatever health care provisions are available are usually found in the urban areas. Since these health providers usually practice fee-for-service medicine, the poor and the disadvantaged often do not receive appropriate care.

Those living in rural areas are denied access to health care because of geography just as the urban poor are denied because of economics. Even though there is a pattern of movement to urban centers from rural areas, millions of people still reside in the small towns, villages, and hamlets of the world. Health care facilities are seldom located in these outposts, and the small-town inhabitants rarely venture to larger cities for treatment.

Numerous strategies have been introduced in an effort to meet the needs of these people. Some nations require all physicians, nurses, and other health care providers to serve in these rural settings for a specific period of time upon completion of their education. This measure helps to meet some health needs, but the health personnel seldom remain in the rural areas once the required service is fulfilled. The

At the China Medical College, traditional Chinese herbal medicines are prepared, studied, and used. The students enrolled in the traditional medical curriculum learn what herbal preparations are effective for specific health problems. Research is conducted to ascertain in what ways the herbs have healing properties.

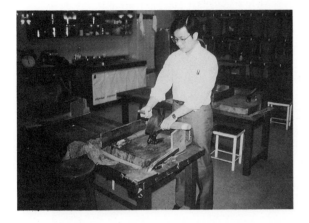

urban centers, with their modern health care facilities, specialized medicine, and greater income potential, are far more attractive to the physicians, nurses, and other health care personnel than the impoverished rural areas of their nation.

There are other reasons, too, for the health care providers to immediately return to the city after their required service is completed. They sometimes see their roles as medical administrators in the clinical setting where direct clinical services are not priorities. Personnel seldom venture from the clinic to administer medicine directly to the people in the small villages. Many times there are cultural and linguistic differences between the health care providers and the rural people. This creates a feeling of distance and of distrust and sometimes results in failure to provide optimum health care.

As a result, in spite of governmental efforts to provide adequate health care in rural areas, most rural Third World residents do not have access to needed health provisions. For many people the principal health care provider is still the traditional village healer who has learned his or her skills and techniques from long apprenticeship with an older healer, quite often a parent or other relative.

Traditional medicine makes use of different herbs, spices, and procedures in the healing process. Many times the healing concepts are rooted in religious beliefs and practices. Traditional medicine has been looked upon by many modern medical practitioners as basically unacceptable medical practice. Modern medicine has tended to ignore and to reject these traditional health systems and procedures. As a result, when modern medicine is introduced into a locality, the people are often urged to turn from the traditional ways of healing.

In recent years it has been suggested that traditional healing systems have much to offer in providing health care to many of the world's population. One important reason for traditional medicine's effectiveness is that many rural, Third World citizens trust, understand, and can afford this form of medicine whereas modern medicine is mistrusted and the facilities and work force are too costly. Also, people do not have to be educated to seek the healer's help; he or she is a visible presence in the community. For these reasons, with the support of governments and the World Health Organization, modern medicine is encouraged to cooperate with and to integrate traditional healers in health care programs. Measures have been taken in many countries to use the best of traditional medicine along with basic concepts of more modern medical care. In fact, some traditional healers have even been given training in the rudiments of modern medical practice.

A second development, which has gained widespread interest, is the use of village health workers as providers of primary health care among the poor, particularly rural people, of the Third World. Primary medical care skills are taught to a person selected from a village. This individual continues to live in his or her village and acts as the basic health care provider. This concept, popularized during the 1970s, is based on the barefoot doctor programs of the Peoples Republic of China. The village health worker provides the same services that the barefoot doctors did.

The village health workers—*promotores del salud* as they are known in many parts of Latin America, or medical *montris* as they are called in

These village dental workers, known as dental montris, in Irian Jaya, Indonesia, are trained to perform extractions and to do simple fillings. They provide the only dental care to thousands of people living in the rural communities of Irian Jaya.

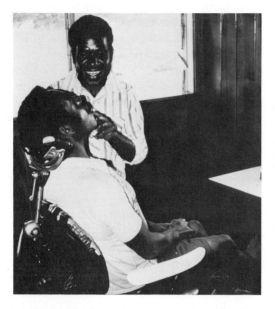
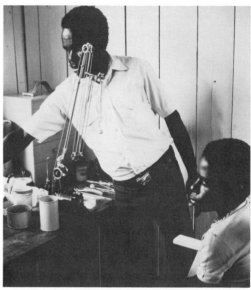

Indonesia—are able to give basic first aid, diagnose certain diseases and provide some medicines, deliver babies, and often help in elementary preventive health strategies. More advanced skills may include nursing and midwifery.

These health workers play an important part in many integrated rural health, agriculture, and economic development projects.[10] Such programs make available a broader base of health personnel for primary health care than a program employing only medically trained physicians and nurses.

In an attempt to meet the health needs of rural people, community development has also become a goal in many Third World nations. The community development concept is based upon two premises: (1) there are not enough health care providers in rural settings so village people can be trained to help meet certain needs, and (2) health problems relate to agriculture, education, and economics, as well as to medicine.

World Health Problems in the Latter 1980s

If you were asked the following hypothetical question, "If you could solve one world health problem that would positively affect the greatest number of people, what would it be?," how would you respond? Before you can consider such a question, however, you must be aware of some of the major world health problems. Initially, world hunger comes to mind. Millions in the world today are starving to death or are seriously malnourished. Population growth is another concern, particularly in parts of South America, Africa, and the Orient. Overpopulation in these areas is an obvious reality. Communicable diseases, though not as extensive a problem as in the past, still cause debilitation and death. The lack of a pure water supply in some 70 to 80 percent of the world causes many of these diseases. Illiteracy, urbanization, pollution, and political and economic systems are yet other obstacles to the health of the world populations.

Compounding these individual problems is the fact that most of them are interrelated. World hunger is often the result of political upheaval, creating a flood of poor, homeless, and hungry refugees. Increased population growth leads to greater pollution problems as well as to urban sprawl. Impure water results in various communicable diseases. Illiteracy is interwoven into nearly all of these problems.

Each of these concerns demands thorough and intensive examination. Here, however, we will examine three problems that are paramount in the twentieth-century world: (1) worldwide hunger, (2) population growth, and (3) lack of a pure water supply.

World Hunger Crisis

The pictures of starving children in Ethiopia, of hungry families in Southeast Asia, or of young children with bloated stomachs suffering from *kwashiorkor* and other protein deficiency diseases in Central America are not pleasant reminders to those who live in North America. Not only are they displeasing pictures to view, but they can, and should, make us feel guilty about our own excessive food consumption. Even more unsettling is the knowledge that such pictures can be multiplied millions of times throughout the world. Malnutrition, hunger, starvation, and resultant death are increasing problems in the world. Estimates suggest that 500 million people (one in eight) in the world today are hungry or malnourished.

Famine is not new to our world; records tell of many such occurrences throughout history. Food shortages have been recorded as far back in history as ancient Egypt, Rome, Greece, and biblical times. In India in 1837 famine took some 800,000 lives. And only a century ago, millions of Chinese died during a three-year famine.

Today the world food crisis is more significant because there are many other related problems. Population growth makes movement to new lands impossible when agricultural fields become too impoverished for food production. Mass migration to urban areas from rural localities to search for jobs and economic prosperity compounds the problem.

The lack of adequate fresh water in many parts of the world is also related to malnutrition and hunger.

The present world hunger crisis has evolved over a period of time. The conditions that have led to the present lack of adequate food supplies and related worldwide hunger have been developing for years. However, several human-made and natural occurrences in the early 1970s seem to have accelerated the crisis. At the beginning of the 1970s, there was a surplus of grain in the world. Many developed nations had enough grain to feed their own populations, help nations with serious food-related problems, and still retain a measure of reserves. But in the past decade, this surplus of world grain has been seriously depleted.

Worldwide economic inflation has contributed to the food crisis. In many poor nations of the world, people spend as much as 80 percent of their income on food. With the escalating costs of importation, fertilizer, and fuel, food costs have more than doubled in the past decade. As a result, the poor cannot afford to pay for adequate food.

The price of oil has been particularly disastrous to people living in poor, underdeveloped nations. Since the Arab boycott of oil production in the early 1970s and the companion rise in crude oil costs, nations that must import oil have had to pay exceedingly high prices for food production. Many of the Third World nations must import oil in order to operate irrigation pumps, cultivation machinery, and produce-transport vehicles; and for use in heating and cooking. Fertilizers and pesticides, which are oil-based, have also risen in price. As a result, the quality of planted grains has decreased and insect loss increased.

Weather patterns have also played a part in the grain shortage and thus the world food crisis. During the early 1970s several regions of the world suffered serious drought. The Sahel region of Africa was especially hard hit. Thousands of acres of marginal farming land were destroyed through desertification. Many people in these areas, previously able to raise enough food for survival, became dependent on food supplied by external sources.

Another contributing factor to the present world food crisis is the food consumption pattern of developed nations. Meat products, particularly beef, are widely consumed in the United States, and cattle are usually fed grain to fatten them before they are butchered. It has been estimated that beef cattle in the United States eat forty million tons of grain per year—enough grain to feed 200 million people for a year at the basic level of four hundred pounds of grain per person per year.

Fertilizers are very important for farmers in the Third World, as their use can produce better qualities of grain. For example, one pound of fertilizer stimulates production of five to ten additional pounds of grain. Yet each year millions of pounds of fertilizer are used in North America on lawns, flower gardens, and golf courses. If even this amount of fertilizer were allocated to impoverished nations, there would be a significant improvement in food production.

Population growth has clearly contributed to the world food crisis. Each year there are 75 to 80 million more people in the world than the previous year. This means more mouths to feed but less available land on which to raise adequate food supplies. This relationship of population increase to food production has been discussed for years. As long ago as 1798, Thomas R. Malthus wrote a classic essay on this topic entitled *Essay on the Principle of Population, 1798.* Malthus's basic thesis was that population increases more rapidly than resources. He held that food production would not keep up with the ability of the human race to reproduce. Malthus hypothesized that population, if unchecked, increases in a geometric ratio, while food production increases only arithmetically. In spite of opposition to Malthus's ideas and the continuing research efforts to increase food production, population growth is still outstripping the available food supplies in many nations of the world.

As nations become more industrialized, the citizens desire eating patterns similar to those in developed countries. Their diets change from vegetable to animal protein, increasing the demand for meat products. As consumption patterns of the developing world follow the consumption behaviors of the more affluent societies, the food crisis will become even more pronounced.

Landownership patterns in many Third World nations also contribute to the world food crisis. Many poor, landless farmers are forced to pay much of their food-production profit to the landowner. Many tenant farmers owe the landowner money for the purchase of seed, fertilizer, and other items needed to plant and grow the crops. Thus, there is little motivation for landless peasants to increase food productivity when the landowner absorbs the profits. In many countries, landowners constitute only a fraction of the entire population but are usually wealthy, well fed, and have the political clout to continue the manipulation of landless peasants and food products prices.

In Central America, as in other parts of the world, the problems of hunger and malnutrition are worsening. One important factor in this situation is that agricultural products are exported to developed nations rather than being used to feed the local population. This process has been termed *export cropping* and has been an important basis of Central American economy for years. Coffee, cotton, sugar, beef, and bananas account for the majority of Central American exports. Unfortunately, export economy has not resulted in benefits for the majority of people in these countries. The large landowners and the rich have benefited, and the peasants are faced with higher food prices.

Beef exportation from Central America to the United States shows how American eating patterns can affect malnutrition and hunger in another part of the world. Since the 1950s beef exporting from Central American ranches has increased. The beef usually is cut-rate because of the low production costs. However, in the years since 1960, beef consumption by Central Americans has actually fallen by 20 percent because less beef is available for them. Since the majority of the meat is exported to the United States, there is often an inadequate supply in the shops and markets of many towns and villages.

The cost of beef in Latin America has risen dramatically because the ranchers would prefer to sell to markets in the United States where they can get a higher price. The poor peasant in Central America cannot afford the inflated prices and the local landowner will not lower the price if there are greater profits in exporting. As a result, meat consumption drops, an important source of protein is lost, and malnutrition increases. In the meantime the poor workers and their families, without an adequate amount of protein, spend their days working to supply the food tables for the overfed in the United States.

The problem of hunger is a cyclical matter. The human body needs food for physiological growth, repair, and for energy to keep the body systems functioning. The necessary minerals, vitamins, fats, carbohydrates, and calories can only be obtained from eating a balanced diet. The inability to obtain food results in limited functioning—or malfunctioning—of the human body and mind. When the body systems do not function properly, disease invades the body, muscles become thinner, and every body organ focuses its efforts simply upon keeping alive. As starvation sets in, the mind is dominated by a desire for food; other matters have little importance. Obviously, then, as social and environmental conditions reduce food sources, people are unable to work or to function optimally, and greater debilitation occurs.

Food Aid

In recent years a broad range of activities has focused upon the world's hungry and starving. Various television specials conducted by different private, volunteer organizations (PVOs) have been used to raise funds to provide food for world hunger.

The work of an American group of recording artists known as USA for Africa has been instrumental in providing grants to organizations and agencies to combat famine and to provide direct food supplies to many hungry and starving people in the world. This group in 1985 recorded the hit song "We Are the World." Probably the best-known activity under the direction of this group was the Live-Aide

Concert of 1985. Many rock and pop artists in Europe and the United States conducted an international concert to raise money and the consciousness of the world regarding the hungry. Through the efforts of USA for Africa, nearly $100 million have been raised. In 1986 another project, Hands Across America, focused specifically on the needs of the poor and hungry in the United States.

Numerous world agencies have made food available to help those in need. Food aid takes a variety of forms. The food aid program of the United Nations is the World Food Programme based in Rome. The primary priority of this program is to provide food to victims of natural and human-made disasters. Other program work occurs through the provision of grants to private organizations as well as to international agencies working in areas of severe hunger.

Many problems must be overcome in channeling food to people in need. (1) Logistics is one problem that is very difficult to solve. Often roadways are poor and make it nearly impossible to transport food and grain from the docks and the cities to rural isolated villages. As a result thousands of people have flocked to the cities where it is their hope that food might be obtained. (2) Many localities do not have adequate food storage facilities. All too often food aid "rots" or is infested with rodents or is stolen before it gets to those in the most need. Obviously adequate storage facilities must be planned and constructed as part of any food aid program. (3) The food that is "imported" is often not compatible with traditional food habits of the people for whom it is intended. Foods should be provided that are local staples rather than surplus food from the sending nations.

Food aid is more than raising funds and "sending" the hungry something to eat. It involves all of these dimensions which are relevant to community health.

Population

Is there a problem of overcrowding in the world? Do you consider population growth to be an issue in need of resolution during the latter part of the twentieth century? Most Americans would respond to these two questions with a very emphatic yes. Indeed, population growth is viewed as a very serious concern by most informed Americans.

The population explosion is evident in the crowded streets of Asian cities. The stress created by population problems in such localities as Mexico City; Jakarta, Indonesia; and Calcutta, India; plus literally thousands of other cities throughout the world, convinces most westerners of the seriousness of this problem. But it hits closer to home as American farmland, woods, and natural beauty spots give way to expanding cities, suburbs, factories, and shopping centers.

In spite of our seemingly obvious concern about population growth, literally millions of people throughout the world fail to agree that there is a population problem. At a worldwide conference on population sponsored by the United Nations and held in Bucharest, Romania, in 1974, there was disagreement about whether or not the world is actually experiencing a population problem. As a matter of fact, some nations, including those of Eastern Europe, expressed a desire for *increased* population in their countries.[11]

Other nations suggested that the population problems as identified by many of the developed nations are really economic matters. They felt that the unequal distribution of the world's resources and wealth significantly contributes to population problems and that economic equality must be achieved by the redistribution of these resources. When this happens, fertility will decline as the natural result of social and economical development.

Still other nations viewed the concern over population as nothing more than a continuing effort by the nations of the capitalist, developed world to exploit Third World nations. Developing nations are very suspicious that the industrial world does not wish to have additional countries industrialized. There are racial overtones in these fears in addition to economic considerations. Since much of the Third World lies in black Africa and oriental Asia, some see population control as an attempt by the white, European, or North American world to keep the black or oriental populations "in check."

In spite of differing nationalistic, political, and regional views relating to the issue of population growth and control, the accumulated data clearly indicates an increase of people. As we review this data, it is important to question just how many people the Earth can accommodate. Resources are not infinite and are being depleted at a seriously rapid rate.

The present world population is slightly more than five billion people, having reached that figure in 1987. By the turn of the century, this number is expected to increase to over six billion. The present doubling rate, or the amount of time that will elapse at the present growth rate before the number of people doubles, is about thirty-five years.[12]

The most dramatic increase of the population growth rate has occurred in this century. There were only a quarter of a billion people in the world from the beginning of humankind until the end of the fifteenth century, when the Americas were discovered. Population doubling to a half billion did not occur until more than 150 years had elapsed (about 1650). It took nearly two centuries, until about 1850, for the world's population to double again, reaching the one billion mark. The doubling period for the next billion was only eighty years; the two billion figure was reached about 1930. The world's population reached four billion in the mid-1970s, and five billion in 1987 (fig. 4.1).

Many concerns must be considered in analyzing the problems of population growth. The regions of the world with the greatest population growth rate are also the poorest and most economically undeveloped. In some African and Asian nations the growth rate surpasses 3 percent per year. In some instances there is a doubling rate of under twenty years. In most of these nations, this population growth is compounded by illness, poverty, and a lack of resources vital to healthful and productive living.

Another problem is that in much of the Third World the population is very young. Nearly half the population in Latin America, Africa, and Asia is under twenty-one years of age. This means that a large sector of the population is of childbearing age.

Figure 4.1 The population of the world has skyrocketed in the past century. There is little evidence that this growth will subside in the near future.

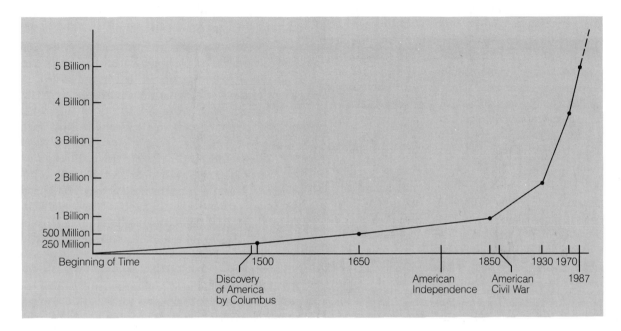

Even with major efforts at population control in these nations, an overall population leveling will not occur until well into the twenty-first century. Unless the average number of children per family is dramatically reduced, the worldwide population explosion will not abate in the near future.

It has been estimated by the United Nations Fund for Population Activities that in spite of the decline in world population rate, zero population growth cannot be reached worldwide until the year 2110.[13] There are several reasons for this continued population growth. Longevity has increased in many parts of the world, especially in the developed nations. With increased longevity and lower death rates, population rises.

Less than a century ago the infant mortality rate in the United States surpassed one hundred per one thousand live births. Today this statistic is less than eleven per one thousand. Improved communicable disease control measures, better infant and child health care services, and better nutrition have all contributed to the reduced levels of infant mortality in the United States. As a result, population growth has accelerated. This pattern has occurred in all of the nations of the industrial, developed world.

Until the mid-1800s death rates were high, the result of many different diseases. But with the identification of specific disease-causing microorganisms and the germ theory of disease, death rates have been greatly reduced. Today smallpox, diphtheria, and many other communicable diseases are either eradicated or significantly reduced as a result of immunization programs for young children.

It is no easy task to develop population control programs because there are barriers to their success. In many areas of the world, children form a kind of "social security" as old age approaches. People wish to have a number of children so that they will have help in farming the land and thus provide increased economic security.

Another reason that family planning is relatively ineffective is that in many Third World nations the infant mortality rate is still very high. Many parents see as many as one-half of their children die from disease, hunger, or other conditions before reaching the age of five. If they are to have the size of family believed to be necessary and desirable, it means having many more children. These additional children are "insurance" that there will be enough hands to do the work. Therefore, it is nearly impossible to achieve family planning among these people.

Religious teachings and practices are yet another barrier to population control, especially in countries where the Roman Catholic and the Islamic religions are practiced. The Roman Catholic faith prohibits the use of artificial birth control measures. This presents serious problems in many already overcrowded areas of the world where the Catholic faith is strong, as it is in the Latin American countries. The teachings of the Islamic religion also oppose birth control measures. This can lead to the population doubling in many Middle Eastern nations within twenty years.[14]

In many countries governmental policy is supportive of population growth. These countries see population expansion as an overall part of the economic growth of the nation. Additional numbers of people are actually desired. In a study conducted by the Population Commission of the United Nations Economic and Social Council, most nations in the world felt that a higher rate of population growth was desirable or that the current rate was satisfactory. Only one-third of the nations considered a lower population growth rate desirable.[15]

Another very important barrier to population control programs is illiteracy. Teaching illiterate people to practice effective birth control measures is very complex since the reproductive process must be explained. In spite of many relatively easy-to-learn birth control procedures, getting poor, illiterate, people to understand and practice these measures requires effective communication and learning strategies.

Pure Water Supply

In thousands of rural villages scattered throughout the world the source of water is a watering hole shared by both people and animals; it is a slow-moving stream polluted by sediment and human and animal excretion; or it is located several miles from the place where people live. Not only are these water sources often contaminated, but in many arid regions of the world, sufficient water is too expensive for the very poor. As a result, a great number of people have no access to an adequate, pure water supply.

The World Health Organization, through extensive studies, has estimated that in many of the world's poorest nations, over 80 percent of the population lack a fresh water supply.[16] In some Third World nations the percentage is less, but in most instances it still means that more than half of the population lack pure water.

Millions of people throughout the world suffer from disease caused by impure water. The problem is so widespread that the World Health Organization has estimated that impure water supplies cause nearly 80 percent of all diseases in the world.[17] Many of these diseases are the result of ingestion of microorganisms found in the water. For example, gastroenteritis, typhoid, and cholera are commonly found in the areas where water is contaminated. Usually contamination of the water is due to poor sanitary practices—the failure of people to use sanitary latrines.

Parasitic diseases are often endemic to areas having poor water supplies. Many parasites live in water and, without proper water purification, are ingested by the local inhabitants. Parasites are also able to burrow through the skin and enter the bloodstream of individuals who walk barefoot in the water. Examples of two such parasitic diseases are schistosomiasis and dracunculiasis. Schistosomiasis is carried by snails that reside in slow-moving or stagnant water; dracunculiasis is carried by the guinea worm.[18]

Communicable diseases are also transmitted by impure water. An example is trachoma, which causes blindness in thousands of individuals who wash in the dirty water.

A common cause of many health problems is the contamination of water. (a) Cattle are found in a river. (b) The same watering hole is later used by a man as a water source for himself and his family.

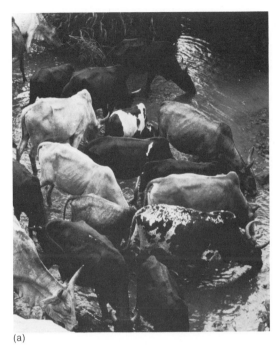

(a)

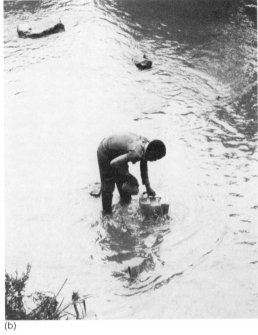

(b)

Another contributing factor to the problem of impure water is that mosquitoes, which are carriers of malaria, breed in stagnant water such as ponds, open sewage systems, or water in outdoor cooking pots. At one time (the 1950s) it was felt that malaria would be eradicated with the use of the pesticide DDT. But today malaria is at epidemic proportions in many areas of the world. Mosquitoes have built up a resistance to DDT, and their breeding grounds—stagnant waters—are still common.

Any effort to improve the pure water supply in a community must include measures to stop the pollution of the water source. Sanitary latrines must be introduced as an alternative to the streams and rivers. However, in communities where latrines have been introduced, the people frequently do not use them. They fail to understand the relationship between improper sanitation, impure water supply, and disease. These people must be taught the appropriate behaviors necessary for good health and well-being.

Another reason water supplies are polluted is that they are used as garbage "dumps." Many times the garbage from the local village is emptied directly into the river or stream. Unfortunately people living downstream draw their drinking water from this same source. This demonstrates that an improved water supply is not the task of a single isolated community. The efforts of all who use the same water supply must be coordinated from village to village, city to city, and country to country.

The problem of a pure water supply has no easy solution. National and international conferences have been held to develop resolution strategies. These conferences have been less than effective overall, but improvements have occurred in some countries.

A pure water supply can improve the health of many Third World inhabitants. For these little girls in a squatter settlement in Colombia, a communal tap represents a big step forward. For them and their families, it means better health.

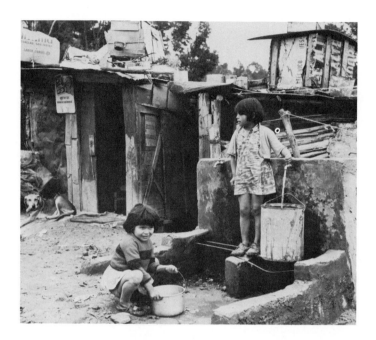

Where positive action has taken place, the people of the area have been educated about and convinced of the need for pure water as a means to prevent disease, sickness, and debilitation. The government, too, has seen the need for action and has been committed to pure water programs.

As mentioned earlier, the 1980s were designated as the International Water Supply and Sanitation Decade by the United Nations Water Conference in 1977. The goal of this effort was to make available fresh water for all people in the world by 1990. By mid-point in the decade some 150 different activities in over eighty Third World nations had been implemented.[19] Many nations had demonstrated a commitment to the idea of improved water supply for the people of their communities by establishing goals for 1990. However, their intentions were seldom matched by the necessary funding to carry out the plans.[20]

How successful such an effort will be remains to be seen. It requires the cooperation of many multinational organizations and agencies. Governments must set water supply as a high priority, both programmatically and economically. Also, creative measures need to be designed to educate people.

This program to improve the quality of the water supply will not be effective unless similar efforts are made to improve sanitation. Sources of drinking water must be free from contamination both by humans and by animals.

Lack of fresh water is closely related to the problem of malnutrition and hunger. Physiologically, the human body needs water just as it requires food. Hunger and malnutrition reduce the body's resistance to disease and infection. Thus, a malnourished body is more susceptible to the illnesses caused by impure water. Diarrhea often accompanies many of these diseases and results in a loss of body fluids, compounding the problem of malnutrition.

If the goal of providing safe drinking water (safe both chemically and bacteriologically) were achieved, the immediate result would be healthier, more productive people. There would be less mortality and morbidity. A safe water supply would virtually eliminate all pathogenic conditions that are the result of impure water contact. Improved health status and productivity would no doubt play an important role in the social and economic stability of the nation.

Desertification

Each year about six million hectacres of land are turned to desert and about twenty million hectacres are reduced to zero economic productivity. One in five people in the world lives in the path of the advancing desert.[21] This process of desert encroachment and land deterioration is known as *desertification*. Desertification causes land to become so denuded that it cannot sustain agriculture or human habitation.

Desertification occurs on all the world's continents. In North America, sheep farming on the Navajo Indian Reservation, combined with poor range management, has destroyed much of the marginally productive land. In South America, the Atacama Desert in Chile has expanded and today cacti are found where more tropical vegetation used to be. This, too, has been caused by overgrazing of cattle and sheep.

Possibly the most widespread encroachment of desert lands has taken place in the Sahara Desert of North Africa. All along the southern boundaries of the Sahara, the desert has shifted. Aerial photography has shown that these boundaries have shifted southward an average of ninety to one hundred kilometers (fifty to sixty miles) since the late 1950s.[22] This desert movement has affected all countries immediately south of the Sahara known as the Sahel: Gambia, Niger, Sudan, Chad, and Upper Volta. For example, in Sudan, large concentrations of Acacia trees were common around the capital of Khartoum in the mid-1950s. Today it is necessary to travel at least ninety kilometers south to find similar stands of this tree.[23]

Drought caused by desertification forces these women to pick leaves for food from one of the few green trees along the Mali-Upper Volta border, the Sahel region. The carcass of a cow is in the foreground.

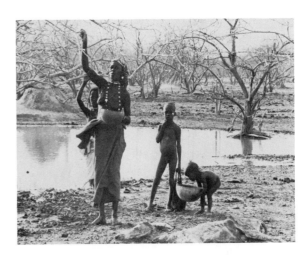

Desertification compounds the problems of food and hunger. In many arid areas of the world the inhabitants are nomads. With the loss of productive land for growing crops, the people either must go without adequate food or are forced to leave their nomadic life-styles and move to urban areas. In the cities, they live in already overcrowded conditions, and few have the skills to make a decent living.

The continuing loss of productive land has broader implications. This situation often means that a nation becomes dependent upon other nations to feed its population. This creates an inflationary food cost spiral so that many people cannot afford even basic nutrients. The outcome, of course, is malnutrition and hunger.

There are several causes of desertification. (1) *Shifting rainfall patterns* have caused drought in many parts of the world in the past two decades. Hundreds of thousands of cattle and other livestock have been lost; some estimates suggest that as many as 25 percent of all cattle herds starved to death. Thousands of people have lost their lives and many were forced to flee to relief camps where food was provided by other nations.

(2) An *increase in livestock* contributes to desertification. Cattle, sheep, and other grazing animals can rapidly destroy marginal grasslands (fig.

Figure 4.2   Cycle of desertification

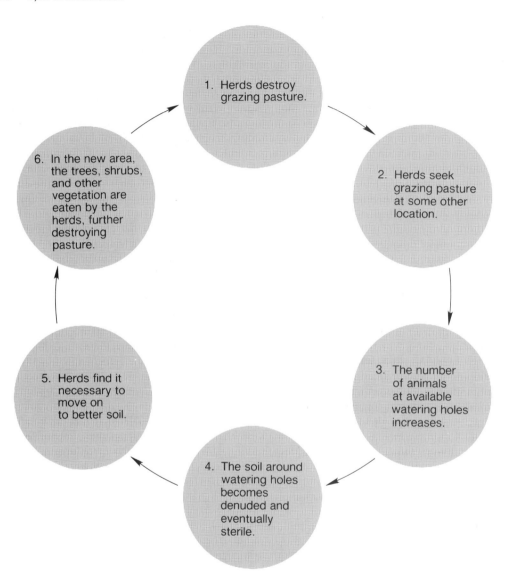

1. Herds destroy grazing pasture.

2. Herds seek grazing pasture at some other location.

3. The number of animals at available watering holes increases.

4. The soil around watering holes becomes denuded and eventually sterile.

5. Herds find it necessary to move on to better soil.

6. In the new area, the trees, shrubs, and other vegetation are eaten by the herds, further destroying pasture.

4.2). In one province of Sudan the livestock population has grown sixfold in the past twenty years. This is due in part to the increased demand for meat products by people in the Third World.

Goats present a serious problem in arid localities. A small herd of goats can destroy large areas of vegetation in a relatively short period of time.

Feeding upon any foliage found in drought-stricken areas, goats have even been found jumping up into low trees.

Cattle, sheep, goats, and other animals, like humans, need water to survive. Often in the desert regions the only water available is a watering hole. The animals come to these spots to drink and soon eat all vegetation surrounding the hole. The land is left denuded, erosion results, the watering hole becomes polluted, and, since the vegetation renewal cycle is very slow in arid regions, the area is destroyed for future productivity. Therefore, the cattle are moved to another productive watering hole and the unfortunate cycle repeats itself.

(3) Another cause of desertification is *human population growth*. After several years, traditional farming procedures deplete the land of needed nutrients and the farmers move to another location. The vacated fields stand idle and are renewed with shrubs, grasses, small trees, and other vegetation. With increased numbers of people, the available land is diminished so farmers cannot move on to new, more fertile fields. Overgrazing and overcultivation occur, leaving no opportunity for the land to replenish itself and resulting in decreased crop production and the eventual destruction of the already low-quality soil.

Whether the process of desertification can be slowed, halted, or reversed is uncertain. Most experts suggest that the root cause is human-made.[24] If this is true, then people must seek ways to solve the problem. In 1977, a United Nations conference on desertification took place in Kenya. Many ideas, theories, and suggestions for solutions were discussed. However, many of the possible solutions only create other environmental problems which, in turn, contribute to the original problem of desertification. No major successes have been noted and the deserts continue to advance. The effects upon food production and human well-being continue to be negative, with little hope for resolution in the near future.

Issue—Case Study "Lifeboat" Ethics

Hunger, overpopulation, disease, infant mortality, poverty—the world health problems are overwhelming. It seems as though there is little room for optimism. One college student, after study of the many issues relating to world health, concluded that it seemed as though the world was "going to hell." In the face of such a gloomy forecast, an individual might be tempted to accept the theoretical concepts of lifeboat ethics.[25]

Lifeboat ethics suggest that the poor, underdeveloped nations should not be helped by the industrial, developed world. In short, lifeboat ethic proponents suggest that each developed country is a lifeboat. These countries have limited resources and will only be able to survive if these resources are kept and used for those in "the lifeboat." Only those "in the boat" will survive and live; all others will be lost to starvation, hunger, and death. The United States and other industrialized nations should not try to feed the entire world, nor provide health care to the poor of the Third World, nor spend time and money to help the needy.

Lifeboat ethic theorists point out that improvement of certain problems will only compound the problem in the future. For example, any efforts to control communicable diseases, to reduce infant mortality, or to reduce death rates will result in greater numbers of people. This, in turn, will cause more food shortage, greater incidences of hunger, and more poverty. This theory raises many questions. If you have ever visited, lived in, or worked in a Third World nation, you may find it hard to accept the idea that the people you have come to help and befriend might be those doomed to "sink" in the sea of life.

Can you look on the world scene from your lifeboat of luxury and resources and permit little children, your friends and acquaintances, or just simple well-meaning people to drown? Does the concept of "lifeboat" ethics have any meritorious features in your judgment? What would be the ultimate outcome in the world if the concepts of lifeboat ethics were applied? Would world conditions improve or get worse?

Summary

A review of health conditions in the world reveals some seemingly insurmountable problems. Disease, lack of adequate and appropriate health care, hunger, malnutrition, overpopulation, lack of pure water supplies, and environmental pollution are but some of the serious problems faced by humanity. Throughout history, numerous conferences have been held and many organizations and programs designed to improve the health of people have been established. These efforts have met with varying degrees of success.

In 1948, the World Health Organization was founded as an agency of the United Nations. Through WHO's programming, with its six regional offices, some positive measures have been taken. For example, a major worldwide program, organized and conducted by the World Health Organization, has eradicated smallpox; has established international standards for foods, drugs, and vaccines; and has educated many health professionals, particularly from Third World nations. Although the World Health Organization's priorities and program efforts change as new situations and problems arise, not all of their programs are successful. Malaria is still a worldwide problem in spite of efforts to eradicate it.

In most Third World nations, health care providers and facilities are not made available to the poor. Various attempts to correct or improve this condition have not been particularly successful.

Changing concepts have led the World Health Organization to place greater emphasis on primary health care. This emphasis resulted in an international conference at Alma-Ata, USSR, in 1978. This conference produced a document that now serves as an important guide to the World Health Organization and to other international agencies and organizations. The document assists in setting program goals, priorities, and efforts throughout the world.

An important reason for health problems in many nations of the world is the lack of adequate health care facilities and work force. This is particularly true in rural areas and among the poor in urban localities. Governmental efforts to combat the problem have included mandatory service in underserved regions by physicians, nurses, and other health providers. The integration of traditional medical healers with modern medicine has also received increasing support. Another approach at meeting the health needs of the world population has been the integration of health care strategies with community development efforts, where the village health worker is a primary health care provider.

Though there are many world health problems, three are especially critical: world hunger, population growth, and the lack of pure water sources. Each of these three negatively affects the health, well-being, and life-style of millions of people throughout the world. None can be totally isolated from the other, although international efforts, conferences, and programs have been designed to focus upon improvement of each.

The world's resources are not infinite and nowhere is this more obvious and relevant to world health problems than in the availability of land for agricultural purposes. In many countries of the world, climate affects the land used for growing crops. Each year the deserts continue to encroach upon marginal farmland, leading to an uprooting of millions of people, particularly those living in the Sahel of Africa. Desertification has also contributed to the problems of hunger, malnutrition, and starvation.

Discussion Questions

1. Explain the relationship of the World Health Organization to the United Nations.
2. Describe the organizational structure of the World Health Organization.
3. Provide some examples of World Health Organization programming.
4. Why has it not been possible to develop successful malaria eradiction programs throughout the world?
5. What has been the value of the declaration of the conference on international health at Alma-Ata?
6. Give an illustration of the meaning of primary health care.
7. Explain the significance of the 1982 statement of UNICEF on the state of the world's children.
8. What have been the results of use of oral rehydration therapy?
9. What can be learned from using cardboard growth charts?
10. Do you feel it is possible to integrate the practices and concepts of traditional medicine with those of modern medical practice? Explain your position.
11. What are some of the things that a village health worker can do that contribute to improved health in his/her community?
12. Explain some of the causes of the present world food crisis.
13. Identify some of the problems associated with getting food aid to the people who are most in need of it. How can these problems be solved?
14. What was the basic position expressed nearly two hundred years ago by Malthus regarding food, hunger, and population?
15. In your view, is there a world population crisis? Explain the reasons behind the position you have taken.
16. Why do some nations desire not to encourage population reduction?
17. What are some of the problems that result from impure water supplies?
18. Discuss the relationships between water supply and sanitation of the local environment.
19. Describe the process of desertification.
20. What position do you take regarding the concept of lifeboat ethics?

Suggested Readings

Numerous articles on issues related to international health can be found in the following three World Health Organization publications: *World Health, World Health Forum,* and *World Health Chronicle.*

Anderson, Alastair. "Oncho: A Concerted Effort." *World Health* (March, 1986): 14–15.

Bannerman, R. H. "Traditional Medicine in Modern Health Care." *World Health Forum* 3, no. 1 (1982): 8–13.

Brown, George F. "Conference Report: United Nations International Conference on Population." *Studies in Family Planning* 15, no. 6 (November/December, 1984): 296–302.

Dondero, Timothy J. "Nutrition and Health Needs: in Drought-Stricken Africa." *Public Health Reports* 100, no. 6 (November/December, 1985): 634–38.

Ellis, William S. "Africa's Sahel: The Stricken Land." *National Geographic* 172, no. 2 (August, 1987): 140–79.

Forman, Martin J. *Nutritional Aspects of Project Food Aid.* Rome: Food Policy and Nutrition Division, FAO (1986).

Gorchev, H. Galal, and Ozolins, G. "WHO Guidelines for Drinking-Water Quality." *WHO Chronicle* 38, no. 3 (1984): 104–08.

Howard-Jones, Norman. "The World Health Organization in Historical Perspective." *Perspectives in Biology and Medicine* (Spring, 1981): 467–82.

International Conference on Primary Health Care, Alma-Ata, USSR. *Primary Health Care.* Geneva: World Health Organization, 1978.

Ofosu-Amaah, Virginia. *National Experience in the Use of Community Health Workers: A Review of Current Issues and Problems.* Geneva: World Health Organization (1983).

Paulino, Leonardo A., and Mellor, John W. "The Food Situation in Developing Countries." *Food Policy* (November, 1984): 291–303.

Sanderson, Fred H. "World Food Prospects to the Year 2000." *Food Policy* (November, 1984): 363–73.

Skeet, Muriel. "Community Health Workers: Promoters or Inhibitors of Primary Heath Care?" *World Health Forum* 5 (1984): 291–95.

World Health Organization. *The Work of WHO, 1984–1985: Biennial Report of the Director-General.* Geneva: World Health Organization, 1986.

Endnotes

1. "Sessions of the WHO Regional Committees." *WHO Chronicle* 39, no. 6 (1985): 223.

2. Henderson, Donald A. "Smallpox—Epitaph for a Killer." *National Geographic Society Magazine* 154, no. 6 (December, 1978): 800.

3. Ibid., 797.

4. Anderson, Alastair. "Oncho: A Concerted Effort." *World Health* (March, 1986): 14–15.

5. World Bank. *Health: Sector Policy Paper.* Washington, D.C.: World Bank, 1980: 10–46.

6. Report of the International Conference on Primary Health Care, Alma-Ata, USSR, *Primary Health Care.* Geneva: World Health Organization, 1978: 24–25.

7. UNICEF, State of the World's Children Report. New York: UNICEF, 1982.

8. U.S. Agency for International Development, *AID Highlights* 3, no. 1 (Winter, 1986): 2.

9. The subject of breast-feeding and infant formula is discussed in chapter 16.

10. Newell, Kenneth W., ed. *Health by the People.* Geneva: World Organization, 1975.

11. "A Report on Bucharest." *Studies in Family Planning* 5, no. 12 (December, 1974): 362–64.

12. United Nations Fund for Population Activities, *Population Facts at Hand.*

13. United Nations Fund for Population Activities, *World Health* (November, 1981): 31.

14. Raymond, M. Susan Ueber. *Health and Policymaking in the Arab Middle East.* Washington, D.C.: Georgetown University, 1978, p. 47.

15. United Nations Fund for Population Activities, *Population Facts at Hand,* 6.

16. Guest, Iain. "The Water Decade 1981–1990." *World Health* (January, 1979): 3.

17. Ibid.

18. Parasitic diseases are discussed in more detail in chapter 9.

19. World Health Organization, *The Work of WHO 1984–1985.* Geneva: World Health Organization, 1986: 144.

20. Ibid., p. 145.

21. Tolba, M. K. United Nations Environment Programme, New York: United Nations reported in *The Futurist,* Vol. XX, no. 4 (July/August, 1986): 5.

22. Eckholm, Erik, and Brown, Lester R. "The Spreading Desert." *War on Hunger* 12, no. 8: 4.

23. Ibid.

24. Tolba, Mostafa Kamal. "Desertification: A Man-Made Process." *World Health* (July, 1977): 2–3.

25. Hardin, Garrett. "Lifeboat Ethics: The Case Against the Poor." *Psychology Today* 8, no. 4 (September, 1974): 38–43, 123–26.

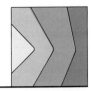

UNIT TWO

Resources of Community Health

5

Health Personnel and Facilities: The Resources of Health Care

The health care industry is no small enterprise. In terms of personnel, the health care field is the third largest industry in the United States. Some 5 percent of the total nation's labor force—nearly six million people—are involved in health care in some way.[1] The growth in the health care industry has been exceptional in the past two decades. One in seven new jobs created during the past decade was related to health care. The number of people employed in the industry has risen to nearly six million in the mid-1980s from 4.2 million in 1970—a growth rate three times faster than that of the total employment field.[2]

In spite of this growth in the number of individuals involved in the health professions and related health activities, problems do exist in the health work force. One area that has received widespread discussion, debate, and evaluation in the past decade concerns the adequacy, in terms of number, of health personnel. Are there enough physicians, dentists, nurses, and related health professionals to meet the health demands of the American population? How can health care providers be more equitably distributed on a geographical basis? Can a greater number of minorities be brought into the health care industry as health care providers?

When the matter of health personnel is discussed, the number of physicians is often the first focus of interest, yet other health professionals must also be considered. In recent years a group of non-physician health care providers has developed: physician's assistants and nurse practitioners. In addition to these individuals, numerous other health workers are found in the various health-related professions.

Medical Education Programs

During the 1960s and 1970s increased federal financial support resulted in greater numbers of health professional school graduates and in the expansion of existing professional programs. Numerous new medical, dental, nursing, and allied or related health schools and training programs plus schools of public

Physicians

Date	Number
1960	275,000
1965	305,000
1970	348,000
1975	409,000
1980	487,000
1983	542,000

Source: U.S. Bureau of the Census, *Statistical Abstracts of the United States: 1986* (106th Ed.), Washington, D.C., 1985.

health were developed. For example, by the beginning of the 1980s there were forty-three more medical schools, seventeen more dental schools, and three more schools of optometry than in 1950.[3]

Physicians

Since 1960 the number of medical school graduates has increased significantly. By the mid-1980s there were over 540,000 physicians in the United States.[4] Present consensus seems to be that the existing medical schools will prepare an adequate number of health professionals for the future. It has been projected that physician supply will continue to increase into the 1990s. Then the projections are that the growth percentage will slow down; however, it will continue to exceed the growth of population. The ratio of physicians to population is projected to increase from 198.8 per 100,000 population in the early 1980s to 234.5 in the early 1990s.[5]

The Graduate Medical Education National Advisory Committee (GMENAC), commissioned by the Department of Health and Human Services, analyzed the distribution of physicians by specialty and recommended strategies for determining the future need for physicians in the United States. This committee was appointed by and reported to the Secretary of the Department of Health and Human Services.

Medical Schools	
Date	*Number*
1960	91
1965	93
1970	107
1975	123
1980	140
1983	142

Source: U.S. Bureau of the Census, *Statistical Abstracts of the United States: 1986* (106th Ed.), Washington, D.C., 1985.

Foreign Medical Schools— Percent of Newly Licensed	
Date	*Percent*
1960	17.7
1965	16.7
1970	27.3
1975	35.4
1980	18.7
1983	23.1

Source: U.S. Bureau of the Census, *Statistical Abstracts of the United States: 1986* (106th Ed.), Washington, D.C., 1985.

Their final report, presented in 1980, contained 107 recommendations. One important recommendation about the medical work force was that by the year 1990 there would be a surplus of seventy thousand physicians in this country. Three reasons were cited for this projected surplus: (1) the increase in medical school students in the 1970s, (2) the influx of physicians who graduate from foreign medical schools and come to the United States to practice medicine, and (3) the increasing number of people relying upon nonmedical health care providers for primary health care needs. The GMENAC recommended in their report that there be no new medical schools and no increase in the size of enrollment in already existing schools.[6]

There is general agreement that an adequate number of physicians is available in the United States. But what continues to be a problem is an inadequate distribution, both geographically and by medical specialty, of existing medical personnel. If you have ever been in need of a physician and have been unable to find one, you have some idea of the problems of health care access. There is a significant shortage of primary care physicians in the United States. Approximately 38 percent of the nation's physicians are in primary care or general practice.[7] The majority of all physicians (over 60 percent) are specialists who practice specialized medicine and are not available for routine medical care and treatment. The number of these medical specialists has continued to increase in recent years.

The reduction in available primary care physicians has resulted in shortages in certain localities. Shortages are particularly acute in rural communities and in the inner-city areas. This shortage becomes a serious burden for the nation's economically disadvantaged living in these localities. It is a seemingly never-ending circle. The medical provider chooses not to live in these localities for several reasons, one being that the poor are less likely to pay for health care. As the poor individual is not as likely to have resources to pay for preventive health care, the chance becomes greater that the services of a physician will not be sought. The services provided by local health departments often are the principal source of medical care for many of these individuals.

Foreign Medical School Graduates

As the GMENAC reported, the physician educated in another country who immigrates to the United States to live and practice medicine has had a significant impact on the health care system in recent years. In the early 1960s, foreign medical school graduates constituted approximately 17 percent of the total number of physicians in the United States.

By the latter 1970s this figure had risen to 33 percent of the newly licensed physicians in America.[8] In 1977 the federal government passed legislation that has reduced the influx of foreign-educated physicians into the United States.

The foreign physician, however, has provided health care to underserved populations or in those localities with large numbers of economically disadvantaged persons. These are areas where needs for health care providers exist; therefore, many foreign medical school graduates often locate and in turn provide primary health care in rural areas or inner-city locations.[9]

Another factor relating to the increase in number of foreign-trained physicians concerns foreign medical study by Americans. Often these individuals have been unsuccessful in getting admitted to a medical school in the United States. These American-born, foreign-trained medical school graduates often lack equivalent clinical and educational experience to that of the American medical school graduate. They may find it difficult to get into residency programs in United States hospitals.

Other Health Professions

The supply of other health care providers, such as dentists, optometrists, podiatrists, and pharmacists, appears to be adequate. The problem of geographic distribution of these health providers is similar to those of physicians. Urban areas tend to have the greatest concentration of providers.

Today there are sixty dental schools throughout the United States compared with fifty-three just a decade and a half ago. There are over 138,000 dentists in the United States. Nearly two-thirds of the total dental care work force are auxiliary personnel, dental hygienists and dental assistants, who provide many dental services.[10]

There are thirteen schools of optometry, five schools of podiatry, and seventy-two colleges of pharmacy. Due to the increasing number of professional schools and the increased enrollments in already existing schools during the past decade, there

Dentists

Date	Number	Dental Schools
1960	105,000	47
1965	112,000	49
1970	116,000	53
1975	127,000	59
1980	141,000	61
1983	150,000	60

Source: U.S. Bureau of the Census, *Statistical Abstracts of the United States: 1986* (106th Ed.), Washington, D.C., 1985.

	Female	Nonwhite
Dentists	6.2%	.9%
Pharmacists	28.5%	2.9%

seems to be no need for the establishment of additional health professional schools in the immediate future.

In spite of this assumed adequate supply and projected future oversupply, there is an imbalance of both race and sex in these health professions. Over 90 percent of dentists, optometrists, podiatrists, and pharmacists are white males.

Admission to these professions has been limited for many minority groups, such as blacks and the Spanish-speaking population. Minorities have been poorly recruited, have historically received a general denial of access into medical and dental schools, and have had, in general, inadequate academic backgrounds. These factors combined with the existence of few minority role models have often created a lack of awareness among black adolescents of the opportunities in medicine.

Other Medical Practitioners

The medical doctor (MD) is educated in what is known as the allopathic medical model. Thousands of people receive treatment every day in the United States by medical practitioners other than these. Best known are the osteopathic physician (D.O.) and the doctor of chiropractic medicine.

Osteopathic Medicine

The underlying philosophy of *osteopathic medicine* originated in the late 1800s with the concepts of Andrew Still. According to this philosophy of medicine, impairment of nerve function—pinching of the nerves as they leave the spinal column—results in musculoskeletal disturbance and places stress on the body. Manipulative therapy is used to restore "structural integrity" of the skeletal system.

Osteopathic medicine has gradually modified many of its original concepts. Today the doctor of osteopathic medicine uses the same methods of treating disease and injury as the allopathic physician. This includes the use of drugs, surgery, radiation, and other physical modalities plus manipulation of the musculoskeletal system.

Osteopaths are licensed to practice in all fifty states after passing the same examination as is given to the medical doctor. Most D.O.s practice in osteopathic hospitals. However, increasing numbers now have medical staff appointments in general community hospitals.

Chiropractic Medicine

Another healing modality that attracts many patients every year is *chiropractic medicine,* which is based on a theory originally put forth in 1895 by Daniel Palmer. This theory is that health is determined by the "structural integrity" of the bones of the vertebrae. Disease results from improper alignment or derangement of the vertebrae, known as spinal subluxations. These derangements cause a disturbance of the nervous system that "is often a primary or contributing causative, provocative and extending factor in the pathological process of many common and at times seemingly intractable human ailments."[11]

The doctor of chiropractic medicine uses manipulation or adjustment to return the vertebrae to proper alignment. These procedures restore nerve transmission and normal functioning of body parts. The chiropractor uses X ray to detect subluxations and also employs clinical nutrition, physical therapy, basic hygienic practices, and other measures directed toward the prevention and treatment of disease.

Historically, chiropractic medicine has been opposed by allopathic medicine. However, in 1980 the American Medical Association approved the referring of patients to chiropractors. This measure was taken in part by the threat of lawsuits claiming monopolistic practices by medical doctors in the health care field. Most health insurance companies reimburse for chiropractic services.

Nontraditional Medicine

There are several other nontraditional medical practitioners. The *naturopath* uses a system of healing that uses therapies of sunlight, manipulation, exercise, water, air, organic foods, nutrition supplements, and naturally occurring drugs in the promotion or restoration of normal body processes. The *homeopath* treats diseases by giving drugs in small doses. The *naparapath* subscribes to a system of therapeutics based on the theory that diseases are caused by connective tissue and ligament disorders. The *Christian Science practitioner* makes use of religious concepts and beliefs in healing modalities.

The ancient Chinese art of *acupuncture* has received increasing interest in the United States. Acupuncture is the procedure of treating diseases by the insertion of fine needles into the human body at specific points. Research is ongoing to learn how acupuncture works in the relief of pain and the treatment of disease.

Registered Nurses

Date	Number	Nursing Programs
1960	517,000	1,128
1965	621,000	1,182
1970	750,000	1,340
1975	961,000	1,362
1980	1,273,000	1,385
1983	1,404,000	1,466

Source: U.S. Bureau of the Census, *Statistical Abstracts of the United States: 1986* (106th Ed.), Washington, D.C., 1985.

Nursing

Nursing has a rich heritage in the United States. It is estimated that there are nearly 1.5 million actively employed registered nurses in this country.[12]

Working in a variety of settings, nurses are found in any inpatient health care facility and in most outpatient clinical settings. They care for patients in hospitals, nursing homes, and other institutions. Many nurses also work in the industrial setting, as public health nurses in our communities, as well as in schools, providing very important services to school-age children. Registered nurses are also found in doctors' offices.

Whether there are an adequate number of registered nurses is open to question. It is more important to consider whether an adequate number of nurses with specific skills work in certain clinical settings. In spite of the fact that 70 percent of nurses work in hospitals, there is little question that a shortage of nurses willing to work in the hospital setting exists. This is obvious from the job advertisements in the newspapers where many openings for nursing employment are listed. This shortage has been noted by the American Hospital Association

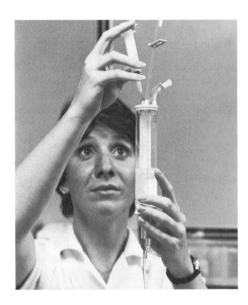

Nurses provide both physical and emotional care for patients. Here a nurse adds medication to an intravenous administration set, which dispenses the drug directly into the patient's vein.

and the National League of Nursing. It appears that this shortage will get worse in the immediate future—the result of a number of factors. The turnover of nurses in the hospital is very high and so contributes to a lack of continuity in work relationships. In spite of the increase of males entering the nursing profession, it has basically been females who are nurses and many do not stay in the work force for extended periods of time. It is still common for nurses to leave the active practice of nursing when their children are young, or work only on a part-time basis during the years that their children are at home. Increasingly, nurses are finding work opportunities in settings other than hospitals.

A perceived lack of status and input about hospital working conditions causes many nurses to find work in other settings, such as in public health, in industry, or in schools. Nursing has been striving for a greater shared responsibility with physicians in the practice of medical care in the hospital and in other inpatient facilities.

Nursing education has gone through a variety of changes in recent years. The number of nursing graduates and nursing schools has greatly expanded in the past two decades. This increase is due in part to the several different training programs for nurses. The hospital-based programs as well as the associate-degree programs prepare the nurse primarily for institutional nursing service. Most hospital-based programs are two or three years in duration, and expose the student to a variety of clinical experiences in the hospital setting. These programs are being phased out throughout the country because of cost factors on the part of the hospital and the present feeling in the nursing profession that all nurses should hold either the associate degree or the bachelor of science in nursing (BSN) degree.

The associate-degree program is a two-year program usually offered by a junior or community college. The curriculum emphasis in this program tends to be more academic than clinical. Though there are clinical learning experiences, they are limited compared to the hospital-based programs.

A third type of nursing education program is the baccalaureate-degree program. This program usually combines a strong hospital-based clinical experience with the educational requirements of a four-year degree institution. In addition to the registered nurse degree, graduates of these programs receive the BSN (Bachelor of Science in Nursing). This educational program, like most baccalaureate-degree programs, is a four-year educational experience.

The general trend in nursing education today is toward the four-year degree program. This is in part due to the increased need for an in-depth education and also the prestige that a degreed individual has in American society. Also, the degreed nurse is usually able to command a greater salary than the non-degreed individual.

Nurses with advanced degrees, such as the MSN or the PhD, remain in short supply. These individuals are needed to fill teaching positions in nursing education programs, for administrative work both in the academic world and in the institutional setting, as well as to conduct research in the field of nursing.

Nonphysician Health Care Providers

Most health problems of people who seek primary care can be managed by nonphysician health care providers. These individuals are trained to perform services that traditionally were offered only by physicians, and have been active in areas where there is a critical shortage of physicians. Two types of nonphysician health care providers have developed since the mid-1960s: (1) the physician's assistant (PA), and (2) the nurse practitioner (NP). A third type of nonphysician health care provider, a sub-group of the nurse-practitioner, is the nurse-midwife.

Physicians' Assistants and Nurse Practitioners

These nonphysician health care providers are trained to perform selected tasks that were, in the past, usually performed by physicians. These tasks are actually an extension of the nursing role. But in addition to the regular nursing duties, various primary care medical services are performed.

The physician's assistant and nurse practitioner provide primary care in a variety of settings. They have been useful in meeting the need for health care personnel in the inner cities and in other medically underserved localities. The physician's-assistant program has been somewhat successful in servicing small communities. Three-fourths of all physician's assistants are working in primary care, and half of these are in rural communities. The nurse practitioners are not as likely to settle in rural areas, preferring the larger cities.

Both the physician's-assistant and nurse-practitioner programs originated in 1965. The first physician's-assistant program was introduced at Duke University. The nurse-practitioner program began at the University of Colorado when a nurses' training program expanded the scope of practice to develop the pediatric nurse practitioner. The early physician's-assistant programs included many former military corpsmen and medics who had completed their military duty. Back in civilian life they found it difficult to use the skills developed in the

The nurse practitioner is important to many occupational health programs. Here a nurse practitioner conducts an eye examination as part of the health evaluation for each Kimberly-Clark employee in the company's Health Management Program.

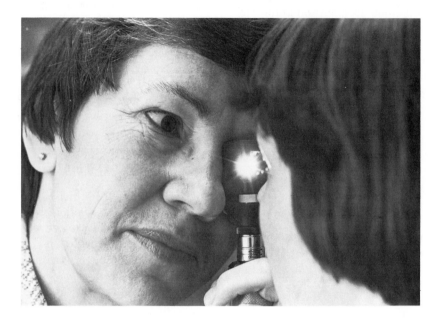

military in any productive capacity. Today there are some 250 training programs for these nonphysician health care providers throughout the United States. It has been estimated that there are approximately sixteen thousand nurse practitioners and forty-three thousand physician's assistants.[13]

The training programs for these occupations differ in both curriculum and program-completion time from one institution to another. Physician's-assistant programs range anywhere from one to two years in duration. Nurse-practitioner training usually is one year in length in addition to the normal nurses' training program.

Duties

As stated earlier, the nonphysician health care provider performs a number of services that were formerly physician responsibilities. These services include taking a health history, performing routine medical examinations, and providing emergency medical care.

In addition to traditional advanced nursing duties, both the physician's assistant and nurse practitioner are able to perform some diagnostic procedures, assess health status indicators, perform health maintenance tasks, and, generally, better assist sick patients. Because these individuals are active in health care, ambulatory care services can be extended to more people. Some of these providers are even trained to perform minor surgery such as suturing. They are also found providing various types of rehabilitative medical services.

Patient education and health counseling are other important roles played by the nonphysician health care provider. If the patient is informed of his or her problem and shown how to cope with it, a better sense of wellness and adaptation results.

Since the primary duties of the nonphysician health care provider involve caring for the well and treating minor illnesses, the physician should be able to spend more time with, and so better care for, the chronically and more seriously ill.

Specialties

Both the physician's assistant and the nurse practitioner may be trained in a number of specialized roles. The family nurse practitioner serves mothers and children. This practitioner is able to deal with infant diseases, as well as injuries and most emergency situations involving infants and children.

Other nurse-practitioner specialists include the gerontological nurse practitioner who works with the elderly in both private and public settings. In addition, a number of school districts throughout the country employ a school nurse practitioner. The pediatric nurse practitioner cares for expectant mothers and children, and advises parents in telephone conversations about home management of minor pediatric problems.[14] He or she also provides care and assistance for newborn infants and their parents. Most of the problems dealt with by the pediatric nurse practitioner are not serious enough for the child to be seen by the physician, yet still require the input of a medical person. Physician's-assistant specialists can be found in a broad range of medical practice.

Issues

A number of issues and concerns have developed over the physician's-assistant and the nurse-practitioner programs. One important concern is whether the consumer will accept this new health care provider in place of the physician. Would you go to a physician's assistant or receive the services of the nurse practitioner rather than seeing a physician? For the most part, people in the United States are so philosophically oriented to the physician as the predominant and sole health care provider that acceptance of the nonphysician provider has been limited. In spite of this reluctance to accept this new type of medical care provider, the nurse practitioner has proven to be an effective provider of primary care.[15] As patients have more exposure to these individuals as a source of medical care, they have become more receptive to them.[16]

In order for the nurse practitioner and the physician's assistant to be even more widely and effectively employed, it is important that they receive greater physician acceptance. Many physicians do not understand the role or responsibilities of this type of health provider. Some physicians even view the nonphysician health care provider as a threat to their practice, both economically and professionally. Perhaps, though, exposure to these new health professionals during medical training will encourage physicians to accept them.[17] The future physician needs to learn the value of the nurse practitioner and the physician's assistant and can develop an appreciation of the interactive roles they can play in the provision of health care. Physicians who employ nurse practitioners have come to value them.[18]

A number of legal questions have been raised concerning this new type of health care provider. The appearance of the nonphysician health care provider has forced many states to reexamine and change state statutes regarding medical practice and procedures. Medical supervision of both groups, especially the physician's assistant, is necessary. However, the definition of acceptable supervision has been controversial. Must the physician's assistant work in direct proximity to the physician? All states require some type of direct supervision. The question as to whether the nurse practitioner is practicing medicine without a license has gone to court in one state.[19] That court ruled that they were. Obviously many difficult and unanswered legal questions still exist in various localities.

Reimbursement

Pay for services provided by the nonmedical health care provider also presents problems. For example, the nurse practitioner should receive greater reimbursement than the traditional RN or BSN nurse. The training is more extensive and the individual is capable of performing a much broader range of services to the patient. However, many medical clinics and physicians do not employ nurse practitioners for that reason, choosing instead to pay the lower salaries of traditional registered nurses.

The services of the nonphysician health care provider should reduce costs to the patients. In theory, certain health care should be provided by a nonphysician in the outpatient, clinical, or office setting at a reduced price. However, in practice, when the nonphysician health care provider is employed by a physician or group practice, it is not uncommon for the costs to be greater. This is because the physician's assistant or nurse practitioner is considered a member of the health care team and, as such, the cost of his or her employment must be passed on to the consumer. There is no evidence that the nonphysician health care provider has helped to reduce health care costs.

Nurse-Midwives

A registered nurse who has completed additional education and training beyond the basic nursing program may be a nurse-midwife. This additional education prepares the nurse to provide health care for women and their babies during pregnancy, labor, delivery, and the postnatal or postpartum period. They also provide gynecologic care for nonpregnant women.

The nurse-midwife provides such prenatal care as the early diagnosis and initial physical examination of pregnancy. The nurse-midwife is also involved in all aspects of managing a normal delivery, including staying with the patient until the delivery is over. Other important services offered by the nurse-midwife include family-planning advice and health counseling.

The nurse-midwife works in association with physicians, usually with an obstetrician/gynecologist or general practice physician. The physician must permit the nurse-midwife to perform those tasks for which he or she is prepared to handle—most cases of pregnancy and childbirth; but a patient with high-risk complications is referred to the physician.

Nurse-midwifery was first introduced into the United States in 1925.[20] The first educational program to train the nurse-midwife was established in 1931 in New York City.[21] Presently, there are twenty-one nurse-midwife educational programs in the United States. There are more than three thousand certified midwives in the United States with the greatest numbers residing in California, New York,

and Florida.[22] Though some nurse-midwives work in private practice, most are affiliated with hospitals or with public health facilities.

Midwives have traditionally been found in localities where there is a lack of physicians to serve the economically disadvantaged. In recent years their services have been sought by middle and upper class couples desiring more personal involvement in the pregnancy and birthing process.

The nurse-midwife is not as common in the United States as in other countries throughout the world. In fact, in some European countries, most deliveries are managed by the nurse-midwife.

There are still a number of unanswered questions about the future role of nonphysician health care providers. Since an important reason for their existence has been to make health services available in medically underserved areas, it will be important to observe whether they remain in these geographical localities. Will they continue to work and live in the rural communities or the inner cities, or will they seek employment in medically overexposed areas as doctors have? It seems that the appearance of these new health care providers is timely, since their services will increase the availability of health care for the needy in this country.

Allied Health Personnel

Included in the allied health professions are various health technologists and technicians, therapists, laboratory workers, administrators, dieticians, and nutritionists. Technical advances in the health care field have led to the establishment of many new health occupations. The increasingly sophisticated technology of health care has created a demand for better-trained and more knowledgeable workers. Technologists, such as inhalation and respiratory therapists, are trained to operate diagnostic and monitoring equipment and to perform rehabilitative services. Increasing need for rehabilitation services has resulted in growing demand for occupational and physical therapists.

The physical therapist helps the injured, handicapped, and disabled person to regain physical movement if possible and to adapt to the handicapped conditions. Here a VA hospital physical therapist assists a disabled veteran in preparing for the National Veterans Wheelchair Games, one of the recreational services sponsored by the Veterans Administration and other veterans service organizations.

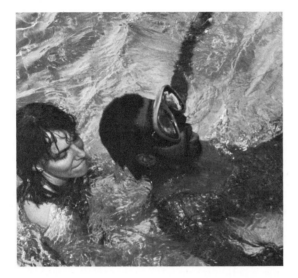

Increased Demand for Allied Health Professionals, 1982–1995 (Projected)

Clinical Laboratory Technologists and Technicians
Dental Hygienists
Dietitians
Electrocardiograph Technicians
Electroencephalographic Technologists
Health Record Technicians
Licensed Practical Nurses
Occupational Therapists
Physical Therapists
Physician's Assistants
Radiologic Technologists
Respiratory Therapists
Speech Pathologists and Audiologists
Surgical Technicians

Source: Bureau of Labor Statistics, Health Professions Report, Washington, D.C.: Bureau of Labor Statistics (August 8, 1984).

Allied health personnel constitute a majority of all persons working in the health care profession. These individuals work in a multiplicity of health care settings, such as physicians' and dentists' offices. The allied health worker has specific skills to contribute to the care, treatment, and rehabilitation of the health consumer.

Some allied health personnel perform tasks that in the past were the responsibility of physicians, dentists, or nurses. For example, dental hygienists today clean teeth, perform initial examinations, and take X rays. They play an important role in preventive dental health.

There are over one hundred occupational titles in the health field. Some 3.5 million health workers, or approximately 66 percent of all health personnel, are considered allied health personnel.[23] In spite of the different titles, nearly 90 percent of the total personnel employed in the allied occupations are among the following.[24]

1. dental assistants
2. dental hygienists
3. dental laboratory technicians
4. dietitians and dietetic technicians
5. health and medical-record technicians, assistants, and aides
6. medical-laboratory technologists, technicians, and assistants
7. occupational and physical therapists
8. radiology technologists, technicians, and assistants
9. respiratory therapists
10. speech pathologists and audiologists

The demand for increasing numbers of individuals in the allied health professions depends upon a number of variables. The past decade has witnessed significant need in most of the professions. Projections indicate that this need will continue to be greater than what has been the case in the late 1980s.

Education and Training

The professional education and training of allied health personnel take place in many different settings including hospitals, vocational schools, and colleges. The emphasis, however, has been on academics lately rather than on training in health service facilities. The trend has been away from the hospital setting and toward the colleges and universities. The number of college and university allied health programs has grown from two thousand to 6,900 since the mid-1960s.[25]

Many allied health training programs are offered by two-year colleges. The student receives clinical experiences in the hospital or other health care facilities, but the basic academic education takes place in the college or university setting. Some programs are hospital-based throughout the entire training period. The allied health programs most frequently found in hospitals include clinical laboratory, radiologic technology, administration, mental health, and dietetic and nutritional services.[26]

Some allied health training programs are offered by vocational training institutions. Usually, the programs found in these settings train students in medical office assistance, dental assistance, nursing aid, dental and medical laboratory technology, and radiologic technology.[27]

Many medical schools have departments of allied health. Here allied health personnel receive education and degrees beyond those offered by the two-year college program. In some instances, graduate degrees are earned at these institutions.

Licensure and Certification

Some allied health students must obtain either state or national, or both, credentials before they are able to practice. Usually these credentials are in the form of either a license or a certificate. These indicate that the individuals have fulfilled certain educational and skill requirements and are endorsed to work in a given locality. Some allied health fields require formal registration as well as certification.

Licensing for some allied health professions is performed under the mandates of state law. Dental hygienists, physical therapists, physician's assistants, and occupational therapists provide examples of this pattern of licensing. Medical record administrators and technicians, dietitians, respiratory therapists, and cardiopulmonary resuscitation technologists are certified by their respective professional societies.

Another method by which the student obtains state or federal permission to practice is through the accreditation of the educational institution or training program. An institution or a training program must meet specific standards established for the academic curriculum, the faculty, institutional resources, and facilities. An evaluation team from the accrediting agency visits the institution at regular intervals and either approves the program or makes recommendations for change. The approval is granted for a specific period of time and then recertification is required. All students graduating from the program will have the necessary credentials to practice. The process of obtaining credentials, whether on an individual or institutional basis, results in a degree of standardization from one locality to another throughout the nation.

Professional Associations

The various health professions are represented by a number of professional health associations. These associations are usually national in scope, often having state and local affiliates, and play several different roles. In-service education and updating of knowledge and skills are major concerns of a variety of meetings that are conducted for the association membership. These professional meetings provide opportunities for presenting research of interest to the profession and for the membership to debate and approve policy statements and professional resolutions.

A number of the professional associations have established standards of training and certification and/or licensing for those entering the specific health profession. For example, such standards have been

Selected Professional Health Associations

American Dietetic Association
840 No. Lake Shore Drive
Chicago, Illinois 60611

American Hospital Association
840 No. Lake Shore Drive
Chicago, Illinois 60611

American Optometric Association
7000 Chippewa St.
St. Louis, Missouri 63119

American Osteopathic Association
212 E. Ohio St.
Chicago, Illinois 60611

American Psychological Association
1200 17th St. NW
Washington, D.C. 20036

National Association of Sanitarians
1550 Lincoln St.
Denver, Colorado 80203

National Dental Association
5506 Connecticut Ave. NW
Washington, D.C. 20015

National Medical Association
1012 Tenth St. NW
Washington, D.C. 20001

established for physicians (American Medical Association, 535 No. Dearborn St., Chicago, Ill. 60610), nurses (National League of Nursing, 10 Columbus Circle, New York, N.Y. 10019), and dentists (American Dental Association, 211 E. Chicago, Ill. 60611), to name just a few.

The scope and interest of a professional organization may be quite broad. The principal professional health association for those involved in community health is the American Public Health Association (APHA, 1015 15th St., Washington, D.C. 20005). Membership in this association includes representation from all fields working in community health—physicians, nurses, environmentalists, sanitarians, health planners, dietitians, plus a host of others. The annual meeting of the American Public Health Association provides hundreds of sections from which the membership can choose to attend. The major publication of the American Public Health Association is the *American Journal of Public Health,* published monthly. In an attempt to keep the membership updated of current happenings in community health, a monthly newspaper, *The Nation's Health,* is made available to all members.

Many of the professional health associations provide a much narrower span of professional interest. For example, the American Academy of Pediatrics (P.O. Box 927, 141 NorthWest Point Road, Oak Grove Village, Ill. 60007) has basically one objective: to improve the health of children. The American Physical Therapy Association (1156 15th St. NW, Washington, D.C. 20005) is the professional association for those certified in physical therapy.

Many of these associations have played important roles in affecting change in community health. The American Dental Association, for instance, has been a leading proponent in support of community programs for fluoridation of public drinking water.

Federal Support of Health Personnel Programs

During the 1960s and the 1970s the federal government became increasingly involved in financing the training of health personnel. This support funded the development of new health professional schools, the renovation and expansion of existing programs, and provided loans, stipends, and fellowships for students. Federal monies were the primary stimulus for the growth of these institutions.

Several federal programs were developed in an attempt to help solve the problem of health personnel maldistribution and shortage. Three such programs are: (1) the National Health Service Corps, (2) the Area Health Education Centers Program, and (3) the Health Professions Educational Assistance Act of 1976.

National Health Service Corps

In an attempt to increase the accessibility of health personnel in underserved localities, the United States Congress established the National Health Service Corps in 1971. The federal government identifies shortage areas based upon the number of health care providers in a given geographical location, the number of people living in the area, their health needs, and their ability to obtain health care. The designation enables a region to receive National Health Service Corps personnel. These individuals, representatives of various health professions, are stationed in the locality for specific periods of time. Physicians, dentists, nurses, pharmacists, optometrists, medical and dental assistants, and health administrators are some of the personnel who have been active in this program. Even though personnel from different health professions are included, physicians comprise the greatest number of those involved in the program.

National Health Service Corps participants receive a government-paid medical education. In return, the individual contracts to serve a given period of time in a selected medically underserved locality after completion of medical school. The amount of time varies from two to four years, depending upon the length and amount of support received during the professional education. Upon completion of the required obligation, the health provider may elect to leave the National Health Service Corps but remain in the underserved community as a private practitioner, or the individual is free to move elsewhere to establish a medical practice.

A long-range objective of this program is for the health personnel to remain in the community in private practice after the government obligation has been fulfilled. However, studies have shown that this objective has not met with much success.[28] Physicians usually leave the communities after the obligation is completed and return to more favorable settings to practice medicine. Often they enter some type of specialty training, leaving the general practice of medicine.

Local communities wishing to become involved with the National Health Service Corps make a request through either the state or the local health department for the specific personnel needed. If a physician is needed, the community is expected to provide office or clinic facilities. People who receive health care from Corps personnel pay a service charge, but it is returned to the federal government since National Health Service Corps personnel are salaried by the government.

Area Health Education Center Program

Owing its conception to a Carnegie Commission Report issued in 1970, the AHEC program began in 1972. The Carnegie report pointed out the need for better health care in the United States. Commission recommendations called for an increase in the number of health care personnel, an improvement in the geographic distribution of personnel, an increase in governmental support of health care professional education, and an increased use of allied health personnel in the health care field. The report also called for the establishment of area health education centers. Such centers would help to solve health personnel shortages in certain geographical settings.[29] In 1971 Congress passed the Comprehensive Health Manpower Training Act, which gave legislative authority to the AHECs.

The purpose of the AHEC program (and other federal government programs) has been to improve the distribution of health care providers in medically underserved areas. This includes efforts to improve the quality and utilization of health personnel. It also encourages those in professional preparation schools to practice in medically underserved areas and urges those already practicing in these areas to remain there.

AHEC support of individuals enrolled in professional education programs in medicine, nursing, dentistry, pharmacy, and the allied health professions has been available. The emphasis of AHEC is upon education and not upon the direct provision of health services to a community. The federal government, through the Health Resources and Services Administration, contracts with the medical school to provide care in medically underserved areas. The medical students who are being supported by this program receive some of their professional training in communities where there is a shortage of medical care providers. Clinical and internship assignments are performed in a hospital or clinic in the community that has contracted to help finance the individual's medical expenses. This training usually develops the primary care skills that are needed in the particular setting. In addition to learning skills useful to a medically underserved area, the student becomes familiar with the community, its people, and the environment. He or she is able to observe diseases and diagnostic and treatment procedures that are unique to the specific community.

As stated earlier, the primary contract for this program is made by the government with a medical school. The medical school is required to pay a minimum of 25 percent of the costs of the program. A variety of professional and economic relationships then develop between the educational institution, the agencies within the community where placement will occur, and the specific students.

Health Professions Educational Assistance Act

This 1976 act provided federal support for the training of physicians, dentists, and related health personnel. A particular goal of this program was to increase the number of primary care physicians, particularly those in family practice, internal medicine, pediatrics, and general practice. An important result of this funding was an increase in student enrollment in professional schools and the development of a number of health professional and public

health schools in the 1970s. Funding under the provisions of this program has been curtailed in the 1980s.

Effect of Federal Programs

In spite of the programs providing an increased number of health personnel, the availability of health services in medically underserved areas has not appreciably improved. New practitioners have not located permanently in these areas. As a result, many government officials have recommended a reduction in or elimination of such programs.

The future of these federal government support programs is doubtful. Federal grants for education and training in the health professions have received minimal support in the 1980s. There is a strong likelihood that by the end of the 1980s federal financial support for these programs will all be eliminated. Many feel that the original goals have not been effectively achieved. The current thinking of many is that the federal government should not continue to be involved with federal support programs such as these. As with so many health programs in which the government has been involved, the future is unclear.

Health Care Facilities

Health care diagnosis and treatment is generally performed in the office of a health care provider (physician, dentist, podiatrist, optometrist, etc.), in a clinic that is funded and operated by public monies (local health department, community health center, etc.), or in hospitals. The private office may be a single operation where the physician, dentist, or other provider works on an independent basis. But an increasingly common development is an arrangement where the health care provider merges with other providers to form a group clinic. The provision of health care is still on an individual practice basis. However, administrative overhead costs, facility costs, and other expenditures are pooled for economic benefit.

Most local and state health departments provide health care in public clinics that are funded by tax monies. The type and extent of services provided in these clinics vary from one locality to another. During the 1960s and 1970s, a number of community health centers and other public health service facilities were established to provide health care, particularly in medically underserved areas. These facilities included neighborhood health clinics, short-term surgery centers, emergency treatment centers, and comprehensive mental health centers. Though available to all persons, the economically disadvantaged usually make the most use of these facilities.

Hospitals

In the United States, hospitalization most often takes place in community hospitals—any nonfederal hospitals that provide both short- and long-term general and specialized care. When patients are hospitalized for care and treatment, it is known as inpatient care. When the patient receives medical care in a hospital but is not lodged in the medical facility, it is referred to as outpatient care.

Community hospitals account for more than 98 percent of all short-term hospitalizations in the United States.[30] There are three classifications of these hospitals, determined by ownership and management: (1) private, nonprofit; (2) public owned; and (3) proprietary.

The private, nonprofit hospitals provide health care for the general public. These hospitals are usually governed by a board of trustees and are operated by religious organizations, community nonprofit corporations, or philanthropic agencies. Private, nonprofit hospitals provide 70 percent of all hospital beds, even though just over half of all community hospitals are so operated.

The nonprofit hospitals qualify for exemption from federal taxation. This tax exempt status permits the hospitals to solicit and accept contributions that are deductible by donors. The nonprofit hospitals are also faced with financial pressures to raise operating capital. They cannot raise money for capital expenditures as can the proprietary hospitals, but must rely on philanthropy, governmental grants, or other measures in the private sector.

The prospective pay system (DRGs) is causing increasing budgetary pressure and competition on all hospitals, particularly the not-for-profit facilities. It appears that, with the rise of economic competition in health care, these hospitals will have to undergo substantial changes in the late 1980s and into the 1990s.

Government-owned hospitals are tax supported and operated by local or state health agencies and offer a range of services. Often they are found in large cities and provide the only health care for large segments of the poor population. Due to financial restrictions, these hospitals are often understaffed. They provide 22 percent of all hospital beds in the United States.

The proprietary hospital is privately owned and is established as a profit-making organization. It is managed by a board of directors and policy is determined by the owners, who are often stockholders who have invested in the corporation.

Prior to the 1980s, for-profit health care facilities were usually rather small and localized. These facilities were often owned by a group of physicians. However, in the 1980s a significant change has occurred. The health care industry has been increasingly seen as a growth industry with investment potential. Ownership of for-profit health care facilities has been increasingly taken over by large multihospital, investor-owned corporations. These hospital management companies include—in addition to hospitals—ownership in nursing homes and ambulatory care facilities.

The largest investor-owned hospital corporation is the Hospital Corporation of America. Other well-known health care corporations are Humana Health Corporation, National Medical Enterprises, and the American Medical International Corporation. Investor-owned corporations have moved beyond the provision of direct health care services into areas of research and new product development. For example, the Humana Health Corporation has done much work on the development of artificial heart surgery.

Many people today go to outpatient ambulatory care centers for medical care. Hospitals now provide outpatient services in a variety of different settings. (a) This facility is housed in a renovated gasoline station. (b) Free-standing emergency trauma centers, separate from any hospital, are rapidly developing facilities in many cities.

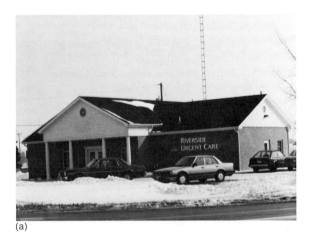

(a)

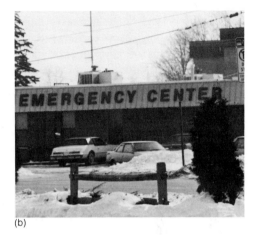

(b)

Obviously monetary profit is a principal goal of such corporations. Some estimates are that by 1990 close to half of all health care in the United States will be performed in investor-owned corporation facilities. As a result profit will be an increasing factor in the future shape of the United States health care delivery system. These large corporations will increasingly purchase smaller hospitals and other health care facilities as they grow larger.

Those who support the expansion and growth of the for-profit health care delivery system suggest that investor-owned health management companies provide a more efficient delivery system. They are able to attract capital for expansion, development, and growth. It is felt that better quality health care is able to be provided and that industrial management principles will assure better health care.

On the other hand, opponents of this development question the basic motives of the for-profit movement. Should the motive of provision of health care be monetary return on investment? It is felt by many that everyone's health needs cannot be met adequately by corporations seeking a profit motive. Those individuals who cannot afford the costs of the investor-owned facilities will be forced to go to public and voluntary hospitals for their health care. This will add serious pressures to this segment of the health care delivery system. Public hospitals could become health care facilities basically for the economically disadvantaged population. How will funds be raised to meet the demands of such a development? Will the quality of health care be similar for the economically disadvantaged to that found in the for-profit facility, or is this leading to a "two-track" health care system in the United States?

Cost Containment Strategies and Hospitals

With the increase in health care costs during the past two decades, hospitals have been experiencing increasing pressures to hold down costs. This has resulted in a number of major changes in medical care as it relates to all health care facilities, particularly hospitals.

One important change has been the decrease in use of hospital inpatient services and the corresponding increase in outpatient, ambulatory health care. Procedures which in the past would have meant inpatient hospitalization of a couple of days are now often performed on an outpatient basis, the result being less cost to the consumer. In two years during the mid-1980s hospital admissions were down more than 8 percent.[31] Outpatient visits alone rose four-fold in one year—1985.[32] The increased interest in outpatient services has been encouraged by cost containment patterns of governmental insurance programs, by hospital insurance coverages provided by business and industry, and by insurance companies.

Advances in medical technology have also been a factor in the growth and expansion of ambulatory surgical health care. For example, cataract removal used to require several days of immobilization. This surgical procedure now takes less than a half hour because of new technologies that eliminate most of the radical cutting and suturing.

This switch from inpatient care has resulted in a lower hospital occupancy rate. Hospitals have been forced to reduce bed facilities and staff. Staffing reductions have involved both part- and full-time personnel. In one year the reported reduction nationally in full-time personnel in community hospitals was seventy thousand.[33]

In spite of this change in hospital inpatient care, overall hospital costs have continued to rise. With individuals having minor problems receiving outpatient care, those patients being cared for in hospitals tend to have more serious problems and need more expensive, technologically sophisticated procedures. Increased malpractice insurance premium costs have also added to the financial stresses on hospitals. As a result many smaller hospitals have been forced to close, to form alliances with larger urban hospital centers, or have been bought out by for-profit health care corporations. Nearly half of all hospitals in the United States are small or rural facilities with less than one hundred beds.[34] Many of these smaller hospitals are in rural settings and have been the primary source of health care for many people living in a broad geographical region.

In order to be competitive and to be able to survive economically, hospitals are making numerous changes in their operations. Departments are having to be cost effective; failure has led to the elimination of certain departments in many hospitals.

Increased marketing of services is now seen. Hospitals are developing new or expanded services, many of which are designed to make use of facilities no longer occupied at full capacity. Programs are being developed that will result in economic profit such as health promotion programs, alcoholism treatment, and substance abuse rehabilitation programs. Today, one sees advertisements in the mass media and on community billboards for various hospital programs. This was unheard of several years ago.

Diversification is occurring in many hospitals, particularly the smaller ones. Facilities previously used for acute care have been converted to provide such services as long-term care, ambulatory care, and retirement housing. Another idea is to place nursing homes near hospitals so that hospital patients who require long-term care can be transferred to the nursing home. If an acute episode arises the patient can quickly be returned to the hospital.

Another competitive force that has had an effect on hospital use and the cost of health care is the development of for-profit outpatient care facilities. For example, in many communities there are free-standing surgicenters where outpatient surgery can be obtained, ambulatory care centers where emergency and other primary care services are provided, and home care programs. All of these have played a role in changing the shape of health care provision in the mid- to latter 1980s.

Summary

The health care industry is the third largest industry in the United States. Close to six million persons are employed in some profession or occupation related to the provision of health care. Physicians and other health care providers account for about one-third of these employees, while nearly two-thirds are allied, or related health personnel.

In spite of growth in the health care industry, some still question the adequacy of the number now employed in the field. Are there enough physicians, dentists, nurses, and other health care personnel? What is an adequate number? Most studies of health personnel report that the supply of health providers has greatly increased in the past two decades and, projecting into the future, a surplus will result in most fields.

The majority of all persons in the health care industry are allied health personnel. There are over one hundred occupational titles that fall into this category, with over 3.5 million employed persons.

These persons are trained to contribute to the care, treatment, and rehabilitation of the patient. The education and training of allied health personnel have become more academic, and a number of allied health fields now have state and national standards for obtaining credentials. Most of the health professions have some type of professional association for membership of those certified in the given field.

Health personnel generally work in medical offices, clinics, and other outpatient facilities, or in hospitals and other inpatient settings. Most hospitalization in the United States occurs in community hospitals. The trend in hospital development in recent years has been toward larger, more comprehensive facilities, with many being owned by for-profit health care corporations. Increasing economic stresses have had an impact on the operation of most hospitals in America in the 1980s.

Discussion Questions

1. What have been some of the issues in the 1980s concerning physician manpower?
2. Discuss some of the conclusions that the GMENAC Report addressed regarding the future medical work force needs in the United States.
3. What are some reasons for the shortage of nurses interested in working in the hospital clinical setting?
4. Identify and discuss the trends in nursing education as seen in the 1980s.
5. Explain the impact that foreign medical graduates have made on the American health care system.
6. What are some of the issues that surround the employment of the nonphysician health care provider?
7. Discuss the legal status of the nonphysician health care provider.
8. What is a nurse-midwife?
9. Discuss the role that the allied health manpower personnel play in the American health care system.
10. What are some of the differences between the National Health Service Corps program and the AHEC program?
11. Identify some of the factors that have contributed to the growth of the for-profit hospitals.
12. What are some of the questions raised about the increase in operation of hospitals by large, for-profit, health care corporations?
13. How has the interest in cost containment of health costs affected the hospitals in the 1980s?
14. What is diversification as it relates to hospitals?

Suggested Readings

Batey, Marjorie V., and Holland, Jeanne M. "Prescribing Practices among Nurse Practitioners in Adult and Family Health." *American Journal of Public Health* 75, no. 3 (March, 1985): 258–62.

Diliberto, Rosemary A. "The AHEC Contribution to Social Work Education." *Public Health Reports* 101, no. 2 (March/April, 1986): 187–91.

Gessert, Charles E., and Smith, Daniel R. "The National AHEC Program: Review of Its Progress and Considerations for the 1980s." *Public Health Reports* 96, no. 2 (March/April, 1980): 116–20.

Hayes, Eileen. "The Nurse Practitioner: History, Current Conflicts, and Future Survival." *Journal of American College Health* 34, no. 3 (December, 1985): 144–47.

Henry, Marie O. "How Many Nurse Practitioners are Enough?" *American Journal of Public Health* 76, no. 5 (May, 1986): 493.

Kernaghan, Salvinija G. "The Nurse Shortage: How Can We Turn the Exodus Around?" *Hospitals* 56, no. 3 (February 1, 1982): 53–56.

Luft, Harold S. "For-Profit Hospitals: A Cost Problem or Solution?" *Business and Health* 2, no. 3 (January/February, 1985): 13–16.

McNutt, David R. "GMENAC: Its Manpower Forecasting Framework." *American Journal of Public Health* 71, no. 10 (October, 1981): 1116–24.

Pattison, Robert V., and Katz, Halliem. "Investor-owned and Not-for-Profit Hospitals." *New England Journal of Medicine* 309, no. 6 (August 11, 1983): 347–53.

Report to the President and Congress on the Status of Health Professions Personnel in the United States. Department of Health, Education, and Welfare, Public Health Service, Bureau of Health Manpower, DHEW Publication No. (HRA) 8-53, 1980.

Rosenblatt, Roger A., and Moscovice, Ira. "The National Health Service Corps: Rapid Growth and Uncertain Future." *Milbank Memorial Fund Quarterly, Health and Society* 58, no. 2 (1980): 283–309.

Schlesinger, Mark. "The Rise of Proprietary Health Care." *Business and Health* 2, no. 3 (January/February, 1985): 7–12.

Tootelian, Dennis H., and Gaedeke, Ralph M. "The Changing Role of Pharmacies in the 1990s." *Journal of Health Care Marketing* 6, no. 1 (March, 1986): 57–63.

Endnotes

1. U.S. Bureau of the Census, *Statistical Abstracts of the United States, 1986* (106th Ed.), Washington, D.C., 1985.

2. Statistical data and analysis in this paragraph are from data provided in various publications of the Bureau of Health Manpower, Department of Health and Human Services, Washington, D.C.

3. Department of Health and Human Services, *Health, United States, 1979* (Washington, D.C.: U.S. Government Printing Office, 1979): 152.

4. U.S. Bureau of the Census, *Statistical Abstracts,* p. 103.

5. "Projections of Physician Supply in the United States." Bureau of Health Professions, Health Resources and Services Administration, Rockville, Md.

6. Department of Health and Human Services, *Report of the GMENAC to the Secretary,* DHHS Publication No. (HRA) 81-857 (1981): 23.

7. Department of Health and Human Services, *Health, United States, 1980* (Washington, D.C.: U.S. Government Printing Office, 1980): 80.

8. U.S. Bureau of the Census, *Statistical Abstracts.*

9. *Report of the GMENAC to the Secretary,* 1–5.

10. National Health Insurance Association, Source Book of Health Insurance Data, p. 77.

11. National College of Chiropractic, *Fact Sheet on Chiropractic,* (Lombard, Illinois: The College): n.d.

12. National Health Insurance Association, Source Book of Health Insurance Data, p. 77.

13. U.S. Bureau of the Census, *Statistical Abstracts.*

14. *Report of the GMENAC to the Secretary,* 20–21.

15. Mauksch, Ingeborg G. "The Nurse Practitioner Movement—Where Does It Go from Here?" *American Journal of Public Health* 68, no. 11 (November, 1978): 1074.

16. Henry, Marie O. "How Many Nurse Practitioners Are Enough?" *American Journal of Public Health* 76, no. 5 (May, 1986): 493.

17. Weinberger, Morris, et al. "Changing Nurse Staff Attitudes toward Nurse Practitioners during Their Residency Training." *American Journal of Public Health* 70, no. 11 (November, 1980): 1206.

18. Henry, Marie O. "How Many Nurse Practitioners?" 493.

19. Hayes, Eileen. "The Nurse Practitioner: History, Current Conflicts, and Future Survival." *Journal of College Health* 34, no. 3 (December, 1985): 145.

20. Rooks, Judith Bourne, and Fischman, Susan H. "American Nurse-Midwifery Practice in 1976–1977: Reflections of 50 Years of Growth and Development." *American Journal of Public Health* 70, no. 9 (September, 1980): 990.

21. Ibid., 990.

22. Information provided by the American College of Nurse-Midwives.

23. Department of Health, Education, and Welfare. A Report on Allied Health Personnel, DHEW Pub. No. (HRA) 80–28, PHS, Health Resources, Administration, Bureau of Health Manpower, 1980: I–1.

24. Ibid., II–2.

25. Ibid., III–1.

26. Ibid., III–5.

27. Ibid., III–6.

28. Rosenblatt, Roger A. and Moscovice, Ira. "The National Health Service Corps: Rapid Growth and Uncertain Future." *Milbank Memorial Fund Quarterly, Health and Society* 58, no. 2 (1980): 300.

29. Carnegie Commission on Higher Education, *Higher Education and the Nation's Health.* New York: McGraw-Hill Book Co., 1970.

30. Department of Health and Human Services, *Health, United States, 1980* (Washington, D.C.: U.S. Government Printing Office, 1980): 87.

31. The Hospital Research and Educational Trust, *Economic Trends,* Chicago, Ill.: American Hospital Association, (Spring 1986): 2.

32. Ibid., 2.

33. Ibid., 2.

34. Ibid., 1.

6

Epidemiology: Counting and Analyzing for Planning and Programming

What Is Epidemiology?

Historically, the study of the occurrence of diseases in human populations has been known as epidemiology. The term *epidemiology* is derived from two Greek words *epi* and *demos, epi* meaning "among" and *demos* meaning "people." Hence, the work of epidemiology looks at such factors as the distribution of disease and injury and the determinants of these conditions among people. The basic concern in epidemiological study is focused upon groups of persons, not separate individuals.

Investigation of disease occurrence is not new. It is likely that mankind first began to study disease causation and distribution by asking simple questions. What is causing sickness in our family? Why is there an increase in illness among our people? Is there a reason why adults do not get certain illnesses they had when they were children?

The more formal development of epidemiology came about as a result of study of the great communicable disease epidemics of the past, such as smallpox, yellow fever, cholera, the plague, and numerous other infectious diseases. The primary emphasis has been on identifying the *etiology* or cause of specific diseases.

The findings of epidemiological study can be used for many purposes. One use is to determine the magnitude of diseases or other conditions, and their impact on certain populations. Information gathered from the epidemiological process can be used in setting community health program priorities, in evaluating the effectiveness of current programs, and in determining what type of treatment facilities may be needed in the future.

Through the years the procedures of epidemiology have been applied to a broad range of problems other than infectious diseases. For example, early studies in this century looked at problems of malnutrition. Lack of certain nutrients among population groups resulted in such conditions as scurvy and pellagra. More recently the procedures and techniques of epidemiology have focused on chronic illnesses, such as malignant diseases, cardiovascular diseases, diabetes, the various types of arthritic conditions, and a host of other chronic ailments. The process of epidemiological study has been applied to safety causation and prevention. It has been used widely in occupational safety and health studies, in studies of health services needs, in the measurement of health risks, and in health planning. Epidemiologic methods are also applied to family planning, congenital defects, mental illness, and drug addiction.

Epidemiology asks what characteristics that seem to contribute to a given disease can be identified within a population group. It also looks at the role that environmental factors play in certain people getting a specific disease or injury. Epidemiology looks at frequencies of diseases in groups of people and identifies factors that influence these frequencies.

The Epidemiological Model

The epidemiological model involves the interaction of three different factors influencing disease: (1) the *causative agent,* (2) the *host,* and (3) the *environmental factors.* Epidemiological research is directed toward one, two, or all three of these factors with the hope of breaking the "chain of infection." In noncommunicable disease studies, a change in any of the three components can affect the factor under study.

Chain of Infection

In the case of infectious diseases, a host may be an individual, an animal, or a plant. Our concern is primarily with diseases where humans are the host. Pathogenic microorganisms, or pathogens, leave the host reservoir through a route of discharge, known as a *portal of exit.* Portals of exist are discharges from the mouth and the nose by coughing, sneezing, breathing, and speaking. Other portals of exit are fecal wastes, saliva, blood, mucous membranes, semen, open wounds, sores, and insect bites.

Figure 6.1 The chain of infection

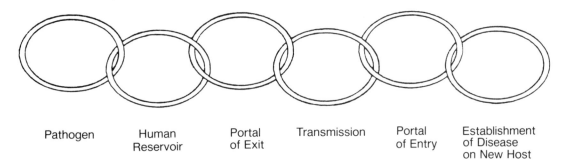

Pathogen   Human   Portal   Transmission   Portal   Establishment
    Reservoir   of Exit   of Entry   of Disease
                                                                on New Host

Figure 6.2 Pathogen transmission from host to host

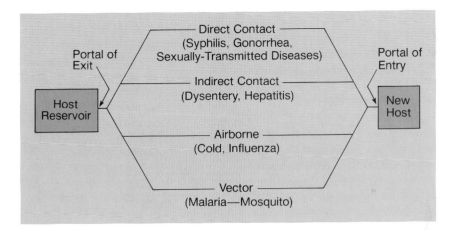

Once the pathogen comes into contact with a new host, it enters by what is known as a *portal of entry*. Usually the portal of entry and portal of exit are part of the same body system. For example, microorganisms that leave a host reservoir by way of the nose and mouth, such as by a cough or sneeze, enter another host who breathes the air droplets containing the pathogen. Pathogens that leave a host by way of human feces work their way back into the food or water chain and so into the digestive system when food or water are ingested. This communicable disease chain of infection is pictured in figure 6.1. Communicable disease control measures are effective if they break any one of the links in this chain of infection.

Pathogenic microorganisms are transmitted between the host reservoir and a new host in several different ways: by direct contact, by indirect transmission, by airborne transfer, and through the action of a vector (fig. 6.2).

Direct contact transmits disease when a new host comes into contact with the infected skin or mucous membrane. This is the case in sexually transmitted diseases in which the microorganisms of syphilis, gonorrhea, and AIDS are transferred through the direct contact of sexual partners.

Indirect transmission involves an intermediate object as the mode of transmission between hosts. Diseases that are spread by the ingestion of contaminated food, milk, and water are considered to be the result of indirect transmission. This is also the case when the pathogenic microorganism is present on towels, bedding, hypodermic needles, and other objects—all known as *fomites*—which are used by a diseased person. The disease is transmitted to another individual who uses the same objects. Serum hepatitis is an example of an indirectly transmitted disease. The microorganisms remain on hypodermic needles so that when drug addicts share unsterile utensils the disease is transmitted from one host to another.

Another means of communicable disease transfer between hosts is through *airborne transfer*. Disease organisms are spread either on air droplets or dust from one locality to a host. The common cold and influenza are spread in this way.

Vectors are arthropods that transmit pathogenic microorganisms from one host to another. Many insects spread disease by biting the host and transferring the pathogen. Others carry the pathogenic organisms on their body and contaminate food ingested by hosts. The fly is a common vector of disease.

The most widespread communicable disease in the world is malaria. This disease is caused by a parasite, a one-celled protozoan, and transmitted by the Anopheles mosquito. This parasite spends part of its life cycle in human red blood cells and the other part in the female Anopheles mosquito.

Communicable Disease Control

The control of communicable disease requires action to break the chain of infection. This action may involve the human host, as when an individual is immunized before being exposed to a disease, or it may mean taking drugs for protection against the pathogens, as when individuals take chloroquine as protection against malaria.

Several factors come into play in developing control programs for malaria. Malaria can be controlled by destroying the mosquitoes and their breeding places. This is not an easy task. Swamps must be drained, breeding places must be sprayed with pesticides to destroy the larva, or all sources of standing water must be eliminated.

Malaria transmission occurs primarily between dusk and dawn. This is because of the nocturnal feeding habits of Anopheles mosquitoes. Therefore, individuals need to stay in well-screened areas, use mosquito nets, and wear clothes that cover the entire body.

Chloroquine is the primary drug of choice to treat attacks of malaria. It is used both to cure and to provide protection against malaria. In some areas of the world the mosquitoes have become resistant to chloroquine. Since 1982 the Centers for Disease Control has recommended combined use of chloroquine and Fansidar for those traveling in chloroquine-resistant areas.

There are risks of adverse reactions for individuals using Fansidar. Individuals who have known histories of reaction to sulfa drugs should not use this drug.

Control measures may be taken to reduce the possibility of pathogen transmission between hosts. For instance, a condom can be used during sexual intercourse to protect against the spread of sexually transmitted diseases. In addition, any disease control program administered by a community health agency is usually designed to reduce or eliminate disease vectors.

In determining the needed communicable disease control measure or measures, it must first be decided where the focus would be most effective: on the host, the reservoir of infection, the microorganism, or the means of transmission. Economy, effectiveness, education, and available resources are all factors in this decision.

Noncommunicable Disease Applications

The application of the epidemiological model is widely used within the community health, health care, and accident prevention fields today. In relation to the increasing use of smokeless tobacco and oral cancers, the epidemiologists might direct attention toward the individual using tobacco (the host), the tobacco itself (the agent), or the means of obtaining the product (the environment). It is first beneficial to ascertain the most efficient focus. For example, programs designed to educate the host of the dangers associated with chewing tobacco products have been developed. It is doubtful if measures directed toward the elimination of the agent, the tobacco, are effective. Some ordinances and regulations have been established to discourage its purchase. However, most disease control professionals have concluded, in using the epidemiological model, that the best way to reduce this "cycle of disease" is to focus on the host.

The epidemiological model has also been used in the study and prevention of accidents. This model was first suggested as an approach in accident prevention in 1948.[1] When the focus is directed toward the person (the host), various actions can be taken to reduce the risk of an accident. For example, the development of driving skills or bicycle skills helps reduce the possibility of accident. The agent of causation of an industrial or home injury may be one of a number of different possibilities. It may be a piece of metal that flies into the eye of an individual running a lathe in a factory or it may be a knife resting in a drawer that cuts a finger when one reaches in. The agent of injury may be the flame from a grill or a fire. Measures need to be taken to reduce the possibility of the causing agent coming into contact with the individual. This may mean purchasing a car with a padded dashboard or a shatter-proof windshield. It means putting sharp tools in storage racks or wearing eye protection devices.

The third factor in the epidemiological model includes a variety of different environmental factors. In highway safety a number of engineering actions and developments have made for safer travel.

The use of break-away sign poles and construction of dual highways are measures designed to protect the host from accident.

Types of Epidemiological Studies

Analysis and study of data leads to the establishment of a hypothesis or several hypotheses about the causative agent. Once the hypothesis is established, it is necessary to test it. Epidemiologists conduct such tests either by observational or experimental study.

Observational Studies

Not involving the manipulation of a population, these kinds of epidemiological investigations focus on events in a field setting, such as a community, hospital, clinic, school, worksite, or other environmental setting. Grouping of a specific population for analysis is on the basis of certain identified characteristics such as age, race, sex, occupation, or other demographic variables.

There are three different kinds of observational studies: (1) prospective, (2) retrospective, and (3) cross-sectional. A *prospective study* begins with a group of people who are free of the disease or problem being investigated and share common experiences. This grouping is referred to as a *cohort*. The individuals vary in the degree of exposure to a given factor being studied. The different groups are followed over a period of time to ascertain the effect of exposure to the given factor. For example, in a study to ascertain the effect on child development of breast-feeding compared with bottle feeding, a specific number of newborn infants will be selected. At a given time, or at various intervals, these babies will be evaluated for the particular growth developments in question. Comparisons will be made between those who were bottle-fed with those who were breast-fed.

A prospective study involves group identification before the disease develops. Though one particular factor is usually designed into the study, often observations of a variety of outcomes can be obtained from this type of study. For example, if a

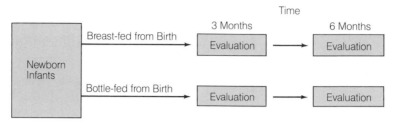

Cohort—Newborn Infants
Factor Under Study—Breast-feeding Compared with Bottle-feeding
    and the Effect on Growth and Development
Time Factor—Selected Time Factors
Evaluation—Weight Gain at 3 and 6 Months
    Physiological Development at 3 and 6 Months

group of young adults were being studied over a period of several years to ascertain the effectiveness of regular exercise in reducing hypertension, it is most likely that a number of measures could also be made relating to such factors as cholesterol levels, triglycerides, and overall weight control.

The prospective study usually is long-term, expensive, and time-consuming. It is often very difficult to maintain controls because there is a need for a large number in the cohort group resulting in rather large-scale projects.

One of the best-known prospective studies in the United States has been the Framingham, Massachusetts, cardiovascular disease study, which was started in 1948 and conducted by the United States Public Health Service. The primary goal was to ascertain the relationship of a number of different factors to the development of heart disease. More than six thousand individuals between the ages of 30 and 62 were initially selected to be studied over a period of twenty years. During this time period all participants were given a physical examination every other year in order to obtain information about factors that are related to heart disease, such as serum cholesterol, blood pressure, weight, and cigarette smoking. Great amounts of information about risk factors and heart disease were acquired.[2] The Framingham Study has been used as a prototype for similar long-term studies in other localities.

A second type of observational study is the *retrospective study*. This type of study looks at population groups that include individuals with or without the disease. The past history of these people is analyzed in order to ascertain what factors, either personal life-style, environmental, or other, might have led to the cause of the health problem under consideration and why others in the study were not affected. In this type of study the individuals who have the disease or problem under examination are referred to as "cases" while those that do not have the problem are "controls."

One might wish to study those factors that contributed to the development of asbestosis among a certain population group. A selected sample of employees who worked with asbestos in the construction industry over a given period of time (maybe from 1955 to 1965) are chosen for the study. These individuals are similar with respect to other factors except for the specific exposure under study. Comparisons are made with regard to the presence of asbestosis at the present time, and conclusions are formulated about what factors might have caused this disease. Retrospective studies are less expensive to conduct and are less time-consuming. It is also possible to look at more than one risk factor in this type of study.

A type of retrospective study often used in epidemiological study is the *cross-sectional study*. In this procedure exposure of two groups being compared is limited to their current situations. The cross-sectional study does not establish a sequence of events leading to findings. It is simply a survey of present status, which is the simplest form of observational study. Survey studies are undertaken to describe the distribution of disease or other factors of concern, are easy to accomplish, and can be done in a rather short period of time. For example, a study might be conducted to ascertain the extent of hearing loss among elderly people living in a given community.

Experimental Studies

Unlike observational studies where the epidemiologist only observes and records, experimental epidemiology involves a manipulation or intervention of human populations. The conditions of the study can be controlled. This type of study seeks to identify cause-and-effect relationships.

In experimental research some action is taken within a population group. It may be the withholding of a treatment, a drug, or other factor from an identified group to ascertain certain relationships and causes. On the other hand, it may be exposing the experimental group to medication, a vaccine, or something that has an uncertain effect. Experimental epidemiology can be divided into (1) clinical studies and (2) community studies.

There are three types of *clinical studies:* (1) therapeutic trials, (2) intervention, and (3) prevention. The *therapeutic study* attempts to ascertain whether a therapeutic procedure is effective in relieving symptoms of a disease or whether its use will improve the specific conditions relating to the disease. Probably the most common type of therapeutic study involves the study of the effects of a new healing modality or a new drug.

The retrospective study

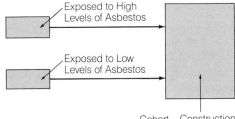

Construction Workers
1955 to 1965

Exposed to High Levels of Asbestos

Exposed to Low Levels of Asbestos

Cohort—Construction Workers Who Worked with Asbestos from 1955 to 1965

Factor under Study— Extent of Cases with Asbestosis among Workers in Mid-1980s

Evaluation—
1. Individuals with Asbestosis
2. Individuals with Other Respiratory Diseases

The cross-sectional study

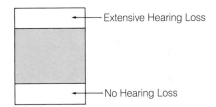

Extensive Hearing Loss

No Hearing Loss

Cohort—Elderly People Living in Town A at Present Time

Factor under Study—Extent of Hearing Loss among Current Residents

Evaluation—Demographic Factors (Age, Sex, Race, etc.) as They Relate to Hearing Loss

Intervention studies involve the application of some intervention modality in an attempt to improve the chances that disease risk can be reduced. For example, many studies have been conducted to ascertain the effect of exercising in reducing risk for cardiovascular disease, hypertension, and stroke.

The *preventive study* involves the application of some measure designed to prevent disease. Probably the most common preventive epidemiological studies are vaccination programs. Vaccines are applied to a population group to prevent diseases such as tuberculosis, malaria, and the childhood diseases.

In medicine and public health, experimental studies are not always feasible. For example, if a study looking at the relationships of chewing tobacco and oral cancer were being conducted, it would be necessary to randomly assign individuals to two groups. One group would be required to chew tobacco for a given period of time, the other would not be permitted to use any tobacco products. Obviously, using human subjects to intentionally cause illness, disease, or debilitation is unacceptable. The random selection to this group would be considered unethical. One can see that many human experimental studies are not possible. Therefore, much experimental research must be performed in the laboratory with animals.

Animal research is also the setting in which many early effects of drugs are first studied. Only where there is a strong possibility of success can human research take place.

The experimental epidemiological research study must be controlled if it is to provide useful information. This type of study involves identifying at least two equally assigned groups. In the development of an experimental study individuals are assigned to specific groups for study. It is important that the groups to be studied are comparable. Two groups are usually identified: (1) the *control group,* which will not be given the particular factor, and (2) the *experimental group,* which will be given the specific treatment under study. The researcher should randomly assign subjects to specific study groups. It is also possible to conduct experimental studies using several groups. In these situations several different types or amounts of the treatment may be tested.

A second type of experimental study is the *community study.* Rather than the subjects being individually selected and assigned to a study group, a population group is selected for involvement in the study. Individuals are studied residing in the community of selection. One of the classic public health community experimental studies was begun in 1945 in New York state to ascertain the effectiveness of preventing tooth decay by placing fluoride in the public drinking water. In that study two communities located about thirty-five miles apart, Newburgh and Kingston, New York, were selected for study. The communities were about equal in population. Sodium fluoride was added to the drinking water of Newburgh while the drinking water of Kingston was left unchanged. For ten years children of various ages were examined for tooth decay in the two communities. It was concluded after ten years of study that the fluoridation of public drinking water is an effective and safe measure for reducing the incidence of tooth decay.

Measurement Used in Epidemiology

Quantitative data is used to identify the incidence of a disease or specific factor being studied in a selected population. Biostatistics, or counts of individuals, are the basic data used in epidemiology.

Presentation of Data

Data that are collected in epidemiological studies must be presented in a useful manner. Initially one has simply a frequency count. For example, one might have a count of twenty persons in the school having influenza, or thirteen teenagers may have sought assistance of the local health department in the past month for treatment for syphilis.

Frequency counts are the simplest, most frequent statistical procedure used in epidemiology, but they are of little value in and of themselves. In order to be useful, data must be presented as proportions or rates, which put data into some perspective in relationship to the population under consideration.

Rates (R) are usually expressed as the number of people with a given problem in relation to the number of persons in the population at risk, and are obtained by dividing the number of cases of the problem under study by the population in the study.

$$R = \frac{\text{Number of Cases}}{\text{Population Under Study}}$$

Data can be presented as the number of persons with a given problem at a particular point in time. This is known as the *prevalence rate*. The prevalence rate indicates the number of people out of the considered population who have the disease at a specific time. The prevalence rate is determined by dividing the number of existing cases by the total population involved in the study. This result should be multiplied by 1,000; 10,000; or 100,000; depending upon what ratio for comparison one wishes to use. When considering prevalence rates the ratio is usually expressed per 1,000 population.

Formula for Prevalence Rate

$$\frac{\text{Number of Existing Cases}}{\text{Total Population}} \times 1000$$

(At a specific point in time)

For example, in a school district with 4,500 students there were 34 absent on January 18 with influenza. The prevalence rate on January 18 was 7.5 (per thousand).

$$\frac{34 \text{ (existing cases)}}{4,500 \text{ (total school population)}} = .0075 \times 1,000 = 7.5$$

Another type of statistic used by epidemiologists is the *incidence rate*. This measures the number of cases that developed over a specific period of time.

It reflects the number of new occurrences that developed in ratio to the total population at risk. The formula for determining incidence rate involves dividing the number of new cases by the number of individuals in the population at risk over a given period of time. This decimal is multiplied by whatever ratio for comparison is going to be used (i.e., 1,000; 10,000; or 100,000).

Formula for Incidence Rate

$$\frac{\text{Number of New Cases}}{\text{Population at Risk}}$$

(Over a given period of time)

For example, in a given community of senior citizens during the months of February and March, thirty-four people developed the common cold to the extent that it necessitated a visit to the physician. The population at risk for this study, senior citizens, numbers 3,252. The incidence rate for the common cold during these two months was 10.5 (per thousand).

$$\frac{34 \text{ cases of the common cold}}{3,252 \text{ senior citizens}} = .01045 \times 1,000 = 10.5$$

Sources of Data

Data that are used in epidemiological work come from a variety of different sources. Much information is available from data collected every ten years in the national census. The recording of vital data by the local and state health departments provides a vast array of information for use in epidemiology. Also, morbidity information can be obtained from many other sources in the community such as hospitals, clinics, physicians, schools, and the courts.

Birth rates, United States: number of live births per 1,000 population

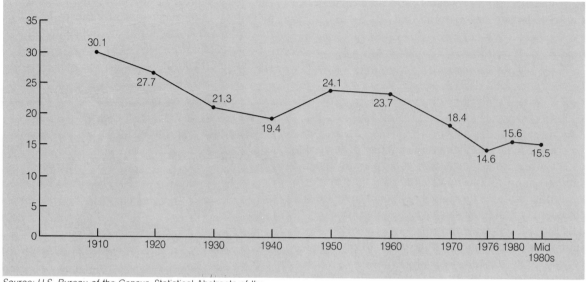

Source: U.S. Bureau of the Census. Statistical Abstracts of the United States, 1986, 106th ed. Washington, D.C.: U.S. Government Printing Office.

Census Data

In the United States a census, gathering information on the entire national population, has been conducted by the Federal Bureau of the Census every ten years since 1790. Census data that are useful to epidemiological studies include age, sex, race, marital status, and other factors such as geographical distribution. Use is made in epidemiology of census data to determine the vital health events as rates.

Vital Statistics

The major source of information about the health of a population lies in the collection of vital statistics. The individual state and local health departments are required to collect and register vital data on citizens within their jurisdictions. These vital statistics include births, deaths, marriages, divorces, and morbidity from various diseases.

Data are collected at local levels and then relayed to the state health department for compilation and statistical analysis. Legal responsibility for registration of vital data lies with the state governments. The vital statistics section of the state health department handles the recording of the data. The official record is filed permanently in that office. When an individual needs to obtain a copy of a birth certificate or other personal document, a copy may be obtained from the state health department.

Statistical information collected by state health departments is transmitted to the National Center for Health Statistics, which in 1987 became part of the Centers for Disease Control in Atlanta, Georgia, in Washington, D.C., where nationwide vital statistics are compiled and disseminated. This center was established in 1960 to provide data—to any agency, organization, or persons needing such data—regarding births, deaths, illnesses, disability, health services, marriages, and divorces. In addition to these data, it now has an extensive body of information regarding health status, utilization of health resources, and health care expenditures in the nation.

DO NOT
WRITE IN MARGIN
RESERVED FOR
ODH DATA CODING

UNCERTIFIED COPY

TYPE OR PRINT IN PERMANENT INK

HEA-2703

V.S. 2
5112.06 REV. 1/78

a. _____
b. _____
c. _____
CHILD
d. _____
e. _____
f. _____
g. _____
h. _____
ATTENDANT
i. _____
j. _____
k. _____
MOTHER
l. _____
m. _____
FATHER
n. _____
o. _____
p. _____
q. _____
r. _____
s. _____
t. _____
u. _____
v. _____
w. _____
x. _____
y. _____
z. _____

DIVISION OF VITAL STATISTICS
CERTIFICATE OF LIVE BIRTH

Reg. Dist. No. _____
Primary Reg. Dist. No. _____
Registrar's No. _____

Birth No. 134 –

CHILD—NAME First Middle Last	SEX	DATE OF BIRTH (Month, Day, Year)	HOUR
1.	2.	3a.	3b. M

HOSPITAL—NAME (If not in hospital, give street and number) | CITY, VILLAGE OR LOCATION OF BIRTH | COUNTY OF BIRTH
4a. | 4b. | 4c.

REGISTRAR—SIGNATURE | DATE RECEIVED BY LOCAL REGISTRAR
5a. | 5b.

I certify that the above named child was born alive at the place and time and on the date stated above. | DATE SIGNED | ATTENDANT—M.D., D.O., midwife, other (Specify)
6a. SIGNATURE | 6b. | 6c.
ATTENDANT—NAME (Type or Print) | MAILING ADDRESS (Street or R.F.D. No., City or Village, State, Zip)
6d. | 6e.

MOTHER—MAIDEN NAME First Middle Last | AGE (At time of this birth) | STATE OF BIRTH (If not in U.S.A., name country)
7a. | 7b. | 7c.
RESIDENCE—STATE | COUNTY | CITY, VILLAGE OR LOCATION | STREET AND NUMBER OF RESIDENCE | INSIDE CITY LIMITS (Specify yes or no)
8a. | 8b. | 8c. | 8d. | 8e.
MOTHER'S MAILING ADDRESS (Street or R.F.D. No., City or Village, State, Zip) (If same as above, enter Zip Code only)
9.

FATHER—NAME First Middle Last | AGE (At time of this birth) | STATE OF BIRTH (If not in U.S.A., name country)
10a. | 10b. | 10c.

INFORMANT'S NAME OR SIGNATURE | RELATION TO CHILD
11a. | 11b.

INFORMATION FOR MEDICAL AND HEALTH USE ONLY

RACE – (e.g., White, Black, American Indian, etc.) (Specify)		ORIGIN OR DESCENT (Italian, Mexican, German, English, Cuban, Puerto Rican, etc.) (Specify)		THIS BIRTH—Single, Twin, Triplet, etc. (Specify)	IF NOT SINGLE BIRTH—Born first, second, third, etc. (Specify)
MOTHER	FATHER	MOTHER	FATHER		
12.	13.	14.	15.	16a.	16b.

PREGNANCY HISTORY Complete each section				EDUCATION—MOTHER (Specify only highest grade completed)		EDUCATION—FATHER (Specify only highest grade completed)	
LIVE BIRTHS (Do not include this Child)		OTHER TERMINATIONS (Spontaneous and Induced)		Elementary or Secondary (0-12)	College (1-4 or 5+)	Elementary or Secondary (0-12)	College (1-4 or 5+)
17a. Now living	17b. Now dead	17d. Before 20 weeks	17e. 20 weeks and after	18.		19.	
Number ____ None ☐	Number ____ None ☐	Number ____ None ☐	Number ____ None ☐	BIRTH WEIGHT IN GRAMS 20. GRAMS	APGAR SCORE 1 min. / 5 min. 21.	MONTH OF PREGNANCY PRENATAL CARE BEGAN First, second, etc. (Specify) 22a.	PRENATAL VISITS Total number (If none, so state) 22b.

DATE LAST NORMAL MENSES BEGAN (Month, Day, Year) | COMPLICATIONS OF PREGNANCY (Describe or write "none")
23. | 24.

DATE OF LAST LIVE BIRTH (Month, Year) | DATE OF LAST OTHER TERMINATION (Month, Year) | GESTATION IN WEEKS CLINICAL ESTIMATE | CONCURRENT ILLNESSES OR CONDITIONS AFFECTING THE PREGNANCY (Describe or write "none")
17c. | 17f. | 25. WEEKS | 26.

COMPLICATIONS OF LABOR AND/OR DELIVERY (Describe or write "none") | CONGENITAL MALFORMATIONS OR ANOMALIES OF CHILD (Describe or write "none")
27. | 28.

NAME OF PROPHYLACTIC USED IN EYES OF CHILD | DATE OF APPROVED TEST FOR SYPHILIS, IF NONE STATE REASON | DATE OF APPROVED TEST FOR GONORRHEA, IF NONE STATE REASON
29. | 30. | 31.

Each year the National Center for Health Statistics publishes an annual report entitled *Vital Statistics of the United States.*

Vital statistics are helpful in community health program planning. From the study of such data, it is possible for the health officials to determine where specific problems exist and to tailor corrective action accordingly.

Live Births By law all live births must be recorded and a certificate of live birth registered. A standard certificate of live birth has been developed by the National Center for Health Statistics. This certificate contains two parts. The first part identifies the name of the child and the parents, and the second part is designed for "medical and health use only." Information in this section—about maternal age, race, birth weight, marital status and education of parents, plus the pregnancy history of the mother—is useful for epidemiological investigations.

The standard statistical datum used for stating birth rates is the *crude birth rate*. This statistic is arrived at by dividing the number of live births during the year by the average population at midyear. In formula it looks like this:

$$\text{Crude Birth Rate} = \frac{\text{number of live births during the year}}{\text{average population at midyear}}$$

The usual factor for expressing birth rate is per one thousand population.

A live birth has been defined as:

. . . the complete expulsion or extraction from its mother of a product of human conception, irrespective of the duration of pregnancy, which, after such expulsion or extraction, breathes, or shows any other evidence of life such as beating of the heart, pulsation of the umbilical cord, or definite movement of voluntary muscles, whether or not the umbilical cord has been cut or the placenta is attached.[3]

This definition, which is based upon the 1950 World Health Organization definition, is used in most states of the United States in determining the start of life. A few states use a shortened definition.

Birth records give some indication of population growth. Birth rates are influenced by a number of variables, the most important of which is the number of women of childbearing age. The birth rate in the United States dropped to an all-time low of 14.6 in 1976, but since then has risen slightly to the present rate of 15.5. The United States Bureau of the Census projects that the number of women of childbearing age will continue to increase into the early 1990s. If this happens, there is a strong possibility that a similar rise in birth rates will occur.

Mortality A statistic that can tell much about the health conditions of a given population is the mortality rate, or number of deaths per one thousand population. This is particularly true if there is a decrease in the mortality rate since a decrease is indicative of overall improvement of the health of a

Rank	Cause	Percent of All Deaths
1	Heart Disease	38.3
2	Malignant Neoplasms	21.2
3	Cerebrovascular Diseases	8.9
4	Accidents	5.5
5	Chronic Obstructive Pulmonary Diseases	2.6
6	Pneumonia and Influenza	2.3
7	Diabetes	1.7
8	Liver Disease and Cirrhosis	1.6
9	Atherosclerosis	1.5
10	Suicide	1.5
11	Homicide	1.2
12	Perinatal Related Conditions	1.2
13	Nephritis, Nephrosis	0.8
14	Congenital Anomalies	0.7
15	Septicemia	0.4
	Other Causes	10.6

Table 6.1 Fifteen leading causes of death, United States

Source: Office of Health Research, Statistics, and Technology, Department of Health and Human Services, 1981.

population. The presence of a large number of elderly individuals in the population produces a rise in the mortality rate. This is one reason that these rates are more valuable when they are age-adjusted or when specific age groups are presented separately.

Mortality rates are often expressed in relation to the specific cause of death. Death rates are published in terms of age, sex, race, cause of death, and geographical location. This kind of data is useful in keeping abreast of causes of death. Ninety percent of all deaths are currently attributable to the fifteen causes listed in table 6.1. Several specific kinds of mortality data are collected and used in analyzing the health conditions of a population. Most of this data concerns mother and child health.

The basic indication of mortality is the *crude death rate,* determined by dividing the number of deaths during the year by the average population at midyear. The crude death rate is expressed in ratio per one thousand population. This rate has continued to decline since the early years of this century to a rate of 8.6 in the mid-1980s.

$$\text{Crude Death Rate} = \frac{\text{Number of Deaths During the Year}}{\text{Average Population at Midyear}}$$

$$\text{Infant Mortality Rate} = \frac{\begin{array}{c}\text{Number of Deaths in Calendar Year}\\ \text{Among Infants Less Than One Year of Age}\end{array}}{\text{Number of Live Births During Calendar Year}} \times 1,000$$

Infant Mortality The number of deaths that occur in infants under one year of age, excluding fetal deaths, is the infant mortality rate. This statistic is one of the most widely accepted measures of estimating the health of a population. The survival of an infant during the first year of life also reflects the health of the mother and the health condition of the newborn's environment.

Infant mortality rates are expressed in terms of the number of incidences per one thousand live births. Currently this rate in the United States is 10.9 (see table 6.2).[4] The Department of Health and Human Services has set as an objective for the nation by the year 1990 an infant mortality rate of nine.[5]

Fetal Death Commonly referred to as *stillbirth,* fetal death is defined formally:

. . . death prior to the complete expulsion or extraction from its mother of a product of human conception, irrespective of the duration of pregnancy; the death is indicated by the fact that after such expulsion or extraction the fetus does not breathe or show any other evidence of life such as beating of the heart, pulsation of the umbilical cord, or definite movement of voluntary muscles.[6]

This definition, like that of live birth, is based on the World Health Organization determination set forth in 1950. Most states use this definition; however, some differences do exist on the length of gestation. United States fetal death rates are shown in table 6.3.

Table 6.2   Infant Mortality Rates, United States, 1940–1985

Year	All	Whites	All Other
1940	47.0	43.2	73.8
1950	29.2	26.8	44.5
1960	26.0	22.9	43.2
1965	24.7	21.5	40.3
1970	20.0	17.8	30.9
1975	16.1	14.2	24.2
1980	12.6	11.0	21.4
1985	11.2	9.7	19.2

Source: U.S. Bureau of the Census. *Statistical Abstracts of the United States.* Washington, D.C.: U.S. Government Printing Office, 1986, p. 74.

Table 6.3   Fetal Death Rates, United States, 1950–1985

Year	Rate
1950	19.2
1960	16.1
1970	14.7
1980	9.2
1980s (mid)	9.0

Source: U.S. Bureau of the Census. *Statistical Abstracts of the United States.* Washington, D.C.: U.S. Government Printing Office, 1986, p. 74.

The official death certificate, as used in most states, includes places to record information about the deceased, the cause of death, and the disposition of the body.

OHIO DEPARTMENT OF HEALTH

DIVISION OF VITAL STATISTICS

CERTIFICATE OF DEATH

DO NOT
WRITE IN MARGIN
RESERVED FOR
ODH DATA CODING

Reg. Dist. No. _____

Primary Reg. Dist. No. _____

State File No. _____

Registrar's No. _____

a. _____
b. _____
c. _____
d. _____
e. _____
f. _____

DECEDENT

| DECEDENT—NAME First | Middle | Last | SEX | DATE OF DEATH (Mo., Day, Year) |
| 1. | | 2. | 3. | |

| RACE—(e.g.,White,Black,American Indian, etc.) (Specify) | AGE—Last Birthday (Years) | UNDER 1 YEAR Mos. Days | UNDER 1 DAY Hours Mins. | DATE OF BIRTH (Mo.,Day,Yr.) | COUNTY OF DEATH |
| 4. | 5a. | 5b. | 5c. | 6. | 7a. |

CITY, VILLAGE OR LOCATION OF DEATH 7b. | HOSPITAL OR OTHER INSTITUTION—Name (If not in either, give street and number) 7c. | IF HOSP. OR INST. Indicate DOA, OP/Emer.Rm.,Inpatient (Specify) 7d.

STATE OF BIRTH (If not in U.S.A., name country) 8a. | CITIZEN OF WHAT COUNTRY 8b. | ORIGIN OR DESCENT (Italian, Mexican, German, English, Cuban, Puerto Rican, etc.) (Specify) 9. | SOCIAL SECURITY NUMBER 10.

USUAL RESIDENCE WHERE DECEASED LIVED. IF DEATH OCCURRED IN INSTITUTION, GIVE RESIDENCE BEFORE ADMISSION ➡

WAS DECEASED EVER IN U.S. ARMED FORCES? (Yes, no, or unknown) (If yes, give dates of service) 11. | MARRIED, NEVER MARRIED, WIDOWED, DIVORCED (Specify) 12a. | SURVIVING SPOUSE (If wife, give maiden name) 12b.

USUAL OCCUPATION (Give kind of work done during most of working life, even if retired) 13a. | KIND OF BUSINESS OR INDUSTRY 13b.

RESIDENCE—STATE 14a. | COUNTY 14b. | CITY, VILLAGE OR LOCATION 14c. | STREET AND NUMBER 14d. | INSIDE CITY LIMITS (Specify Yes or No) 14e.

PARENTS

g. _____
h. _____
i. _____
j. _____
k. _____
l. _____
m. _____

FATHER—NAME First Middle Last 15. | MOTHER—MAIDEN NAME First Middle Last 16.

INFORMANT—NAME (Type or Print) 17a. | MAILING ADDRESS (STREET OR R.F.D. No.) (CITY OR TOWN) (STATE) (ZIP) 17b.

CAUSE OF DEATH

n. _____
o. _____
p. _____
q. _____
r. _____

| PART I. | DEATH WAS CAUSED BY: [ENTER ONLY ONE CAUSE PER LINE FOR (a), (b), AND (c)] | APPROXIMATE INTERVAL BETWEEN ONSET AND DEATH |
| 18. | | |

IMMEDIATE CAUSE (a) _____
DUE TO, OR AS A CONSEQUENCE OF:

Conditions, if any, which gave rise to immediate cause, stating the underlying cause last
(b) _____
DUE TO, OR AS A CONSEQUENCE OF:
(c) _____

PART II. OTHER SIGNIFICANT CONDITIONS: Conditions contributing to death but not related to cause given in Part I (a) | AUTOPSY (Yes or no) 19a. | WAS CASE REFERRED TO CORONER (Specify Yes or No) 19b.

ACC., SUICIDE, HOM., UNDET., OR PENDING INVEST. (Specify) 20a. | DATE OF INJURY (Month, Day, Year) 20b. | HOUR 20c. M | HOW INJURY OCCURRED (Enter nature of injury in Part I or Part II, item 18) 20d.

INJURY AT WORK (Specify yes or no) 20e. | PLACE OF INJURY At home, farm, street, factory, office bldg., etc. (Specify) 20f. | LOCATION (Street or R.F.D. no., city or village, state, zip) 20g.

CERTIFIER

s. _____
t. _____
u. _____

To be Completed by ATTENDING PHYSICIAN Only	To be Completed by CORONER Only
21a. To the best of my knowledge, death occurred at the time, date and place and due to the cause(s) stated.	22a. On the basis of examination and/or investigation, in my opinion death occurred at the time, date and place and due to the cause(s) stated.
(Signature and Title)	(Signature and Title)
DATE SIGNED (Mo., Day, Year) 21b.	HOUR OF DEATH 21c. M	DATE SIGNED (Mo., Day, Year) 22b.	HOUR OF DEATH 22c. M
		PRONOUNCED DEAD (Mo., Day, Year) 22d. ON	PRONOUNCED DEAD (Hour) 22e. AT M

NAME AND ADDRESS OF CERTIFIER (PHYSICIAN OR CORONER) (Type or Print) 23. | (Street or R.F.D. no., city or village, state, zip)

DISPOSITION

BURIAL, CREMATION, OTHER (Specify) 24a. | DATE 24b. | NAME OF CEMETERY OR CREMATORY 24c. | LOCATION (City, village, or county) (State)

NAME OF EMBALMER 25. | (LIC. No.) | FUNERAL DIRECTOR'S SIGNATURE 26. | (LIC. No.)

FUNERAL FIRM AND ADDRESS 27. | (STREET NO.) | (CITY) | (STATE) | (ZIP)

DATE REC'D BY LOCAL REG. 28. | REGISTRAR'S SIGNATURE 29. | DATE PERMIT ISSUED 30. | SIGNATURE OF PERSON ISSUING PERMIT 31. | DIST. No.

V.S. 11
5152 06 REV. 1/78

TYPE OR PRINT IN PERMANENT INK

INFORMATION CONCERNING THE BURIAL OF DECEASED MEMBERS AND FORMER MEMBERS OF THE ARMED FORCES OF THE UNITED STATES

FUNERAL DIRECTORS ARE REQUIRED BY LAW TO FURNISH THE FOLLOWING ADDITIONAL INFORMATION FOR DECEASED MEMBERS OR FORMER MEMBERS OF THE ARMED FORCES.

Name of deceased _____

Date of death _____ Date of birth _____

State of birth _____ Branch of service _____

Date of entry into service _____

Type of separation or discharge from service _____ Date _____

Date of burial _____

Name of cemetery _____

Location of cemetery
    County _____
    Township _____
    Village _____
    City _____

Name or number of section in cemetery _____
Number of lot _____
Number of grave _____

Information relative to a deceased veteran may be secured from the Veteran's Discharge Papers.

Neonatal Death When an infant death occurs within the first twenty-eight days after birth, it is recorded as a neonatal death. Data of neonatal deaths do not include fetal deaths (see table 6.4).

Maternal Mortality The number of deaths of women due to childbirth, the complications of pregnancy, and puerperium (the woman's condition after birth) is referred to as maternal mortality. The National Center for Health Statistics defines maternal death as "death from any maternal condition in which the date of onset of the condition was within one year prior to the date of death."[7] On the other hand, the National Vital Statistics System defines maternal death as "the death of any woman while

Table 6.4	Neonatal Death Rates, United States, 1940–1985
Year	**Rate**
1940	28.8
1950	20.5
1960	18.7
1970	15.1
1980	8.5
1980s (mid)	8.0

Source: U.S. Bureau of the Census. *Statistical Abstracts of the United States.* Washington, D.C.: U.S. Government Printing Office, 1986, p. 74.

Death rates, United States: number of deaths per 1,000 population

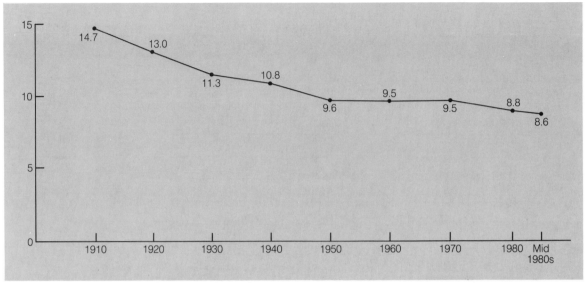

Source: U.S. Bureau of the Census. Statistical Abstracts of the United States, 1986, 106th ed. Washington, D.C.: U.S. Government Printing Office.

$$\text{Maternal Mortality Rate} = \frac{\text{Number of Deaths in Calendar Year Due to Childbirth}}{\text{Number of Live Births During Calendar Year}} \times 1{,}000$$

Table 6.5 Maternal Mortality Rate*, United States, 1940–1980

Year	All	Whites	All Other
1940	376.0	319.8	773.5
1950	83.3	61.1	221.6
1960	37.1	26.0	97.9
1965	31.6	21.0	83.7
1970	21.5	14.4	55.9
1975	12.8	9.1	29.0
1980	9.2	6.7	19.8
1980s (mid)	8.0	5.9	18.3

Source: U.S. Bureau of the Census. Statistical Abstracts of the United States. Washington, D.C.: U.S. Government Printing Office, 1986, p. 74.
*(Per 100,000 live births)

pregnant or within 42 days of termination of pregnancy. . . ." It is for this reason that one often finds differences in maternal mortality rates upon analyzing federal governmental data.

This statistic, unlike other indices of mortality, is expressed as a ratio per 100,000 live births. Maternal mortality was quite common in the early part of this century, but in the 1930s its incidence began to drop. For example, the maternal mortality rate in the 1920s was about seven hundred per 100,000 (700/100,000), but today, the ratio has dropped to below nine per 100,000. This decline has not been equal among the white and nonwhite population.

Maternal mortality in the mid-1980s for the white population was 5.9 while for the nonwhite population it was 18.3. Through the health objectives for the nation, the federal government has established the goal of decreasing maternal mortality by 1990 to five.[8]

The incidences of maternal mortality fall into four major categories: (1) deaths related to pregnancies with abortive outcomes, (2) deaths related to complications of the puerperium, (3) deaths related to complications of the delivery, and (4) deaths related to complications of pregnancy.[9] Deaths from abortive outcome pregnancies tend to be either a result of induced abortions or ectopic pregnancies. Deaths due to illegal induced abortions have been virtually eliminated with the legalization of abortion in the United States: Ectopic pregnancies occur in situations where women have damaged fallopian tubes from gonorrheal infections and the use of contraceptive agents. Deaths in the puerperal period are mainly due to embolisms. The chief cause of fatality among the complications of delivery is hemorrhage, which can be caused by premature separation of the placenta, retained placenta, uterine rupture, or postpartum hemorrhage. Deaths due to complications of the puerperium are mostly attributed to hypertensive diseases such as toxemia.

Abortion States are now required to report induced and spontaneous abortions. For consistency between states, induced termination of pregnancy has been defined as ". . . the purposeful interruption of pregnancy with the intention other than to produce a live-born infant or to remove a dead fetus and which does not result in a live birth."[10]

A spontaneous fetal death is ". . . the expulsion or extraction of a product of human conception resulting in other than a live birth and which is not an induced termination of pregnancy."[11]

The increase in numbers of abortions since 1972, when the Supreme Court legalized abortion in the United States, can be seen by analyzing vital data. In 1972 the rate of abortions per 1,000 women in the United States was 13.2; in the mid-1980s it was 28.8. The rate of abortions per live births in 1972 was 184 compared with a rate of 426 in the mid-1980s.[12]

Marriages and Divorces The record of the number of marriages and divorces is not a direct indicator of the health status of a population. These statistics are more likely to have socioeconomic value. Both are expressed in ratio per one thousand population. Often the number of marriages reflects the age group composition of a locality. A higher marriage rate is often found in a community with a university or college while a retirement community in Florida or Arizona is likely to have a lower marriage rate. The national marriage rate in the mid-1980s was 10.5.[13]

The divorce rate has risen dramatically in the past two decades. The National Center for Health Statistics reported that the divorce rate was 5.2 per one thousand population in the 1980s, a rate nearly two and a half times that of the early 1960s.

Reportable Diseases

In 1878 Congress passed legislation which required the Public Health Service to collect morbidity reports on certain diseases.[14] At that time the diseases of concern were cholera, smallpox, plague, and yellow fever. In order to be able to develop these reports, it was necessary for the individual states to submit data to the federal government. However, it was not until 1925 that all states were reporting on a regular basis information about certain diseases.

Today these data are submitted to the Centers for Disease Control. This information is compiled and published on a weekly basis, and a summary of reportable diseases is published annually.

The responsibility for initiating the reporting of these diseases is the individual health care provider and medical facility. The physician and the hospital or clinic staff are required to report to the local health department all instances of these diseases. This information is reported to the state health department, which then reports to the Centers for Disease

The state health department has been collecting data on the number of industrial workers reported absent from work due to influenza. In one northern county of the state, 286 cases were identified and reported to the state department. Another region reported 198 cases, and in the southeastern section of the state only 162 cases were reported.

While analyzing the population densities of the regions, the state recognized that the northern county has two major cities with a combined metropolitan population of 258,000. The southeastern section included two and a half counties. All villages in this area were small towns, with an estimated total population of 62,000 people. The other region under consideration was the eastern half of one county, which has a combined population of 159,000.

As you analyze these reports, what conclusions can you draw? Which localities within the state would you recommend for immediate aid or programming? Why?

Notifiable Diseases in the United States

Acquired Immune Deficiency Syndrome (AIDS)
Amebiasis
Anthrax
Aseptic Meningitis
Botulism
Brucellosis
Cholera
Diphtheria
Encephalitis
Gonorrhea
Hepatitis
Legionellosis
Leprosy
Leptospirosis
Malaria
Measles
Meningococcal Infections
Mumps

Pertussis
Plague
Poliomyelitis
Psittacosis
Rabies
Rheumatic Fever
Rubella
Salmonellosis
Shigellosis
Syphilis
Tetanus
Toxic-Shock Syndrome
Trichinosis
Tularemia
Typhoid Fever
Typhus Fever
Varicella (Chickenpox)

Source: Centers for Disease Control. ''Annual Summary 1984: Reported Morbidity and Mortality in the United States,'' *Morbidity and Mortality Weekly Report*, 33, no. 54 (March, 1986).

Control. The Epidemiology Program Office of CDC has the responsibility of bringing together all the data and publishing the information for the public.

Data are also collected on a number of nonreportable diseases. These diseases may be no less serious, but for various reasons they have not been added to the required reportable list. The diseases included in this nonreportable category include diseases such as infectious mononucleosis, Reyes syndrome, histoplasmosis, pelvic inflammatory disease (PID), and a broad range of occupational diseases.

An Interdisciplinary Team

The work of epidemiology necessitates the expertise and input of a number of different fields of study. The skills and contributions of basic biological scientists, anatomists, physiologists, and microbiologists are necessary to disease-related work. Pathology and immunology are also necessary since much epidemiology study of disease causation centers around immunization. Also, clinical medicine and preventive medicine are important as groups of individuals are studied. Studies are of little meaning without analysis of statistical data. The skills of biostatistics and research methology must be a part of any epidemiology work.

Summary

The study of occurrence of diseases in human populations is epidemiology. Epidemiological study attempts to identify the cause of diseases. The procedures of epidemiology historically were directed toward solving the epidemics of infectious diseases. In more recent years the procedures of epidemiology have been applied to a broad range of problems in community health other than infectious diseases.

Epidemiological study involves use of the epidemiological model. This model looks at the interaction of three factors influencing health and well-being: (1) the causative agent, (2) the host, and (3) the environmental factors.

Two basic methods are used in epidemiology: observational study and experimental study. Observational studies may be prospective or retrospective. Prospective studies start with a group of individuals who are followed for a period of time to ascertain the effectiveness of a factor being studied. The retrospective study examines the historical records of a population group to ascertain what factors might have led to the cause of a given health problem under study.

Experimental studies are different in that the epidemiologist is able to manipulate the study population. The study population is placed into two equal study groups: the control group and the experimental group. Experimental studies may be clinical or community-involved examinations.

Analysis of data collected in epidemiological studies must be presented so as to be useful. The basic collection of data is placed into ratios which then can be used for comparisons and projections. Data that are important in community health are obtained from many different sources. Census data, vital statistics, and data of reportable diseases are all widely used in epidemiological work.

Epidemiology makes use of a number of different professional fields. All must work together in order that the effectiveness and value of epidemiological investigations are useful.

Discussion Questions

1. Discuss the concept of "epidemiology."
2. Explain in what ways epidemiology is useful in community health.
3. Discuss the relationships of the host, the causative agent, and the environmental factors as they relate to a given disease problem.
4. If you were responsible for developing a malaria eradication program, to which component of the epidemiological model would you direct the major resources? Explain your answer.
5. In what ways is the epidemiological model useful in accident prevention programs?
6. Explain the basic differences between the prospective study and the retrospective study.
7. What is the cross-sectional epidemiological study?
8. Describe how the experimental study differs from an observational study.
9. Explain some of the ethical issues concerning experimental studies.
10. How does the incidence rate differ from the prevalence rate?
11. In an industry with 2,341 employees, 16 were absent from work on March 3 due to respiratory illnesses. What is the prevalence rate in this company for this disease? State the rate in relation to 1,000 population.
12. What use is made of census data in epidemiological studies?
13. Describe the various uses of vital statistics.
14. What kind of information is found on a birth certificate? a death certificate?
15. What can one learn from reviewing the statistical data on marriages and divorces?
16. Explain the differences between infant mortality, fetal death, neonatal death, and maternal mortality.

Suggested Readings

Ahlbom, Anders, and Norell, Staffan. *Introduction to Modern Epidemiology.* Chestnut Hill, Mass.: Epidemiology Resources, Inc., 1984, 97 pp.

Fox, L. P. "A Return to Maternal Mortality Studies: A Necessary Effort." *American Journal of Obstetrics and Gynecology* 152, no. 4 (June, 1985): 379–86.

Friedman, Gary D. *Primer of Epidemiology.* New York: McGraw-Hill Book Company, 1980, 288 pp.

Kaunitz, A. M.; Hughes, J. M.; et al. "Causes of Maternal Mortality in the United States." *Obstetrics and Gynecology* 65, no. 5 (May, 1985): 605–12.

Lilienfeld, Abraham M., and Lilienfeld, David E. *Foundations of Epidemiology.* New York: Oxford University Press, 1980, 375 pp.

"Maternal Mortality: Helping Women Off the Road to Death." *WHO Chronicle* 40, no. 5 (1986): 175–83.

Mausner, Judith S., and Kramer, Shira. *Epidemiology—An Introductory Text.* Philadelphia: W. B. Saunders Company, 1985, 361 pp.

Novick, L. F.; Greene, C.; and Vogt, R. L. "Teaching Medical Students Epidemiology: Utilizing a State Health Department." *Public Health Reports* 100, no. 4 (July/August, 1985): 401–05.

Rochat, R. W. "Maternal Mortality in the United States of America." *World Health Statistics Quarterly* 34, no. 1 (1981): 2–13.

Smith, J., and others. "An Assessment of the Incidence of Maternal Mortality in the United States." *American Journal of Public Health* 74, no. 8 (August, 1984): 780–83.

Thompson, W. Douglas. "Statistical Criteria in the Interpretation of Epidemiologic Data." *American Journal of Public Health* 77, no. 2 (February, 1987): 191–99.

Waters, W. E. "Ethics and Epidemiological Research." *International Journal of Epidemiology* 14, no. 1 (1985): 48–51.

Endnotes

1. Gordon, J. E. "The Epidemiology of Accidents." *American Journal of Public Health* 39, no. 4 (1948): 504–15.

2. Dawber, T. R.; Meadors, G. F.; and Moore, F. G., Jr. "The Epidemiological Approach to Heart Disease: The Framingham Study." *American Journal of Public Health* 41 (1951): 279–86.
   Gordon, T., and Kannel, W. B. "The Framingham, Massachusetts Study, Twenty Years Later." In *The Community as an Epidemiologic Laboratory: A Casebook of Community Studies,* edited by I. I. Kessler and M. L. Levin. Baltimore, Md.: The Johns Hopkins Press, 1970, 123–46.
   McGee, D., and Gordon, T. *The Framingham Study: The Results of the Framingham Study Applied to Four Other U.S. Based Epidemiologic Studies of Cardiovascular Disease.* Washington, D.C.: U.S. Government Printing Office, (1976).

3. Department of Health, Education, and Welfare. *Model State Vital Statistics Act and Model State Vital Statistics Regulations,* 1977, Revision, Pub. No. (PHS) 78-1115.

4. An in depth discussion of infant mortality is presented in Chapter 16.

5. Department of Health and Human Services. *Promoting Health, Preventing Disease: Objectives for the Nation.* Washington, D.C.: U.S. Government Printing Office, (Fall, 1980): 17.

6. Department of Health, Education, and Welfare. *Model State Vital Statistics.*

7. Smith, Jack C., and others. "An Assessment of the Incidence of Maternal Mortality in the United States." *American Journal of Public Health* 74, no. 8 (August, 1984): 780–83.

8. U.S. Department of Health and Human Services. *Promoting Health, Preventing Disease: Objectives for the Nation.*

9. Rochat, R. W. "Maternal Mortality in the United States of America." *World Health Statistics Quarterly* 34, no. 1 (1981): 267.

10. Department of Health, Education, and Welfare. *Model State Vital Statistics.*

11. Ibid.

12. United States Bureau of the Census. *Statistical Abstracts of the United States, 1986,* 106th Ed. Washington, D.C.: U.S. Government Printing Office: 66.

13. United States Bureau of the Census. *Statistical Abstracts.* 79.

14. "History of Morbidity Reporting and Surveillance in the United States." *Morbidity and Mortality Weekly Report, Annual Summary, 1984,* 33, no. 54, (March, 1986): ix.

7

Health Care: Economic Dynamics and Cost Containment

National Health Expenditures

Date	Total (in billions)	Per Capita	Percent GNP
1960	$26.9	$146	5.3
1965	$41.9	$207	6.1
1970	$75.0	$350	7.6
1975	$132.7	$591	8.6
1980	$247.5	$1049	9.4
1984	$387.4	$1580	10.6

Source: U.S. Bureau of the Census, *Statistical Abstracts of the United States: 1986* (106th Edition), Washington, D.C., 1985.

"Medical care, once seen as outside the realm of public health . . . is increasingly seen . . . as part of our fabric, integral to public health responsibility."[1]

Cost of Health Care

It is obvious that health care costs in America are increasing. A visit to a physician's office with a minor problem such as a cold or rash may cost as much as fifty dollars. The cost of a hospital room in many communities exceeds $300 to $400 a day. The national average hospital room cost is $411.10 with an average hospital stay of 6.5 days.[2] Minor surgery followed by a few days of treatment and inpatient care can result in a bill of over $5,000. The costs have continued to rise through the 1980s in all areas of health care: hospital expenses, physicians' costs, the cost of pharmaceuticals, rehabilitation services, and both inpatient and outpatient services.

This steady, often dramatic, rise in health care costs is illustrated on the accompanying graph. The national expenditures for health care in the United States rose from a total of $12.7 billion in 1950 to over $425 billion in the mid-1980s.[3] That is an expenditure of more than a billion dollars a day for health care.

Analyzing this sum into a more personal figure, the per capita outlay for health care costs was $1,721. The percent of the Gross National Product (GNP) spent on health care in the mid-1980s was 10.8 percent, up from 4.4 percent in 1950.[4] Hospital costs, the largest expenditure, account for 41.4 percent of the health care costs. Another 27.8 percent pays for professional physician and dental services.[5]

Third-Party Payment

If an individual were forced to pay out-of-pocket for all health care costs, some would become bankrupt and many would find it impossible to seek and obtain needed care. Most Americans do not have the cash on hand to cover the cost of necessary health care. Because of this, the role of the third party, or health insurance carrier, takes on major significance in the lives of most Americans.

Approximately one-fourth of all health care costs is paid for out-of-pocket.[6] The remaining three-quarters are paid for through some program of health insurance. More than eight-hundred private insurance companies in the United States have health insurance programs offering many different kinds of options to the individual.

Eighty-two percent of all Americans have some type of hospital or medical health insurance coverage.[7] In spite of this figure, less than three-quarters (72.8 percent) of all health care costs are

National health expenditures, United States, in billions of dollars

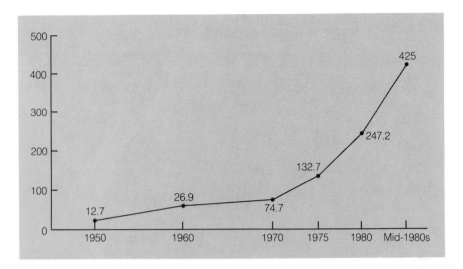

Health expenditures, United States, percent of G.N.P.

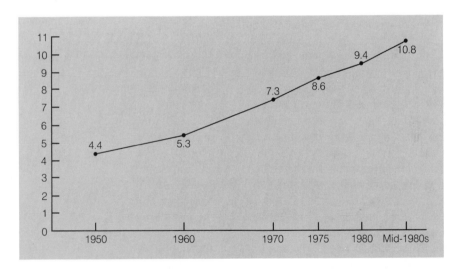

covered by third-party payment. Seventy-nine per-cent of all hospital costs are paid for by health in-surance carriers while only half of all physician's services are covered by third-party payment.[8] Usu-ally those individuals with no health insurance cov-erage are the poor, the less educated, those living in rural locations, the unemployed, or the seasonally employed.

Coverage is provided by a variety of carriers. Some companies are involved only in health insur-ance programs, whereas others offer comprehensive coverage—life, auto, and house insurance, in addi-tion to health coverage. Many people obtain health insurance coverage as part of group health insur-ance programs, which are usually a part of the wage

New technology has contributed to the increased cost of health care. For example, this computerized tomography (CT) scanning machine is an instrument that allows physicians to take a detailed visual slice, or tomograph, of the brain.

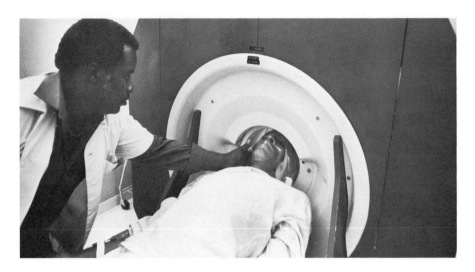

and benefit package provided by the place of employment. Premiums for the health insurance coverage are paid by both the employer and the employee. Other people must purchase health insurance on an individual basis. This is often necessary when one is self-employed or when a group program is not available. There are also health insurance programs that combine group coverage with individual coverage.

The first *accident* insurance plans in the United States were established in the 1850s and 1860s. The first *group health* insurance policy was offered by the Montgomery Ward Company in 1910.[9] Other types of individual, prepaid, hospital benefit plans were established in the 1920s. In 1929 a hospital prepayment plan was started to help public school teachers pay for their health bills at Baylor University Medical Center. The cost for each enrollee was fifty cents per month and provided payment of six dollars per day for twenty-one days of hospital care. This program was established at the beginning of the depression, a time of high unemployment and financial collapse of many economic institutions, and was the beginning of the present Blue Cross program.

Today there are hundreds of health insurance schemes available to the average consumer. In order to make a knowledgeable decision about appropriate insurance coverage, the individual must understand something about health insurance programs and their specific provisions. Regardless of whether the health insurance is an individual or a group program there are several kinds of coverage: hospital, surgical, physician, major medical, income disability, and dental.

Insurance covering the cost of hospital expenses, primarily room and board, is a necessity for most Americans. The type of hospital insurance coverage varies, depending on the services and other supplies the patient receives. With the average length of a hospital stay being 6.5 days per patient, and an average daily cost of $411.10, the average cost of each patient hospitalization is $2,672.15.[10]

Hospitalization insurance is usually sold in combination with surgical insurance. Surgical insurance covers the cost of surgical procedures (including anesthesia) that result from sickness or accident. Usually a schedule of surgical costs will indicate the maximum benefit for each specific type of operation.

Payment for physician services is covered by physician's expense insurance. This covers nonsurgical care that is provided in the hospital or the physician's office. Nonsurgical benefits also include such items as outpatient care and home care. Usually the policy indicates what benefits are covered and the maximum amount of payment provided.

Serious health problems needing expensive long-term care and resulting in large medical expenses can ruin the economic status of most Americans. Major medical insurance is designed to provide protection against such expenses. Maximum benefits are indicated, usually ranging from $10,000 to unlimited coverage. Major medical insurance plans have some deductible provisions as well as coinsurance requirements. Coinsurance refers to a cost-sharing procedure whereby the individual pays a certain percentage of the total cost and the insurance carrier covers the remaining cost. For example, the patient may pay 20 percent of the costs, with the insurance company paying the remaining 80 percent. The coinsurance percentages vary from one policy and type of coverage to another.

Extensive illness often means that an individual is unable to work, creating serious economic consequences. Disability insurance, available on either a short-term or a long-term basis, provides partial replacement of income lost as a result of accident or illness. Short-term coverage is available for a period of up to two years; long-term insurance extends beyond two years to a specified time.

Dental insurance provides coverage for most dental services, including oral examinations, extractions, oral surgery, root canal therapy, and orthodontics. Most dental insurance is provided as part of group health insurance programs. This type of insurance, first made available in 1967, is the fastest growing fringe benefit available to employees today.

Federal Government Involvement

In the United States, health insurance coverage has been a private enterprise activity. The federal government has not become involved in any type of comprehensive national health insurance that is available to the general public. The first federally funded medical care for persons other than those in the military began in 1789 when the Marine Hospital Service provided a compulsory national sickness insurance program for sick or disabled merchant seamen. The Marine Hospital Service later became the Public Health Service.

An early attempt to develop a government-funded health insurance system for a broader segment of the population was made by the American Association for Labor Legislation (AALL) in the first part of the twentieth century. It was then that workmen's compensation laws were passed by the states, providing protection for work-related accidents and injuries. Subsequently, the AALL proposed the establishment of state insurance programs to cover the costs of nonwork-related medical services. Opposition from the American Medical Association defeated such a proposal and so little further action was taken at that time.

Not until the mid-1930s were other attempts made to introduce the concept of national health insurance. Opposition from the private insurance industry and from the organized medical and hospital professions again negated any effective governmental initiative. It was the feeling of private industry, particularly the insurance and hospital industries, that such action interfered with private enterprise. The medical profession considered any type of national health insurance to be "socialized medicine"—unacceptable in a free, democratic society.

Following World War II, President Harry S. Truman proposed the establishment of a national health insurance program to Congress. However, continued opposition by various groups through the 1950s and into the 1960s defeated any such federal legislative proposal.

It was not until the mid-1960s that the federal government passed two medical health insurance programs, Medicare and Medicaid. These programs resulted from increased concern at that time for the social conditions of the economically disadvantaged and the elderly.

Medicare

After years of debate, in 1965 the United States Congress passed legislation establishing a federal health insurance program for the elderly (people aged sixty-five and over). The establishment of Medicare inaugurated the first government payments for health services to a segment of citizens other than federal government employees. The basic purpose of Medicare is to make quality health care available to the elderly. Senior citizens who are entitled to Social Security or railroad retirement benefits are entitled to receive health insurance coverage under this program.

There are two parts to the medicare program: *Part A* provides coverage of hospital expenses, and *Part B* provides medical insurance. The hospital insurance (Part A) pays for inpatient hospital services, for inpatient services provided in a skilled nursing facility, and for services provided by a health agency in the patients' home. The medical insurance (Part B) helps pay for the services provided by physicians, outpatient hospital services, outpatient physical therapy and speech pathology, home health care, and other health services and supplies.

Medicare hospital insurance (Part A) covers all hospital expenses except private rooms, personal comfort items, and doctors' fees. The patient must pay a deductible, but Medicare covers all other costs beyond this initial deductible for the first sixty days. This deductible in 1988 was $540.[11] For the next thirty days of hospitalization (days 61 to 90), Medicare pays for all covered services except for a deductible of $135 per day.[12]

Medicare will pay for up to one hundred home visits. These visits must provide medical services, such as skilled nursing care, physical or speech therapy, or occupational therapy. Full-time nursing care and drugs are not covered by Medicare.

The medical insurance part of Medicare (Part B) is voluntary. An individual chooses to have this coverage, and a monthly premium is deducted from the individual's Social Security check. Upon receipt of covered services, the beneficiary pays a deductible and 20 percent of the remainder. Medicare pays the remaining 80 percent of the medical-surgical charges.

There are several health services not covered by Part B of Medicare: routine physical examinations, eye examinations, eye glasses, and dental care.

Skyrocketing health care costs are a concern for all Americans, but particularly for the elderly existing on fixed incomes. Often the elderly incur charges that require out-of-pocket expenditures since Medicare will not cover them.

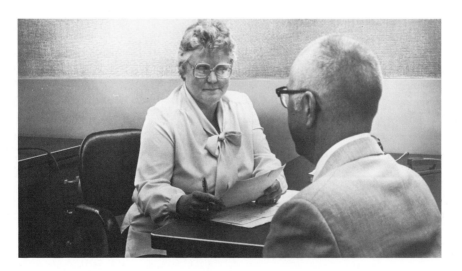

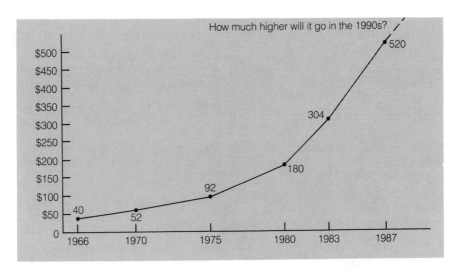

How much higher will it go in the 1990s?

1966	40
1970	52
1975	92
1980	180
1983	304
1987	520

Federal Financial Outlays for Health in Billions of Dollars

Date	Medicare	Medicaid
1967	$4.5	$ 3.4 (1968)
1970	$7.0	$ 4.8
1975	$15.5	$12.2
1980	$35.7	$23.2
1985	$66.0	$32.2 (1983)

Source: U.S. Department of Health and Human Services, Health Care Financing Administration, Office of Research, Demonstrations and Statistics.

Opinions concerning the effectiveness of the Medicare program vary. Without question, it has provided for the health care of many of America's elderly population. However, many problems have been noted by the opponents of Medicare. Since its inception in 1965, Medicare has contributed significantly to the inflationary rise in health care costs. In 1967, $4.5 billion in benefits were paid out. This amount had risen 1466 percent by the mid-1980s, when $66 billion in benefits were paid by Medicare.[13] It has been estimated that this sum will double by the early 1990s.

The individual cost to the senior citizen for Medicare coverage has risen dramatically since 1965. The developers of Medicare established a deductible and copayment provision for Part A and required a premium payment for Part B. When the program started, the monthly payment for Part B was three dollars per month. By the latter part of the 1980s, the premium cost had risen to $24.80 per month, nearly six times what it was when the program started. The deductible portion of Part A has increased more than tenfold in the past decade, from $40 in the late 1960s when the program started to $540 by the latter 1980s.

These increases in deductibles and premium costs have meant that individuals continue to pay more out of their savings or from other resources each year for health care. On fixed retirement incomes, this presents serious problems for many.

Some health providers have abused the Medicare program. Physicians have charged for services not given and for unnecessary surgery. Another reported abuse is "gang" visits to nursing homes, where a number of patients not seen by the physician are billed for a visit. Highlighting the problem of Medicare abuse, Senator Frank Moss testified before the Senate Finance Committee that the Medicare program had been cheated out of $1.5 billion in the previous year by health providers.[14]

In an attempt to combat some of the abuses, the Medicare-Medicaid Anti-Fraud and Abuse Amendments became law in 1977. This legislation was designed to reduce these health provider abuses. Legal penalties for defrauding the government in either the Medicare or Medicaid programs were imposed. Such abuse was considered a felony, with conviction subject to a maximum sentence of five years imprisonment, a $25,000 fine, or both.

Another problem with the Medicare program is that in some localities, physicians will not participate in the program. They refuse to accept Medicare patients. Thus, many senior citizens are unable to obtain needed health care.

Diagnostic Related Groups (DRGs)

In 1983 an amendment to the Social Security Act changed the way Medicare reimbursed hospitals for their services. The basic purpose of this legislative action was to control the increasing costs of health care supported by the federal government through Medicare. The legislation requires hospitals to charge patients at a predetermined rate, which is based on the average cost of treating a particular diagnosis. Prior to this, payment was on a retrospective basis; payment was determined by the bill at discharge. There was no economic incentive to contain costs. The health providers—hospitals and physicians—were reimbursed on a "reasonable" charge basis. They set the fees and Medicare paid the bill.

This prospective payment system provided for the establishment of Diagnostic Related Groups. A rather complicated formula is used to determine the reasonable costs for services offered at health care facilities. The DRG system was derived by taking all possible diagnoses and classifying them into twenty-three major diagnostic categories based on organ systems. These are divided further into 467 different illness categories that are referred to as diagnostic related groups, or DRGs. The DRGs are differentiated by age, principal diagnosis, types of procedures performed, secondary diagnosis, and discharge disposition.

Upon providing service to the patient the hospital is paid a specific amount depending on the specific DRG, regardless of how long the individual must stay in the hospital. DRG cost allowances are predetermined based on the average cost for treating a given illness. If the patient is treated for less cost than the DRG cost allowance, the hospital will make money. On the other hand, if the expenses exceed the DRG cost allowance the hospital will lose money.

When a patient is admitted to the hospital the physician must give an admitting diagnosis. This diagnosis is a preliminary one. As diagnostic and therapeutic results are received the physician will revise the admitting diagnosis and make a secondary diagnosis. A record of surgical procedures is entered, and when the patient is discharged the physician completes a discharge summary. At this point the physician indicates the principal and secondary diagnoses and all surgical procedures performed. Then by way of a coding system the number of the DRG and the preestablished rate are identified.

The Health Care Financing Administration establishes the payment rates for each DRG classification. A variety of factors goes into determining these rates.

This prospective payment system has raised many questions about the quality of care being rendered. Physicians are under pressure to maintain an average length of stay and to utilize an average number of ancillary services. If they exceed these amounts they will need to modify their patterns of practice. Many believe that this system leads to a reduction in the scope of diagnostic testing and therapeutic strategies provided in an attempt to reduce the overall costs.

Diagnostic Related Groups—Illness Categories

Four-hundred-and-sixty-seven different illness categories have been identified. The reimbursement levels for each vary dependent upon the specific diagnosis and treatment needs.

It would be impossible to list reimbursement levels for all groups. The following are several selected categories with reimbursement rates for 1987.

Retinal surgery	$ 2,503.72
Repair of a cleft lip or palate	$ 2,451.91
Coronary bypass with use of a catheter	$18,798.89
Kidney transplant	$16,310.68
Skin graft for an injury	$ 6,320.11
Circumcision	$ 1,335.32

Updated reimbursement levels can be obtained by contacting the local hospital in one's community.

Medicare requires external review organizations to focus on the financial incentives that could cause abuse and negatively affect the quality of care delivered. For the purpose of providing such review, federal legislation passed in 1982 created Professional Review Organizations (PROs). The PRO program replaced the Professional Standard Review Organization (PSRO), which had been in effect since 1972. The purpose of the PROs is to review admission patterns for inappropriate admissions, look at records for unnecessary days and/or services provided, and to verify DRG assignment for accuracy, use, and completeness of information. Penalties may be imposed if clinical information is found to be inaccurate or if other evidences of abuse are noted. The Health Care Financing Administration requires professional review organizations to deny payment to hospitals for medically unnecessary admissions and unnecessary procedures.

Medicaid

Title XIX (Title Nineteen) of the Social Security Act, known as Medicaid, became law in 1965. This provides health insurance for certain economically disadvantaged in America. In order to be eligible for Medicaid benefits, an individual must be on welfare, have dependent children, or receive supplemental security income for the aged, blind, or disabled.

Medicaid does not provide medical assistance to all economically disadvantaged people. Each state determines the eligibility for welfare program participation and, therefore, eligibility for the Medicaid program. This program is administered by each state and is funded jointly with state and federal monies. However, the federal government establishes guidelines and regulations that must be met before federal funds are made available. Federal contributions to Medicaid range from 50 to 77 percent, based on a formula considering the state's per capita income. If a state's per capita income is low, the federal contribution is greater than if the state's per capita income is high. State participation in the Medicaid program is optional.

A number of services must be provided before a state Medicaid program qualifies to receive federal money. An approved state plan must include inpatient and outpatient hospital services, laboratory and X-ray services, nursing services, home health care services, family planning, physicians' services, as well as early and periodic screening, diagnosis, and treatment of children under twenty-one. Each state determines the scope of services covered by its Medicaid program. In some states there are no limitations on inpatient hospital coverage, whereas in others, there are limitations such as length of hospital stay and days of coverage per year.

Payment for physicians' services also varies. Some states limit physician visits to ten per month; another sets a limit of two per month; others set only certain conditions under which reimbursement can be made.

In addition to services that are federally mandated in a state Medicaid program, some states provide additional services. For example, podiatric services, chiropractic services, optometric services, physical therapy, and emergency hospital services are covered in some states but not in others.

Payment for services is made directly to the health provider under Medicaid. The provider must process all forms, submit them for reimbursement, and accept the reimbursement figure determined by Medicaid as payment in full.

The cost of the Medicaid program has risen over 800 percent since its inception. In 1969, the cost was slightly over four billion dollars. By the mid-1980s nearly $34 billion was spent on Medicaid payments. The number of Medicaid recipients has not quite doubled in this same period of time, from about twelve million in 1969 to nearly twenty-two million at the present time.

How effective has Medicaid been? There are a number of responses to this question. Many feel that Medicaid, though effective in providing health insurance to a segment of the American population not previously covered, has been too costly. It, along with Medicare, has played a major role in the escalation of federal government spending for health in the past two decades. Some go so far as to suggest that Medicaid should be eliminated. These individuals consider it too costly and poorly managed. They contend that the federal government should get out of the health insurance business altogether.

Still others feel that Medicaid needs only to be reorganized to make it more efficient. As with Medicare, there have been many instances of fraud and abuse in the Medicaid program. Such health providers have filed for services that were never performed, or have done multiple filing.

Another major problem with Medicaid is the divergence in programs and coverage from state to state. The states with the greatest percentage of the economically disadvantaged population have the least Medicaid coverage. The more industrial and wealthier states tend to have better Medicaid coverage, resulting in a disparity in state Medicaid programs.

Another negative factor concerning Medicaid is that not all poor people are covered. Since only those who are dependent upon public assistance are eligible, and since that determination is a state decision, many individuals are not covered by Medicaid. All too often these same people do not have private health insurance either.

The future of Medicaid continues to remain in question. An acceptable replacement system that would eliminate all of the negative features of the present program is unknown at this time. A number of different ideas and proposals have been discussed by the federal government. Regardless of the form and structure Medicaid takes in the future, it is hoped that the health care needs of the economically disadvantaged will not be ignored. Certainly, with the continued rise in health care costs, their problems will not disappear in the near future.

National Health Insurance

During the 1970s, a variety of national health insurance program proposals was introduced into Congress. The one that would have resulted in the greatest change in the health financing system was sponsored by Senator Edward Kennedy from Massachusetts. Benefit coverage under this proposal would have been compulsory for all citizens and would have covered all health care services. Financing of this program, which would have carried no maximum limits, no deductibles, nor any coinsurance provisions, would have been by payroll taxes and general revenue monies. The program would have been administered by an agency of the federal government created by federal legislation. This proposal would have eliminated the need for private health insurance carriers.

Without question, Senator Kennedy's plan would have resulted in a major change in health care funding in the United States. Also, the role of the federal government in the field of health care would have been greatly enlarged, leading to expanded government regulation and control. The cost of this program to the taxpayers would have been extensive. In spite of these negative factors, all citizens would have been able to obtain health care when needed. Cost would no longer be a limiting consideration. However, this proposal was opposed by the American Medical Association, the insurance industry, the business community, and most conservative economists and politicians.

Another proposal, which would have had a less radical effect on the health care system in the United States, was one sponsored by the American Medical Association. This plan would have used a system of tax credits to encourage the purchase of health insurance from current health insurance carriers. Under provisions of this proposal, Medicare would have remained in effect for the elderly, Medicaid would have been eliminated, and in its place, the government would pay premiums for low-income individuals. Other than these changes, the health insurance system would have remained as it has been. This proposal would have resulted in no change in the delivery of health care.

Between these extremes there were a number of other proposals. One proposal would have encouraged the establishment of health care corporations. The employer would be required to purchase a comprehensive health insurance plan for all employees and to pay at least 75 percent of the premium. If the employee joined a health care corporation, a federal subsidy of a specified percent would apply to the insurance premium. This proposal would have failed to meet the insurance needs of the economically disadvantaged and the unemployed.

Another proposal would have made use of tax incentives to encourage employers to buy health insurance for their employees. This did not—nor did any other proposal—receive widespread public, political, and economic acceptance.

No national health insurance proposal received enough support to be seriously considered for passage by Congress. Many felt that a program of national health insurance would be too costly and unacceptable to the majority of the American population.

In 1976 and 1980 the issue of national health insurance was debated in the presidential elections. The two major national parties held differing views on this issue. In 1976 the Republican party opposed compulsory national health insurance, but supported a program of catastrophic insurance through private insurance companies. Since 1980 the Republican party position has been one of complete opposition to the creation of a national health insurance system. The Democratic party has advocated a national program of comprehensive health insurance, though the particular type of program remains open to debate and discussion.

The issue of national health insurance has been a political issue for years. Since the early 1980s the political consensus throughout the country has generally opposed the development of such a program. As long as the present pro-competition view of health economics prevails in government, it is unlikely that any national health insurance proposals will be entertained by Congress. There is little political support at this point in time for any type of national health insurance except possibly for catastrophic coverage.

The problems encountered in a major health catastrophe have made the need for catastrophic health insurance apparent. Several plans have been proposed in an attempt to help in this type of situation, though presently no plan has been accepted by Congress. However, in 1986 a task-force report of the Secretary of Health and Human Services examined several possible approaches to helping individuals through catastrophic health situations. Principally, all recommendations that were considered involved funding coming from the private sector, not governmental.

For example, employers might be encouraged to purchase health insurance coverage for the catastrophic situation. For the self-employed it was suggested that tax deductions for health insurance premiums be considered. Another idea that has received support is the development of medical individual retirement accounts. These would be tax-favored savings arrangements for the purchase of long-term care insurance.

It remains to be seen what types of catastrophic health insurance programs develop in the near future. The importance of such programs was noted by the Secretary of the Department of Health and Human Services in 1986 when he stated, "All segments of the American population should have protection from the catastrophic financial consequences of illness."[15]

Cost Containment

Most individuals will agree that rising costs of health care as have been experienced in the United States since the end of World War II must be brought under control in some way. Unfortunately there is no simple solution to this problem.

Numerous factors have contributed to increased expenditures for health care. Basic economic inflation has been a major contributory factor. The American public has created a greater demand for health services. The introduction of costlier medical techniques and procedures along with increasing salaries for those employed in health care facilities have added to the problem. Escalating costs resulting from medical malpractice litigation have been passed on to the consumer. Another important factor has been the increase in the elderly population, which results in more people needing long-term care and the presence of costlier chronic diseases.

There has been little reason in the past to control hospital costs, shorten hospital stays, or to limit the use of technology. However, shifts in public sentiment and cost containment have become focuses of public policy. Increasingly the hospitals and physicians are finding themselves confronted with payment systems in which the rate of payment is fixed in advance.

How cost containment of health care can be achieved is a subject open to much debate and discussion. Anyone's answer depends a great deal on his or her political, economic, and social views (as presented in an earlier chapter of this text).[16] No one, quick, simple solution will be found, though several considerations have received attention.

Health Planning

The need for comprehensive health planning is advocated by many who have examined the health care issues in the United States. As has been noted health care costs have risen dramatically as new technology for treating health problems has been developed. Besides being very costly, this technology is often underused and poorly distributed. In many instances duplication of expensive health care facilities, equipment, and services exists. On the other hand, health care services are too often inadequate to meet the needs of the economically disadvantaged, handicapped, those living in rural areas, and minorities. The basic purpose of health planning is to provide coordination at the local and state levels to correct these and other problems related to the distribution and provision of health care.

The original concept of health planning had its beginning in the 1920s.[17] At that time the New York Academy of Medicine issued a report that stated that there was an adequate number of beds in New York hospitals. Other studies looked at the adequacy of hospitals to meet community needs in other localities.

The Hospital Survey and Construction Act, better known as the *Hill-Burton Act,* was passed by Congress in 1946. This legislation, while providing federal funds for local hospitals, also mandated the implementation of planning measures. Each state was required to survey its hospital facilities and to develop a state hospital plan. Before a state could receive federal funds for hospital construction, a survey of existing institutions and a construction plan had to be submitted to the appropriate federal agency.

Between 1946 and the 1960s, all the states developed plans and determined hospital facility construction and renovation priorities. In 1954, the Hill-Burton program was expanded to include nursing homes, outpatient facilities, public health centers, rehabilitation services, and chronic disease facilities. Due to this expansion, over twelve thousand health facility construction and modernization projects were funded by the Hill-Burton program. However, though some planning occurred, there was little effort made to adhere to the Hill-Burton requirements. The activities of hospital facilities and other regional health care facilities were not being coordinated. As a result, the proliferation of health programs during this period only compounded problems.

The Regional Medical Program (P.L. 89–239) came into existence in 1965 as a result of federal legislation. The purpose of this program was to create regional care centers for heart disease, cancer, and stroke patients. This particular program included a planning component that later was integrated into regional health planning legislation.

In 1966 the Comprehensive Health Planning and Public Health Services Act became law. This federal legislation made funds available for comprehensive health planning. It also set in motion planning programs at the state and regional levels. Though efforts at planning increased, there was little authority, other than the power of persuasion, to affect the planning decisions. Thus, some localities had effective planning programs; others did not.

Health planning was not considered successful by the early 1970s despite the Comprehensive Health Planning Act. Both Congress and health industry officials identified the need for local and state planning of health care services. In 1974, another federal law, the National Health Planning and Resource Development Act (P.L. 93–641), was passed. It was hoped that it would succeed where the Comprehensive Health Planning Act had not.

The provisions of the National Health Planning and Resource Development Act were built on experience gained from the planning of the Hill-Burton Act, the Regional Medical Programs, and the Comprehensive Health Planning Program. One important difference from the 1966 legislation (the Comprehensive Health Planning Act) was that the 1974 legislation gave agencies more authority to enforce planning decisions. For example, health systems agencies were given control of federal grant monies for health care services and health resources.

This piece of legislation required that each state governor designate "health service areas." A planning system involving both regional and state health agencies was established. The local Health Systems Agency (HSA) had to develop a regional plan. Also, the state health planning agency was required to develop a state health plan that integrated the various health plans of the HSAs within the state. The state plan then had to be submitted to the governor for approval.

Two hundred and thirteen local health planning agencies, known as Health Systems Agencies, were designated by Congress. Each had its own governing board, the majority of whom had to be consumers. The legislators did not want the HSAs to be dominated by health care providers.

Health Systems Agencies had the responsibility to collect and analyze data concerning health care resources and programs in their regions. The data was reviewed and a health systems plan was written, having long-range goals as well as specific annual implementation suggestions. The plan was to be approved at the state planning level. Through the process of review and comment, the HSA recommended the approval or denial of requests for federal funding applications.

By 1980 most HSAs had developed plans that met minimum federal requirements. Nearly all of these plans addressed the problems of cost containment, health promotion and prevention, and maternal and child health. Four out of five plans included elderly care provisions, and 75 percent included goals for primary health care.[18]

Although many have recognized a need for national comprehensive health planning and extensive efforts have gone into the process in the past, the issue has met with opposition from many government officials and some health care industry professionals. Many of these individuals felt that federal health planning should be eliminated entirely since it had not been effective in containing health care costs. Politicians, medical care providers, and health economists pointed out that there was little evidence of cost effectiveness resulting from the health planning process.

Increased options for the provision of health care services have led to vigorous advertising. The billboards of any large city in the United States reveal numerous options, plans, and programs that are available for purchase.

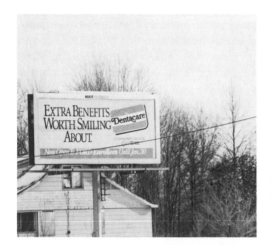

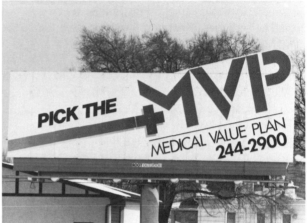

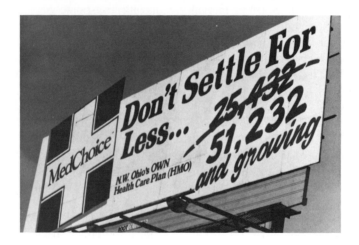

Supporters of health planning still maintained the opposite position. While they admitted that health care costs had not been contained, supporters of health planning pointed out that millions of dollars had been saved by limiting health facility construction and technological facility purchases. Without a planning process it was felt that excessive overbuilding of health care facilities and purchase of expensive technological equipment would have occurred in many communities.

Unfortunately, the real issue in this debate has not focused on the merits of the health planning process. Instead, the focal issue has become that of federal government control, increasing federal expenditures, and government regulatory procedures. In an effort to reduce its involvement in health care and to return control to the states and local communities, the federal government eliminated the federal health planning effort in the early 1980s. This resulted primarily because Congress failed to authorize funding for the program. Whatever health planning is to occur will now be done by the individual states.

State regulatory programs of review and approval by health planning agencies of capital expenditures by hospitals and other health care facilities are known as *certificate of need* programs. Under certificate of need (CON) programming a health care facility cannot build a capital expenditure project without state planning agency review and approval. Individual states now determine to what degree they wish to be involved in health planning. They must determine what will be the functions of certificate of need programs, how they should be structured, and how and to what degree they will be funded.

Since 1982 several states have repealed CON laws. However, a majority of states still have certificate of need programs. This has led to a wide variation of programs by state. For example, in one state reviews are not required where capital expenditures will not substantially affect patient costs.[19] In some states review approval for purchase and operation of expensive medical equipment is not necessary unless the annual costs exceed a given sum of money. A few states have increased their certificate of need review programs.

There has been some thought that the federal government may renew and reauthorize the health planning funding in order to give direction to the structure and scope of state plans.[20] The federal government still sees some need for planning as a cost containment measure for its Medicare and Medicaid programs. It is doubtful that in the near future there will be a return to the type of total federal regional planning that developed in the 1970s. Major planning will be left in the hands of each individual state.

HMOs: An Alternative System

An alternative to the fee-for-service system of health care is the Health Maintenance Organization (HMO). There are two basic types of systems that are referred to as HMOs: (1) the *individual practice association* (IPA), and (2) the *prepaid group practice*.

The basic concept of health maintenance organizations is that payment is made in advance on a fixed contract-fee base by a certain population. This payment (an enrolled family pays an average of $189 per month)[21] is used to cover the costs of a comprehensive range of medical services including hospitals, clinics, and professional and technical personnel.

The individual practice association (IPA) is the result of an agreement between a number of independent physicians to treat patients who are enrolled in a third-party HMO. The health maintenance organization then reimburses the physicians on a fee-for-service basis. Though the consumer prepays, the health care is provided by individual physicians in their private offices as in the traditional fee-for-service system. The HMO management organization markets the plan, collects premiums, and pays the bills.[22] Physicians that are part of an IPA work more independently than those in the group prepaid HMO model and continue to serve non-HMO patients as well.

In contrast, the physicians in the prepaid group practice HMOs are salaried. Their services are provided in facilities that are owned or leased by the health maintenance organization, not in their own individual offices. The providers, who have contracted to work in the HMO for salary, not only provide the normal types of curative health care, but are also encouraged through program incentives to keep the enrollees healthy.

Several principles provide the foundation for health maintenance organizations. An HMO is an organized system of health care. As such, a set of comprehensive services is available to a specifically identified population group. These individuals provide payment on a prepaid contractual basis. Enrollment in the HMO is voluntary. There are specified enrollment periods when a person can join, either as an individual, as a family, or as part of a group. If the HMO has group enrollment, the membership must also have alternative health care options. The employee is then free to select which plan he or she wishes to join. Some HMOs operate on a nonprofit basis, while over half are investor owned for-profit corporations.

The Kaiser-Sunnyside Medical Center in Clackamas, Oregon, is one of thirty medical centers in the Kaiser-Permanente Medical Care Program.

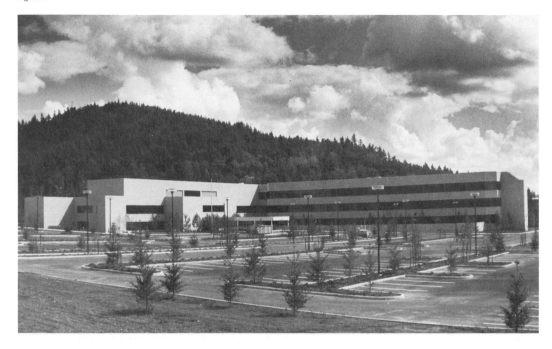

Kaiser-Permanente Medical Care Program

The operation of group prepaid plans is not new. The first such program was started in 1929 in Oklahoma as an extension of farmer cooperatives.[23] Currently, the largest private, prepaid group practice health care delivery program in the United States is the Kaiser-Permanente Medical Care Program. Over 3.7 million people are enrolled in this program.

The Kaiser-Permanente Program operates thirty hospital-based medical centers, eighty-five outpatient medical complexes, a rehabilitation center, a research institute, a school of nursing, and a number of other health care facilities. These facilities are found principally on the West Coast in California, Oregon, and Hawaii, but Kaiser-Permanente centers are also found in Colorado and Ohio. Nearly four-thousand physicians and thirty-five thousand nurses and other related health professionals staff the Kaiser-Permanente facilities.[24]

This particular group prepaid practice program began in the late 1930s when industrialist Henry Kaiser was building the Grand Coulee Dam in the state of Washington. Kaiser felt an obligation to provide health care services for his employees, so he hired a physician to set up a prepaid health care plan for these workers. In time, the program was extended to the families of the workers. Until the end of World War II, the program covered only Kaiser Corporation employees and their families, but in 1945, the plan opened to the general public. Today Kaiser Industries employees constitute only a very small percentage of the total membership.

The setup of the program is quite simple. A member of the Kaiser plan chooses a physician whose geographical location is convenient to subscribers. This physician is salaried and provides services in facilities owned or operated by Kaiser-Permanente. These facilities offer a broad range of health care services, and since there are a number of different plans, the specific coverage will vary. However, all expenses for contracted services are paid for by the plan.

The Kaiser-Permanente Medical Care Program offers a number of services. (a) As an outpatient at Kaiser-Permanente's San Rafael Medical Center in California, one person undergoes transluminal angioplasty, a highly effective and inexpensive alternative to vascular surgery. (b) At the same center, another person is cared for in the intensive care unit.

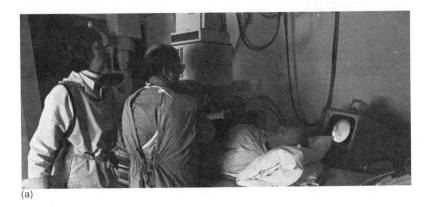

(a)

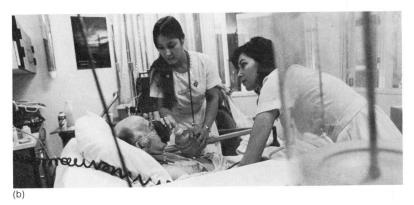

(b)

Federal Government Interest

The federal government became interested in the group prepaid health care concept in the early 1970s during the presidential administration of Richard Nixon. In a message to Congress concerning health in 1971, President Nixon strongly supported the encouragement of and support for the fixed-price contract arrangement for health care services. The term "health maintenance organization" as applied to group prepaid programs was coined early in the 1970s by the Nixon administration.

In 1973 Congress passed the Health Maintenance Organization and Resources Development Act (P.L. 93–222). The act required an HMO to provide its enrollees with a set of specific services having neither time nor cost limitations.

This legislation provided federal funds to groups developing such health care organizations. The funds were to be used for the planning of HMOs and start-up costs. Although these monies were provided, the objective was for an HMO to eventually arrive at a point where it was operationally self-sufficient. Essentially, then, the governmental monies were used for the establishment of new health care businesses.

The HMO legislation was amended in 1976 and again in 1978 for minor operational changes. Several preventive services were included, such as periodic health examinations for adults, voluntary

Services Required by the Health Maintenance Organization and Resources Development Act of 1973

1. Physician services
2. Outpatient services
3. Inpatient hospital services
4. Home health services
5. Diagnostic laboratory and diagnostic and therapeutic radiologic services
6. Preventive health services and early disease detection services
7. Emergency services
8. Prescription drugs
9. Medical social services
10. Vision care
11. Physical therapy
12. Mental health services
13. Prevention and treatment of alcohol and drug abuse and addiction

Source: Health Maintenance Organization and Resources Development Act of 1973, section 1201, (2).

Health Maintenance Organizations

Date	Total	Group (GPP)	IPAs
1976	175	134	41
1980	236	139	97
1984	310	126	184

Source: U.S. Bureau of the Census, *Statistical Abstracts of the United States: 1986* (106th Ed.), Washington, D.C., 1985.

family planning and infertility services, immunizations, and eye and ear examinations for children. Some flexibility on supplemental benefits was also permitted.

One reason the federal government supported this alternative type of health care system was that it would create competition in the field of health care.

With the expansion of HMOs, individuals would have the choice of two kinds of health care organizations. One could select the health maintenance organization (HMO) or continue with the conventional fee-for-service plan with major payment for services made by a third party (the insurance company). Government officials, during the early 1970s, hoped that by 1980, 40 percent of medical care would be delivered by health maintenance organizations. This projection, however, did not come to pass.

This consultation between the surgeon and the radiologist is a primary advantage of the group practice model. Each can utilize the other's specialized medical knowledge.

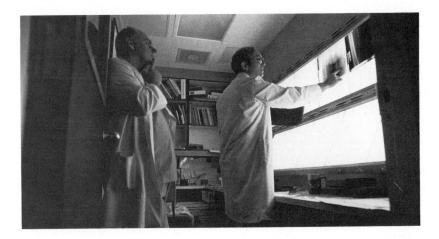

Growth and Expansion of HMOs

In the years since the HMO legislation, the number of health maintenance organizations operating in the United States has expanded from about four million subscribers in the early 1970s to over nineteen million by the mid-1980s.[25] The annual growth rate of HMOs in the 1980s has been over 15 percent, resulting in a doubling of membership every five years.[26] Whereas there were thirty-three HMOs in the early 1970s, today there are nearly four hundred. Two-thirds of the newer HMOs are of the individual-practice association (IPA) model.[27] HMO growth has not been geographically uniform. Over half of all HMO members reside in the western United States with 21 percent of the population in California and 18 percent in Hawaii being enrolled in health maintenance organizations. HMO membership is greater in cities and suburbs than in nonmetropolitan areas.

An important economic principle regarding health maintenance organizations is that unlike traditional fee-for-service health care provisions, HMOs experience financial benefit for keeping people well. If the providers emphasize acute care, expenses will exceed the contracted amount of funds. If, as the result of health preventive measures, expensive health care procedures are reduced, there will be excess funds that can be considered "bonus" money or profits for the staff. Thus the free-market profit motive is employed to help keep people well.

Demographic Profile of the HMO Subscriber

Majority are below forty years of age

Majority are middle class

Majority are employed in an organization with five hundred or fewer employees

Majority have children under eighteen years of age

Source: Louis Harris and Associates, Inc., *A Report Card on Health Maintenance Organizations: 1980–1984*, conducted for the Henry J. Kaiser Family Foundation, Study No. 844003, 1984.

Health Maintenance Organization Enrollment in Millions

Date	Total	Group (GPP)	IPAs
1976	6	5.6	.4
1980	9.1	7.4	1.6
1984	15.1	8.6	6.5

Source: U.S. Bureau of the Census, *Statistical Abstracts of the United States: 1986* (106th Ed.), Washington, D.C., 1985.

Benefits of Enrollment

Why would a person select membership in an HMO? The health maintenance organization provides a broad range of health services in a single setting. The individual is not referred by one physician or clinic to another. With the broad range of comprehensive services provided, the consumer knows exactly where the particular care can be obtained. All records and control of the patient's care are housed in one organization.

Another benefit of belonging to an HMO is that health care is always available. Regardless of the time of day or the day of the week, a subscriber is guaranteed access to a health care system. This type of security is most valuable for those living in medically underserved locations.

Some people join an HMO because they have been unable to locate a physician in their community. For them the health maintenance organization provides access to the health care system. Enrollees are more likely to be mobile, younger families who have not established a patient-physician relationship.[28] Most HMOs have attracted working people and the middle class. The elderly and the poor are not large-scale participants in health maintenance organizations. This is partially due to the location of most health maintenance organizations, as few are located in the inner city or in rural settings. Many HMOs have not accepted Medicare and Medicaid patients in the past, but a number of them are now developing plans to include these patients.

Those who perceive a cost benefit will join HMOs. HMO costs are lower than those in more traditional health insurance programs. Health maintenance organizations have been shown to provide good care at 28 percent less than fee-for-service systems.[29] However, there does not seem to be evidence that the rise in health costs for HMO enrollees is any less than that found in the overall medical care provision.[30]

Membership in health maintenance organizations does result in a savings of money. For example, Ford Motor Company experienced a savings of about five million dollars in premiums through HMO enrollment of only 8 percent of its workforce.[31] Hospital admissions of health maintenance organization patients are about half those enrolled in regular health insurance plans.

"There is very little difference in the overall health status of HMO members and nonmembers of the same age and employment status."

Source: Louis Harris and Associates, Inc., *A Report Card on Health Maintenance Organizations:* 1980–1984, conducted for the Henry J. Kaiser Family Foundation, Study No. 844003, 1984, p. 87.

Problems with HMOs

With a number of benefits that can be identified and with federal legislation designed to encourage the development of health maintenance organizations, it is important to analyze why they have not become as widespread as had been forecast a decade ago. For many people the HMO seems impersonal. There often is no guarantee that an individual will be able to see the same physician with each visit. As a result there is less likelihood that a close physician-patient relationship can develop, though this is somewhat compensated for in the HMO-IPA model.

The health maintenance organization concept has not been accepted by some of the medical profession. Some physicians will not work within this framework. They do not like the salaried concept nor the more structured format of medical practice in a group prepaid program. Their independence is reduced in the group prepaid HMO setting. These negative viewpoints are often overcome with the HMO-IPA model. Growth of the IPAs has led increasing numbers of physicians to join HMOs.

Another major reason for the limited expansion of HMOs in the past had to do with economics. For a health maintenance organization to function economically, it is estimated that there must be a membership of close to thirty thousand. In the early 1980s more than two-thirds of the operational HMOs had ten thousand or fewer enrollees.[32]

Another problem in HMO development has been the high start-up costs. This usually results in large financial deficits during the first few years of operation. These costs are rarely offset by the federal monies made available for HMO establishment.

HMOs: Good or Bad?

What conclusions can be drawn about health maintenance organizations? Conceptually, they appear to be a positive alternative to the traditional fee-for-service provision of medical care. Politically, there has been governmental support for their development. To some degree, there has not been popular support from the public.

A Louis Harris survey conducted in 1984 showed that most HMO members are satisfied with the provision of health care through a health maintenance organization. This report found that 91 percent were basically satisfied.[33] This finding serves to indicate an increased positive view toward health maintenance organizations by those who have joined.

A major concern expressed about HMOs related to the quality of care provided by health maintenance organization providers. Some people view the care received as being inferior to the fee-for-service approach. The quality of physician care and the length of time it often takes to get an appointment were noted. However, some studies have concluded that the quality of care received in HMOs is equal to that received through the conventional plans.[34]

The health maintenance organization approach to receiving health care is a different concept for millions of Americans. As with many things in our society, that which is new, different, and untried often is not readily received by the public. Whether there will be a continuing increase in this form of health care provision in the future remains to be seen. Most projections are that HMO membership will expand through the 1990s, though the estimates vary widely as to what percentage of the total population will eventually be health maintenance organization participants. Nevertheless, they certainly do provide an alternative to the traditional fee-for-service approach to health care.

Preferred Provider Organizations (PPOs)

A relatively new system of health delivery is the preferred provider organization (PPO). The basic concept of the PPO system is rather simple. A self-insured employer, an independent insurance company, or a public organization negotiates a low fee-for-service with selected hospitals and health care providers in a specific area.

Group insurance costs are reduced in exchange for a guaranteed pool of patients. The fee schedule negotiated between providers and consumers is an attempt to create a uniform price for services delivered. Employers looking for an overall cost savings can channel a significant number of employees to cost effective hospitals and physicians. The competitive price for services is possible because the provider charges are discounted by as much as 20 percent.[35]

When employees (consumers) use the PPO facilities and providers they have 100 percent coverage. Should the individual select a hospital or physician that is not on the PPO list, they pay the traditional deductibles and coinsurance rates of the bill.

The only way participating consumers and providers are bound together is through the negotiated fee. The consumers are not required to go to a PPO participant, and each service is handled separately. The consumer retains the right to return to regular insurance coverage at any time.

The first PPOs started in the early 1970s.[36] They were initially designed for hospital employees. Since the early 1970s they have expanded and developed in various ways throughout the country, though there are several common characteristics.[37] For instance, there is a limited grouping of hospitals and physicians who agree to provide services for specified negotiated discounted fees. For the consumer there are no copayments or deductible costs if they receive health care services through the listed providers. A major attraction to hospitals and physicians is the rapid payment of PPO claims. The efficient claims processing of a PPO has made for low administrative costs.

All PPOs have some type of utilization review system. The mechanisms vary with some having physician peer review; others have instituted preadmission certification and concurrent ongoing review.

Utilization review provides assurance that care has been rendered in an effective and cost efficient manner. Proper use of hospital services can result in long-term cost savings.

The concept of the preferred provider organization is so new that there are problems with its administration and operation. Some problems arise due to differences between what the buyer wants for his employees and what the provider is trying to market. The more completely the provider understands the buyer's desires, the increased likelihood of success.[38] The provider must tailor the approach to fit the needs of the consumer. Some hospitals looking at PPOs as a marketing scheme have actually not reduced overall health care costs.

Whether PPOs will increase in development in the years ahead will depend on several variables. Possibly the most important will be whether they will be an effective competitor in the reduction of health care costs. PPOs can be a major factor in health care plans of the future if the corporate world becomes convinced of their cost efficiency and if the employees come to accept the concept of receiving services from PPO providers.

Summary

The cost of health care in the United States has risen consistently during the past two decades. Hospital costs account for the largest percentage of expenses, followed by professional physician and dental service costs. Historically payment for health care has been on a fee-for-service basis.

Payment for health care costs by a third party (health insurance carrier) has increased since the early years of this century. Today many health expenses, including hospital, surgical, physician, major medical, income disability, and dental, are paid by some type of health insurance. The amount of coverage under each category, deductibles, and extent of copayment vary from one health insurance carrier to another.

Health insurance coverage has been provided by private companies. Since 1965 the United States government has funded two health insurance programs, Medicare and Medicaid. Medicare provides hospital insurance and medical coverage for the elderly, while Medicaid covers the cost of health care for certain economically disadvantaged people.

There have been attempts to introduce legislation that would introduce a national health insurance program for all citizens of the nation. However, no program of this nature has been accepted.

Much has been said about taking measures to contain the costs of health care. Various procedures, programs, and activities have been developed with cost containment in mind. One program with this goal has been health planning. Legislation requiring health planning on a local and state level has been passed. Presently the responsibility for health planning rests with the specific state governments.

An alternative to the fee-for-service system of health care is the health maintenance organization. Two types of HMOs, the group prepaid model and the individual practice association (IPA), have expanded in recent years. The largest HMO is the Kaiser-Permanente Medical Care Program. This program serves over three million individuals, primarily on the West Coast.

An HMO is an organized system with an identified population of enrollees receiving comprehensive health care from employed health providers. In the early 1970s, the federal government became interested in supporting and encouraging the development of health maintenance organizations. Since that time increasing numbers of HMOs have come into being throughout the nation.

Another alternative approach to traditional fee-for-service health care is the preferred provider organization (PPO). This organized approach to health care involves providing health services at a prearranged reduced cost factor.

Discussion Questions

1. Discuss some of the factors that have contributed to the continuing rise in costs of health care.

2. What are some of the differences between hospital insurance and major medical insurance?

3. Explain how deductibles and coinsurance are related to the inflation of health care costs.

4. What kinds of coverage are provided under Part A of Medicare? Part B?

5. What incentives that would help to reduce the costs of health care are built into the Medicare program?

6. What groups of people are covered by Medicaid?

7. Do you feel that Medicaid should be changed? If so, explain the changes you would recommend.

8. What have been some of the differing positions regarding the development of a national health insurance program in the United States?

9. Discuss the purpose underlying the establishment of the Diagnostic Related Groups (DRG) program.

10. What is meant by the concept of a prospective payment system of health care?

11. Trace the historical development of health planning in this country.

12. How has the Hill-Burton Act affected federal spending for health since World War II?

13. Identify the similarities and differences between the two different basic kinds of health maintenance organizations.

14. Explain why health maintenance organizations are alternatives to the fee-for-service provision of health care.

15. What are some of the kinds of activities and programs provided for by the Kaiser-Permanente Medical Care Program?

16. Discuss some of the advantages to the consumer of belonging to a health maintenance organization.

17. Would you go to an HMO for your primary source of health care? Discuss the reasons for your answer.

18. Explain how preferred provider organizations (PPOs) might make a contribution to cost containment of health care costs.

Suggested Readings

Averil, Richard F., and Kailson, Michael J. "Development and Interpretation of the Diagnosis Related Groups (DRGs)." *Health Care Financial Management* (February, 1984): 72–82.

Berger, Sally. "Local Health Planning Must Be Revitalized." *Hospitals* 54, no. 13 (July 1, 1980): 54–56.

Dolenc, Danielle, and Dougherty, Charles J. "DRGs: The Counterrevolution in Financing Health Care." *Hastings Center Report* 15, no. 3 (June, 1985): 19–29.

Ellwein, Linda, and Gregg, David D. "Interstudy Researchers Trace Progress of PPOs." *FAH Review* (July/August, 1982): 20–25.

Falk, I. S. "National Health Insurance for the United States." *Public Health Reports* 92, no. 5 (September/October, 1977): 399–406.

Hagen, Ron. "Medigap Insurance: Pitfalls and Progress." *Business and Health* 3, no. 5 (April, 1986): 25–30.

Harris, Louis, and Associates, Inc. *A Report Card on Health Maintenance Organizations: 1980–1984,* conducted for the Henry J. Kaiser Family Foundation, Study No. 844003, 1984.

Jessie, William F., and Sauer, James D. "Physicians and DRGs: Survival Under PPS." *The Hospital Medical Staff* (April, 1984): 2–7.

Luft, Harold S. "Assessing the Evidence on HMO Performance." *Milbank Memorial Fund Quarterly, Health and Society* 58, no. 4 (1980): 501–36.

Manning, W. G., and others. "A Controlled Trial of a Prepaid Group Practice on Use of Services." *New England Journal of Medicine* 310, (1984): 1505–11.

O'Gara, Nellie, and Hickley, Kevin F. "Marketing the PPO." *Hospitals* 58, no. 12 (June 16, 1984): 75–78.

Sapolsky, Harvey M., and others. "DRGs in Theory and in Practice." *Business and Health* 3, no. 7 (June, 1986): 43–46.

Schroer, Kathryn, and Taylor, Ellsworth. "A Survey of PPOs." *Hospitals* 58, no. 6 (March 16, 1984): 85.

Simpson, James B. "State Certificate-of-Need Programs: the Current Status." *American Journal of Public Health* 75, no. 10 (October, 1985): 1225–29.

Wolinsky, Fredric D. "The Performance of Health Maintenance Organizations: An Analytic Review." *Milbank Memorial Fund Quarterly, Health and Society* 58, no. 4 (1980): 537–87.

Endnotes

1. Sidel, Victor W. 1985 Presidential address of the American Public Health Association, November 18, 1985, Washington, D.C. Reported in the *American Journal of Public Health* 76, no. 4 (April, 1986): 373.

2. Health Insurance Association of America. *Source Book of Health Insurance Data, 1986 Update.* Washington, D.C.: the Association, 2.

3. Ibid., 18.

4. United States Department of Commerce, Bureau of Census. *Statistical Abstract of the United States, 1985, 105th Ed.* Washington, D.C.: U.S. Government Printing Office (1985): 97.

5. Ibid.

6. Ibid., 98.

7. Health Insurance Association of America. *Source Book.* 5.

8. *Statistical Abstract of the United States, 1985, 105th Ed.*

9. Health Insurance Association of America. *Source Book.* 91.

10. Ibid. 2.

11. Department of Health and Human Services press release. September, 1987.

12. Ibid.

13. Health Insurance Association of America. *Source Book.* 28.

14. Moss, Sen. F. E., Chairman of the Subcommittee on Long-Term Care, Senate Committee on Aging. Testimony before Senate Finance Committee, July 28, 1976.

15. Quoted in *The Nation's Health* (September, 1986): 5.

16. See chapter 1 for a discussion of pro-competitive debate regarding health care.

17. Braverman, Jordan. *Crisis in Health Care.* Washington, D.C.: Acropolis Books, 1980: 123.

18. Bureau of Health Planning. *Annual Report, 1979.* Washington, D.C.: U.S. Government Printing Office (April, 1980).

19. Simpson, James B. "State Certificate-of-Need Programs: the Current Status." *American Journal of Public Health* 75, no. 10 (October, 1985): 1126.

20. Ibid., 1128.

21. InterStudy Report. Excelsior, Minnesota. Reported in *The Nation's Health* (July, 1985): 3.

22. Harris, Louis, and Associates, Inc. *A Report Card on Health Maintenance Organizations: 1980–1984.* Conducted for the Henry J. Kaiser Family Foundation, Study No. 844003 (1984): VI.

23. "Prepaid Health Care: The Way It Works, What's Being Planned." *U.S. News and World Report* (March 29, 1971): 77.

24. Data provided by Kaiser-Permanente Medical Care Program Annual Report.

25. Harris, Louis, and Associates, Inc. *Report Card on HMOs.* 1.

26. Ibid.

27. Manning, W. G., and others. "A Controlled Trial of a Prepaid Group Practice on Use of Services." *New England Journal of Medicine* 310, (1984): 1505–11.

28. Berki, S. E., and Ashcroft, Marie L. F. "HMO Enrollment: Who Joins What and Why: A Review of the Literature." *Milbank Memorial Fund Quarterly, Health and Society* 58, no. 4 (1980): 625.

29. Manning, W. G., and others.

30. Luft, Harold S. "Assessing the Evidence on HMO Performance." *Milbank Memorial Fund Quarterly, Health and Society* 58, no. 4 (1980): 508.

31. Reported in *Perspective: The Blue Cross and Blue Shield Magazine* 20, no. 4 (Winter, 1985): 9.

32. Braverman. *Crisis in Health Care,* 111.

33. Harris, Louis, and Associates, Inc. Report Card on HMOs. 142.

34. Wolinsky, Fredric D. "The Performance of Health Maintenance Organizations: An Analytic Review." *Milbank Memorial Fund Quarterly, Health and Society* 58, no. 4 (1980): 544.

35. Ellwein, Linda, and Gregg, David D. "Interstudy Researchers Trace Progress of PPOs." *FAH Review* (July/August, 1982): 20.

36. Schroer, Kathryn, and Taylor, Ellsworth. "A Survey of PPOs." *Hospitals* 58, no. 6 (March 16, 1984): 85.

37. Ellwein and Gregg. *FAH Review:* 20.

38. O'Gara, Nellie, and Hickley, Kevin F. "Marketing the PPO." *Hospitals* 58, no. 12 (June 16, 1984): 76.

8

The Private Sector: Of Increasing Importance in Community Health

Programs funded and operated by the government are in the public domain; that is, governmental activity is open to review by the general public. Nongovernmental activity is in the private domain, or private sector. Any organization or agency that is not tax supported is considered "private."

In spite of governmental programs designed to improve the health status of a nation, many activities sponsored, funded, and conducted by the private sector play important roles in community health. Nowhere in the world is this more true than in the United States. Some of the most important medical advances in history have resulted from funding by private organizations. These organizations also provide a number of health services to various segments of society. They are responsible for health promotion efforts targeted at every conceivable audience.

Private sector programs were overshadowed in the 1960s and 1970s by increased governmental programming in the health fields. Legislation, particularly at the federal level, as well as combined federal and state projects, received more attention in most American community health circles than did the private organizations.

During the 1980s a major reversal of this trend has occurred. With reductions in governmental funding for health-related programs and the elimination of many federal health and social service projects and activities, the role of the private sector has assumed increased importance in meeting the health needs of the nation. As a matter of fact, the current political belief, widely accepted by many leading governmental officials, is that health care programs are the responsibility of the private sector, not of government. The result is that many health needs that were the focus of governmental programming in the 1960s and 1970s are now met by private sector programs.

Four community health groupings constitute the private sector: (1) voluntary health organizations, (2) private foundations, (3) corporate health programs, and (4) religious organizations. All but the corporate programs are considered nonprofit.

Each of these four groups can be subdivided into a number of organizations and agencies. Each has a definite focus with specific goals and objectives.

Some programming efforts do overlap, but others are quite specific or unique. Though not coordinated by any central agency, they all play an important role in achieving a healthy United States.

Voluntary Health Organizations

Voluntary health organizations are unique American institutions. Although such agencies can be found in other countries, only in the United States do they play a vital role in society's health programs. These agencies are nongovernmental, non-tax-supported organizations that rely heavily upon volunteer services to accomplish their various program goals.

The voluntary health movement began with the founding in 1892 of the Anti-Tuberculosis Society in Philadelphia. This organization has since been renamed the National Tuberculosis Association, then the National Tuberculosis and Respiratory Disease Association (NTBRD), and later, in 1973, the American Lung Association.

These name changes exemplify the evolutionary process that often occurs within voluntary health organizations. Such organizations usually come into being because of a specific health problem. The resources of the organization, both finances and personnel, are mobilized for the purpose of eliminating or neutralizing that specific problem. When the particular disease is "conquered," the focus of the health organization often changes. Rarely does a voluntary health organization disband when its primary objective has been reached. Instead, it develops new goals.

This is what occurred in the case of the original Anti-Tuberculosis Society. At the end of the nineteenth and the beginning of the twentieth century, tuberculosis was a serious concern in the United States. But when it ceased to pose a serious threat to the health of the general public, the program and objectives of the organization shifted to a broader spectrum. Today the American Lung Association is concerned not only with tuberculosis, but with all lung diseases, including emphysema, pneumonia, silicosis, pneumoconiosis, and asbestosis. Because of the relationship between smoking and lung disease, particularly lung cancer and emphysema, one major program is an antismoking campaign.

Another example of the evolution in voluntary health organizations is seen in the National Foundation for Poliomyelitis. This organization, founded in 1938 by President Franklin D. Roosevelt, had as its original goal the prevention of polio. In the 1940s and the early 1950s, when polio was a great concern, the National Foundation for Poliomyelitis was at the forefront of the "battle against polio." Many researchers, including Dr. Jonas Salk, were recipients of research grants from this organization. After Salk's discovery of the polio vaccine and the elimination of polio as a major health problem in the United States, the National Foundation for Poliomyelitis became known as the National Foundation/March of Dimes. Today the activities of this organization are directed toward the prevention of congenital malformations, commonly called birth defects.

The American Heart Association is an example of a voluntary health organization that has maintained its original emphasis since its formation in 1916 as the Association for the Prevention and Relief of Heart Disease. This agency, which later became known as the New York Heart Association, originally admitted only physicians and scientists as members. By 1924 interest and program had expanded to the point that a national heart association was established, known as the American Heart Association. However, not until 1948 was membership opened to nonmedical persons. Through the years and through these minor changes in membership, the American Heart Association has maintained its original and primary objective, the prevention of heart and cardiovascular disease.

The National Society for the Prevention of Blindness has also had the same emphasis—to reduce needless cases of blindness—since its founding in 1908. Members of this organization believe that half of all blindness in the United States can be prevented. For this reason the activities of the National Society for the Prevention of Blindness are not directed toward blind people, but toward the general public.

Voluntary health agencies range from national or international in scope with large budgets and programs to small, local agencies interested in just one isolated problem. The various voluntary health organizations can be classified according to the specific focus or concern of each agency:

1. Emphasis on a specific disease entity— American Cancer Society, Arthritis Foundation, American Diabetes Association, National Leukemia Association, Cystic Fibrosis Foundation, Multiple Sclerosis Society

2. Health problems affecting specific organs and structures of the body—American Heart Association, American Lung Association, National Society for the Prevention of Blindness

3. Problems of special groups or matters related to a large sector of the population—National Safety Council, Planned Parenthood Association, National Association for Mental Health

Structure

Most voluntary health organizations that operate at the national level have state and local affiliate agencies. Efforts to provide direct local services are more effective when there are these affiliates at the "grass roots" level.

The American Heart Association has fifty-five affiliated heart associations. There is an affiliate in each state except the Dakotas, where one affiliate serves both North and South Dakota. There are also heart association affiliates in the District of Columbia, Puerto Rico, and in the cities of New York, Chicago, Los Angeles, and Cleveland. Each affiliate acts independently, which permits programming tailored to the particular needs of the given geographic location. There are also many Heart Association chapters located in various communities throughout the country, each with specific programs focusing upon the prime objective of this voluntary health organization—the reduction of cardiovascular disease. Each American Heart Association chapter reports to the state or regional affiliate in the area in which they are located.

Volunteer transportation is of enormous value in the American Cancer Society service program. Men and women donate automobiles and time to drive cancer patients to treatments, thus helping to save lives.

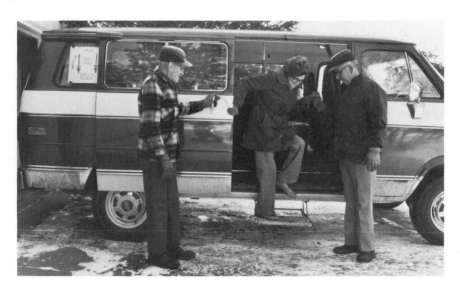

Not all organizations so thoroughly canvas the nation. Whereas the American Heart Association has affiliates in every state, the National Society for the Prevention of Blindness has only twenty-two state affiliates.

Organizations vary from one agency to another. The typical pattern includes a board of directors with a paid executive director, paid professional staff, and volunteer workers. These volunteer workers from all walks of life donate time and talent to the program.

The members of the board of directors usually serve in a voluntary capacity. These people have most likely already provided many voluntary hours, and often many dollars, to the agency. Their responsibility is to establish policy and provide direction for the organization. The board is also primarily responsible for determining how the agency activities will be financed. The executive director, employed by the board and usually a board member, directs the activities of the agency as determined by the board.

Professional personnel are employed by most voluntary health organizations. These individuals carry on the day-to-day work of the organization.

Some staff members have responsibility for program planning and implementation. Since many voluntary health organizations have educational programs and a need to evaluate them, the professional staff usually includes an individual with research skills. This individual develops evaluation designs, conducts statistical analyses, and recommends changes based on the findings.

Volunteer workers help an agency to function efficiently and effectively. They provide professional and supportive services, conduct fund-raising campaigns, and perform a variety of other activities essential to the workings of the agency.

Organizational Activities

There are several kinds of activities in which the voluntary health organization participates: health services provision, research support, sponsorship of educational programs, and service as a lobbying agent in the legislative process.

Services

Various types of health services are rendered by voluntary health organizations. For instance, Planned

A volunteer visitors' service to mastectomy patients called "Reach for Recovery" has been affiliated with the American Cancer Society since 1969. This patient-to-patient service assists breast surgery patients in recovering emotionally, physically, and socially.

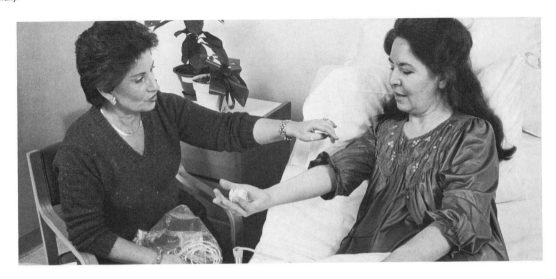

Parenthood services include pap tests and breast examinations for women, blood testing, physical examinations, and male sterilization procedures.

A number of services for cancer patients and their families are provided by the American Cancer Society volunteers. Many, who have themselves been treated for cancer, assist other patients. For example, volunteers are active in the International Association of Laryngectomees, which provides speech training to those cancer patients who have lost their vocal chords. Another volunteer service program is Reach to Recovery, which teaches exercises to mastectomy patients. This program is conducted by women volunteers who have had mastectomies. Ostomy patients receive rehabilitative services.

Personal management of diabetes is very important. Therefore, the American Diabetes Association helps the diabetic to accept, understand, and cope with problems associated with the disease.

The National Cancer Cytology Center furnishes free cyto-sputum test kits for the detection of lung cancer.

The American Lung Association provides respiratory rehabilitation services to individuals suffering from pulmonary diseases. Their services are useful to those with emphysema, chronic bronchitis, and asthma.

A wide range of services is provided by the American Red Cross. Two of the better-known services are (1) those services provided to the families of military personnel and (2) disaster service. When it is necessary for one's family to contact a member of the military on active duty the American Red Cross has the facilities to carry out this function.

In times of natural disasters the American Red Cross undertakes relief activities to help alleviate suffering caused by the disaster. When a disaster occurs the personnel of the American Red Cross are available on a twenty-four-hour-a-day basis providing food, clothing, emergency medical care, and shelter. All Red Cross help to disaster victims is provided at no cost to the recipient. Even though the American Red Cross provides relief assistance when there is a major flood, hurricane, tornado, or other widespread occurrence, most relief actions involve helping victims of fires and accidents in the localized communities.

Research supported by voluntary health organizations is directed at a number of activities although some does not seem related to an ultimate goal. For example, research into improved cardiovascular health has included work with (a) butterflies, (b) freshwater fish, and (c) squid.

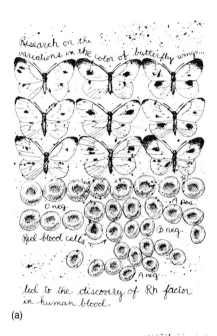

Research on the variations in the color of butterfly wings...

O neg.
A pos.
B neg.
Red blood cells
A neg.

led to the discovery of Rh factor in human blood.

(a)

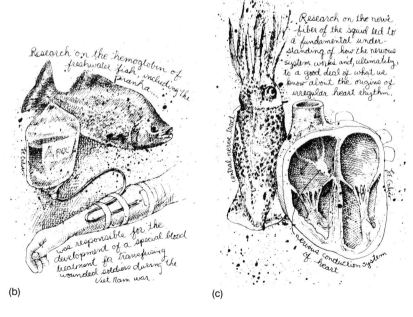

Research on the hemoglobin of freshwater fish, including the piranha...

was responsible for the development of a special blood treatment for transfusing wounded soldiers during the Viet Nam war.

(b)

Research on the nerve fiber of the squid led to a fundamental understanding of how the nervous system works and, ultimately, to a good deal of what we know about the origins of irregular heart rhythm.

central nerve tract

nervous conduction system of heart

(c)

The American Cancer Society supports research such as the interferon project. Here, interferon, a substance that builds the body's defenses against cancer, is being purified and concentrated for use.

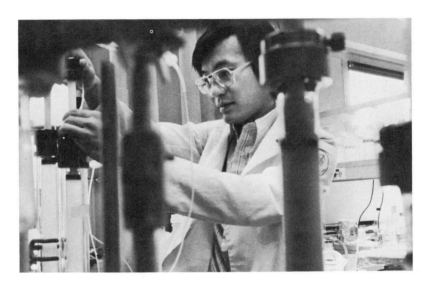

Research

Extensive research efforts are supported by voluntary health organization funds. Millions of dollars have been given to medical and scientific researchers to further their efforts in understanding and curing illnesses.

The American Cancer Society has spent more than $400 million on cancer research since the first funding in 1945. In a current year, $42 million was distributed to medical schools, hospitals, universities, and other institutions for research programs. These programs include molecular biomedical research into cancer and epidemiological studies of large population groups.

The American Heart Association also actively supports research. It has provided nearly $360 million for research since 1949, with over $25 million spent on cardiovascular research in a recent year. An American Heart Association policy is that 60 percent of its national budget must be allocated to such research efforts. Some of these efforts have led to the development of artificial heart valves and pacemakers, as well as the surgical repair of congenital and acquired heart defects. Research into the control of high blood pressure and the relationship of exercise to the prevention of heart diseases has also been conducted.

Research funded by the American Diabetes Association has added to the store of knowledge on the nature and causes of diabetes. Identifying effective methods of treating the diabetic, in addition to research aimed at the prevention and cure of the disease itself, has been important.

The National Foundation/March of Dimes funds have helped identify the causes of congenital diseases and the effective prevention and treatment of birth defects. March of Dimes financial support has also led to the establishment of the Salk Institute in San Diego, California. Here researchers study the growth of both normal and abnormal cells, reproductive biology, virology, and genetics. Grants are made available to young medical students to encourage them to enter careers as medical specialists in birth defects.

Rehabilitation following a laryngectomy is essential for returning patients to active, normal life. The therapist is not only a teacher and supervisor, but also a friend who understands the emotional problems of a patient.

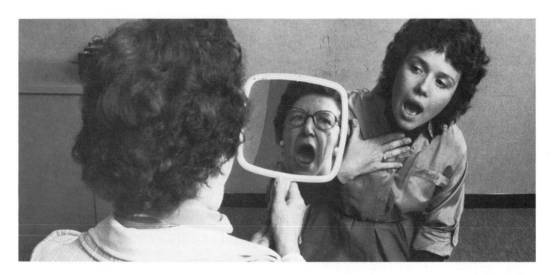

Educational Programs

The most noticeable voluntary health organization activities are educational. Programs designed to promote well-being and to help patients with specific health problems are directed at a variety of audiences. These programs are widely conducted and use many educational strategies—including films, literature, community classes, educational exhibits, and speakers. Radio and television announcements, news releases, and documentaries are also used to inform the public about the concerns of a voluntary health organization.

The American Heart Association conducts public education programs to inform the general population about cardiovascular diseases. Its *Heart Health Education in the Young* is a school program focusing upon the behavioral patterns that contribute to good cardiovascular health. Programs on proper nutrition and the detrimental effects of smoking are also part of the educational activities of the Heart Association.

Another important Heart Association activity has been its cardiopulmonary resuscitation (CPR) training program. This program instructs people to recognize cardiac arrest and to apply CPR skills.

A number of important community educational programs are conducted by the American Red Cross. The American Red Cross is probably best known for its instructional programs in first aid, CPR, and a broad range of water safety programs, including swimming skills, lifesaving, and water safety instruction. In recent years the Red Cross has developed instructional modules relating to nutrition and weight control as well as substance abuse. Other classes include instruction concerning family health and home nursing, stress management, and parenting. All of these educational endeavors are taught by individuals specifically prepared as instructors by the Red Cross.

Some voluntary health organizations offer educational programs for people with a specific health problem. The program objective is to help the individual to cope with the illness, to reverse the problem if possible, and to teach the family how to assist the individual in coping with or reversing the disease. These educational programs are conducted in homes, factories, churches, schools, community clubs, or other appropriate settings; and they employ a number of educational strategies.

Educational programs sponsored by the voluntary health organizations teach skills that will help the individual having a particular health problem to better function in everyday activities. The American Lung Association sponsors swimming instruction for children with asthma.

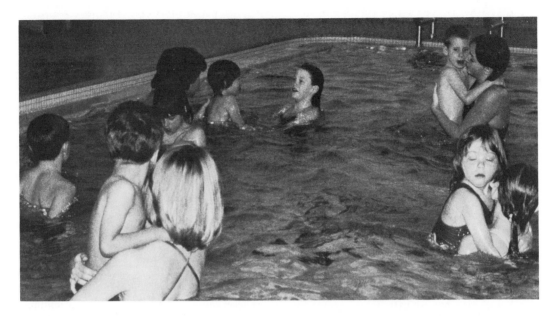

The American Lung Association conducts very effective emphysema and asthma clinics for patients and relatives. The patient learns about the nature of the illness and how to live with the respiratory health problem.

Besides those services mentioned earlier, Planned Parenthood also conducts many rap sessions for sexually active or pregnant teenagers. These sessions instruct the participants in the use of effective birth control or, in the case of the pregnant teenager, in the basics of good prenatal care.

The Glaucoma Alert Program (GAP) of the National Society for the Prevention of Blindness promotes its cause through several activities. For example, one film has been shown on over a hundred television stations. Radio spots, printed literature, and the glaucoma information kit have also been widely used. Well-known personalities have made public appearances on behalf of this educational effort. Television personality Hugh Downs has had a glaucoma tonometry test performed on his syndicated television show.

Many voluntary health organizations provide research data to medical professionals in order to keep these health providers informed of recent developments. Educational workshops, seminars, periodicals, and audiovisual materials are included in professional education efforts of such organizations as the American Lung Association, the American Cancer Society, the American Heart Association, and the National Foundation/March of Dimes. The American Diabetes Association, in addition to conducting seminars and conferences, publishes a monthly professional journal on diabetes. Some national voluntary health organizations have annual conferences where health professionals are informed of the most recent knowledge concerning the specific disease or health problem. The American Cancer Society provides fellowships in chemical oncology for physicians, and scholarships in cancer nursing.

Some agencies tailor their educational programs to a special population group not directly associated with the disease. For example, the American

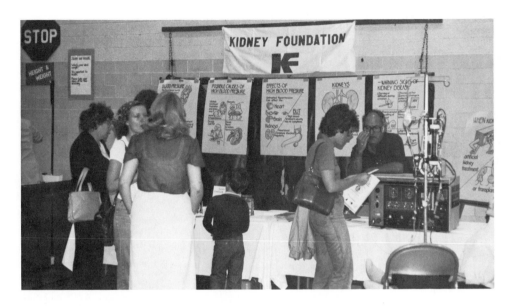

Voluntary health organizations are often involved in community health fairs, using this opportunity to inform citizens of various health concerns.

Diabetes Association has educational programs for teachers, police, and fire personnel. Teachers must know how to cope with the special problems of the diabetic in the classroom. Emergency personnel often deal with diabetics. Failure to recognize diabetic symptoms may result in the false diagnosis of alcohol intoxication. Such an error could be damaging or fatal to the victim.

The American Heart Association also trains teachers, as do the National Dairy Council and numerous other voluntary health organizations. The American Lung Association has been instrumental in the development and dissemination of a health education program for students in grades K through 3 in a number of school districts.

Political Lobbying

The voluntary health organization is often active and frequently effective as a lobby agent. In this capacity, its purpose is to influence legislation that is of specific concern to that agency. One reason that voluntary agencies have been effective at lobbying is that a large number of volunteers with definite interests and concerns can be mobilized successfully.

These volunteers write letters and contact appropriate legislators at both the federal and state levels.

The American Lung Association has been active in lobbying for antismoking legislation. Nationally this organization was also active in supporting the passage of the National Clean Air Act and has been very instrumental in lobbying for reauthorization of this legislation. This interest in clean air relates to the American Lung Association's concern for efficient pulmonary functioning.

The National Society for the Prevention of Blindness has worked for laws that would protect eyes in hazardous environments. The society has also been active in obtaining the government prohibition of a number of potentially dangerous consumer products such as fireworks, toy guns and other weapons, in addition to many toys with sharp edges or projections. The society has also lobbied for the mandatory use of protective eyewear in industrial settings. This concern has now expanded to include the wearing of eyeglasses during sports activities, especially racket sports such as tennis, racquetball, handball, and squash. These increasingly popular sports are a leading cause of sports-related eye injuries.

Financing

The voluntary health agency is financially supported by means other than governmental tax funds. Some agencies provide certain services for which a fee is charged, though support is usually obtained through private contributions and donations.

These contributions come from a variety of sources. Monies are made available to voluntary health organizations from foundation grants, gifts from corporations or estates, memorial gifts, and large and small individual donations. Most of an agency's operating funds are generated by special fund-raising events, including golf and tennis tournaments and exhibitions, bowling contests, running and cycling marathons, and other athletic events.

Fund-raising campaigns are conducted in most communities. The campaign may be either a joint community effort with many agencies participating, or an individual effort of a single agency. There are advantages and disadvantages to both approaches.

The joint venture combines the efforts of the agencies within a community. A specific budgetary goal for each agency is determined. When all agency goals are combined, an overall objective for the entire community fund-raising project is identified, and the community is mobilized in an effort to reach the established financial goal. This joint project, often called the United Way, United Appeal, or Community Chest, eliminates numerous calls on individual citizens during the year. Overhead and administrative expense for the fund-raising effort are shared and as a result reduced.

Some voluntary health organizations do not participate in community fund-raising campaigns. They feel that their specific identity is lost in a joint appeal. These organizations argue that one of the objectives of the fund-raising campaign, in addition to obtaining funds, is to educate the public about the services rendered by the particular agency, and about the health problem with which they are concerned.

Many local voluntary health organizations submit a large portion of their received funds to their state and national affiliate offices. The local community United Way is opposed to this practice.

Nationwide television appeals have been used quite effectively to raise funds. One of the best-known appeals is the "Jerry Lewis Telethon for Muscular Dystrophy" held every Labor Day weekend. In 1987 over $39 million were pledged as a result of this fund-raising effort.[1]

A major portion of a voluntary health organization budget goes directly for program activities. The National Society for the Prevention of Blindness says that over three-fourths of the funds raised each year are used in this way. Less than a quarter is used for administrative expenses. The breakdown is similar for the American Cancer Society.

Problems

The voluntary health organizations provide vital services to the comprehensive community health program. However, they do encounter special problems. Often there is a tendency to duplicate services and programming when a community is served by several agencies. An example is the antismoking program. At least three national voluntary health organizations found in most communities—the American Cancer Society, the American Heart Association, and the American Lung Association—are involved in programs to combat smoking.

Another problem facing the voluntary health agency is economics. As the federal and state governments become involved in health care programs, increased funding through taxation has been necessary. This often results in decreased money being provided by the public. Tax law changes in 1986 which have eliminated tax deductions for contributions to nonprofit organziations for some individuals may have a negative effect on income for the voluntary health organizations.

In spite of the problems facing voluntary health organizations today, they have and will continue to have a vital role to play in the community health programs of our nation. Possibly you, as a citizen, may become involved in a voluntary health organization. Volunteers are always needed, and financial support is never refused by such agencies.

Philanthropic Foundations

There are more than three thousand philanthropic foundations in the United States. These are nonprofit funding foundations in the private sector that support a broad range of educational, humanitarian, social health, and social services. Millions of dollars are distributed annually by these organizations for the support of projects and activities. Health has been the subject of specific interest to several foundations. This interest usually results in the provision of health care to people in medically underserved areas, and in health program planning, development, and research.

The role that foundations play in the support of health and social service programs in the United States has increased as government, particularly the federal government, has reduced its commitment in these areas. Not only are many elected officials unhappy with the level of government involvement, but citizens have also become displeased and frustrated with "big government" and the inability of government programming to meet basic needs. Emphasizing the renewed role of the foundations in this political atmosphere, the president of the Rockefeller Foundation stated in his 1980 annual report, ". . . any substantial withdrawal of government services, or even a markedly increased reluctance on the part of government to provide new ones, will confront foundations with a sharpened need to . . . reassess their priorities."[2] This statement amplifies the important role of the foundations in community health program support and involvement in the years ahead.

Rockefeller Foundation

One of America's largest foundations is the Rockefeller Foundation. Since its establishment in 1913, this foundation has appropriated $1.5 billion in support of projects throughout the world.[3] The principal objective of this foundation is the reduction of human suffering and need.

As a means of achieving this goal, public health measures have long been an important focus of this foundation. The development of public health programs and support of disease eradication programs for such diseases as hookworm, yaws, schistosomiasis, malaria, and yellow fever, were some of the early foundation activities. Today the foundation's scope of interest, plus funding, has broadened to include

the arts, humanities, and international relations. But activities designed to alleviate and solve the problem of worldwide hunger are still vital Rockefeller Foundation programs.

The "conquest of hunger" program involves a number of Latin American and Asian projects designed to increase food production and distribution. In addition, agricultural research focusing upon plant breeding and control of animal diseases is an important part of the hunger program.

The Rockefeller Foundation has long had an interest in the problem of population growth. Presently, the program established to study this problem has three components:[4]

1. research in reproductive biology
2. research on new contraceptive technology, and
3. policy studies to understand the determinants and consequences of fertility and the socioeconomic factors affecting population.

During its seventy years of existence, the foundation has supported a number of programs designed to control diseases. Though communicable diseases are no longer the serious problem they once were in the United States, they still afflict millions of people worldwide, particularly in the Third World. Malaria, trypanosomiasis, and child diarrhea are examples of diseases that this foundation is studying. Specifically, biomedical research to develop a malaria vaccine and to study infant diarrhea in Haiti has been supported by the Rockefeller Foundation.

Particularly in the Third World nations, the foundation has supported educational training programs for such primary health workers as epidemiologists, laboratory technicians, and nurse practitioners. In addition to basic biomedical research and training programs, the Rockefeller Foundation has funded field studies in many parts of the world. These studies have involved pharmacology, biochemistry, and clinical field work.

Henry J. Kaiser Family Foundation

This foundation has supported many programs in health and medicine since it was established in 1948. In fact, the annual fund distribution exceeds $10 million.[5] This foundation was established by industrialist Henry J. Kaiser and his wife out of concern for the unmet health care needs of many in our society. This foundation has set five specific program outcomes for support: (1) research, (2) development of new health care approaches, (3) application of innovative methods of health care, (4) project evaluation, and (5) dissemination of information to improve health care.[6]

Present initiatives of this foundation are to provide support for programs that are designed to improve primary health care. Monies from this foundation are used to encourage the expansion of health maintenance organizations. Scholarships for minority students in medicine and dentistry are made available. In addition, planning, delivery, and improvement of health care receive financial support. Another area of increased support has been encouraging creative efforts focused on health needs of the elderly, particularly the frail elderly. The Henry J. Kaiser Family Foundation usually does not finance institutional construction or laboratory or clinical research activities.

The Robert Wood Johnson Foundation

Supporting projects designed to improve access to health care, this foundation was established in 1972 from the estate of General Robert Wood Johnson. Since its beginning, the foundation has given over $400 million to a variety of institutions and programs.[7] In 1986 alone, over $94.6 million was provided.

The Robert Wood Johnson Foundation funds are allotted to projects having one of three principal interests (figure 8.1):

1. to improve access to personal health care for underserved populations,

Figure 8.1 Funding activity of the Robert Wood Johnson Foundation

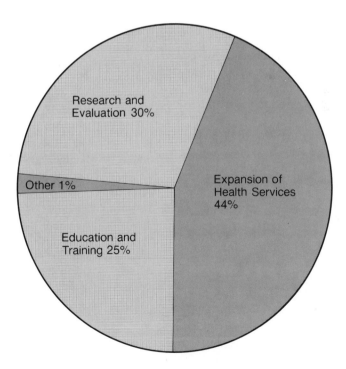

School-Based Programs Supported by Robert Wood Johnson Foundation

National Preventive Dentistry Demonstration Program

$10 million project

School-based preventive dental health project involving 25,000 children in grades 1 through 8 in ten different geographic settings

School Nurse Practitioner Program

$6.5 million project in four different states

Designed to improve children's access to health care by expanding the opportunity for services available at school

Project Results:

1. Medically underserved children gained access to care they did not have before.
2. Much untreated illness was found, such as anemia, ear infection, and scoliosis.
3. Number of fully immunized students increased.
4. Ninety-six percent of health problems identified were followed up with appropriate medical care.

Source: Annual Report, 1985, Robert Wood Johnson Foundation, P.O. Box 2316, Princeton, N.J. 08540

2. to make health care more effective and affordable, and
3. to help people maintain or regain maximum function in their lives.

The goal of improving access to health care has recently been directed toward the chronically mentally ill, the uninsured, and children and the elderly. Funds have also been provided to support community health centers.

The foundation has been interested in research, project development, and demonstration projects as means of attaining these goals. Grants have been made available to a number of hospitals for the purpose of developing primary care group practices. Many people, particularly the disadvantaged, depend on a local hospital as the primary source of health care. The objective of primary care group practices in hospital settings is to offer preventive health care to these individuals.

Research interests have centered upon the health and medical status of black Americans. This foundation has also supported research directed at identifying factors associated with teenage pregnancy.

Another important health need funded by the Robert Wood Johnson Foundation is a program that expands and strengthens the inner-city health service programs developed and operated by municipal governments. Access to health care in rural areas has also received support from this foundation. Efforts to develop nonprofit group medical practices in these medically underserved localities have been financed.

Institutions that train professionals in primary health care have been supported by this foundation. The foundation has supported primary care training programs for nurses—especially faculty education—and for emergency care nurses. It has also encouraged the preparation of rural nurse practitioners, the preparation of physicians for careers in family practice, and training programs for physicians' assistants. Funds have also been generated to help establish a graduate program at a midwestern university to prepare speech and language pathologists to pursue careers in treatment of infants at risk for communication disorders.

In Latin America, community health projects funded by the W. K. Kellogg Foundation are helping to bring medical care to urban and rural communities alike. Efforts are concentrating on infectious diseases, unsanitary living conditions, dental caries, outdated medical curricula and practices, and basic inaccessibility of health services.

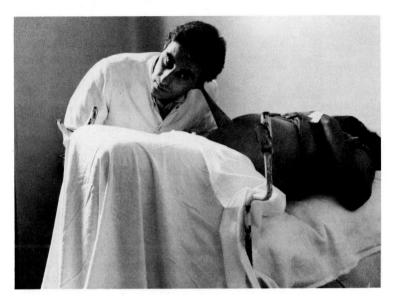

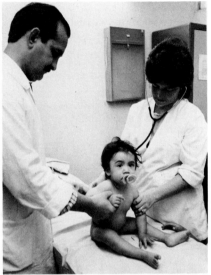

Foundation concerns also include the health needs of children. This interest has resulted in the development of a school health service system, a preventive dentistry demonstration program for school-age children, and a program designed to improve health services activities in the schools in four states.

W. K. Kellogg Foundation

This foundation also supports health programs. W. K. Kellogg, upon creating this foundation in 1930, said that its objective was to "help people to help themselves." The foundation continues to pursue this objective today. Its support is limited to activities in agriculture, education, and health. In addition to supporting programs in the United States and Canada, the Kellogg Foundation funds "help people help themselves" in Latin America, Australia, and selected European countries. The foundation does not fund research efforts; rather, it supports projects that apply existing knowledge to specific needs.

Foundation support for health includes programs that fall into four categories:

1. programs that enhance the comprehensiveness and continuity of health care;
2. activities and projects that are aimed at cost containment and increased productivity of health care;
3. activities related to health promotion, disease prevention, and public health efforts; and
4. efforts to assure quality health care and health professional education.[8]

The programs designed to enhance the comprehensive nature of health care include the establishment of several holistic health centers. Those programs designed to cut costs offer grants to hospitals to combine the skills of several health care providers into a single service.

The foundation's interest in health promotion, disease prevention, and public health has resulted in programs for several different populations. One such project was the development of a secondary school health education curriculum in a New England community. Other projects have involved nursing education and medical school family practice programs. Yet another project supported by the Kellogg Foundation involved the diffusion of health promotion activities to the inhabitants of one midwestern state.

Funds are provided by this foundation for improving access to and availability of health care. One such program supports the continuing education of the nurse practitioners who serve rural regions of the country.

Several health problems are also of interest to the Kellogg Foundation. One project educated physicians on the value of prescribing fluoride supplements for children. This project used film, audio cassettes, and printed literature to inform these physicians about the benefits of fluoride use in preventing tooth decay.

The Kellogg Foundation encourages dental health in foreign countries, too. Foundation-funded programs in Colombia, Brazil, Costa Rica, Mexico, and Bolivia focus on dental education and service in university dental schools.

One can see that this foundation actively supports a number of programs. Some funds help in the establishment of programs. Other monies provide for the enlargement of already existing projects. Demonstration projects, continuing education activities, and curriculum development and improvement are of special interest to this foundation. These programs are costly, too. Since its founding, the Kellogg Foundation has distributed over $532 million.[9] In 1985, expenditures exceeded $74 million, with over 50 percent supporting these health-related projects.

Ford Foundation

Major program focus of the Ford Foundation has been directed at problems of urban and rural poverty. An increasing emphasis of this foundation has been on the problem of teenage pregnancy among the poor, and support of activities designed to reduce infant mortality and childhood sickness. Funds have been provided to develop prevention projects to help children in middle school avoid pregnancy. The emphasis has been upon educational programs that help students make responsible choices about sexual behavior.

The Ford Foundation is currently interested in improving health, nutrition, and intellectual development of poor children in the United States. Community outreach workers contact women early in their pregnancies and help them obtain appropriate health care and nutritional information. For example, in rural Appalachia paraprofessional home visitors are used to advise expectant mothers regarding prenatal care, breast-feeding, and infant development.

The problem of population growth has been another interest of the Ford Foundation. Various programs that are designed to improve family planning and fertility control methods, research to develop new methods of contraception, and information dissemination programs have been supported by this foundation.

In addition, the Ford Foundation has supported field projects in several Third World nations to provide a safe, effective water supply.

Metropolitan Life Foundation

Established in 1976 to support philanthropic organizations and activities, the Metropolitan Life Foundation's only source of funds is the Metropolitan Life Insurance Company. Foundation funding is allocated to several health programs. In 1980, nearly $492 thousand was disbursed to support programs in four health categories: (1) health education, (2) health care planning and cost containment, (3) research and illness prevention, and (4) safety.[10]

The major portion of these funds was used for the medical school education of minority students, for nursing scholarships, and for the growth and development of public health education. Another health education activity funded by this foundation has been the support of college health information and service programs for students. Health topics explored in these programs include alcohol abuse, wellness, and health hazards. Nutrition education—especially in medical schools, in elementary schools, and for the elderly—is also funded.

In a program called "Healthy Me," the Metropolitan Life Foundation has awarded grants to some forty school districts for the promotion of comprehensive school health education programs. This program has emphasized comprehensive health education covering several different grades and subjects, and has encouraged the establishment of positive health habits. These programs have included the development of activity-centered learning settings, emphasis on the development of decision-making skills, the use of computer programs to analyze health practices, and the use of a variety of resources and teaching methods.

The Metropolitan Life Foundation funding in the other three categories (health care planning and cost containment, research, and safety) tends to be less than that for health education. Most grants for programs in these areas are less than five thousand dollars.

Corporate Health Programs

Business and industry are also active in health services and health promotion activities. The basic emphasis of these programs is the improvement of the health and well-being of employees and their families. Therefore, the available services are usually limited to a select group of people associated with the specific company. The employees and their families, not the general public, are the benefactors. These programs include such health promotion activities and classes as smoking cessation, alcohol usage, stress reduction, fitness, hypertension screening, diet and weight control, and other health-related topics. Increasingly, large businesses and industries are developing exercise facilities for employees to use. These facilities include running tracks, weight and conditioning equipment, and aerobic exercise programs. (A more complete discussion of these programs is presented in chapter 18.)

Some companies, however, do provide health-related activities for the general public. In many cases these services are educational, and quite often they are designed to promote a product, as is the case with various food industries. These companies often provide nutrition education materials and programs for the general public or for selected population groups, such as the elderly or school-age children.

Though health promotion is certainly an objective of such programming, product marketing is also accomplished. Regardless of the motive, a number of industries have played a useful role in promoting good health within the community.

National Dairy Council

This organization has been active in developing nutrition education materials and programs. Specific emphasis has been devoted to curriculum development and teaching materials for classroom use.

The National Dairy Council has developed an elementary school curriculum entitled "Food . . . Your Choice," which has been popular in many school districts. This curriculum consists of six sequential levels. Each level presents nutrition education material for the specific grade (1–6), and is designed to provide learning experiences that help the children to make proper nutrition decisions. The National Dairy Council also has three nutrition education programs for use in grades 7 through 10. Each program is prepared to be used in various content subjects: i.e., social studies, home economics, and health.

Metropolitan Life Insurance Company

Another company involved in health and safety education programs is the Metropolitan Life Insurance Company. Many publications and materials have been developed and disseminated by the Health and Safety Education Division of this company. In addition, a number of public service messages on various health and safety subjects are prepared.

A document prepared and distributed monthly by this company is the *Statistical Bulletin*. This publication includes information on such topics as longevity and accidents. The information is useful to many organizations and individuals involved in community health planning and program development.

In communities throughout North Carolina, a project to improve the health of southern blacks is being headed by the General Baptist State Convention of North Carolina, Inc. (GBSC), with support from the W. K. Kellogg Foundation. With the help of the medical profession, the GBSC is training pastors and lay leaders in churches throughout the state to convey vital health information to their congregations.

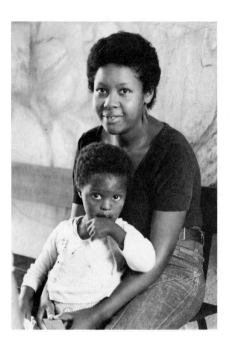

Religious Organizations

Also playing important roles in health programing in many areas are religious organizations. Interest is usually focused on health care in a given locality for a special population group, such as people located in a rural mountain community where there are inadequate resources to meet certain health or other personal needs. Religious organizations have also been active in meeting the social needs of the poor living in inner-city locations. In an attempt to help inner-city teenagers cope with problems of substance abuse, some churches have established drug counseling and rehabilitation programs. In Washington, D.C., with the support of the Ford Foundation funds, one church has operated a community service center. This center was established to help young black males enhance their health, education, and self-esteem.[11]

In addition Ford Foundation grants have been provided to church organizations to prepare materials on teen pregnancy, sex education, and family values. Youth conferences focusing on these matters have also been conducted.

Many relief efforts are designed, administered, and carried out by religious organizations. In situations where a natural catastrophe has occurred, the personnel and services of these organizations move into the area and provide needed medical assistance.

Throughout the United States many hospitals, nursing homes, and other health care institutions are operated by religious groups. The largest number are operated by the Roman Catholic Church. In addition numerous protestant denominations and Jewish religious centers have developed and operate health care facilities.

The increased numbers of homeless individuals in the United States have resulted in the need for increased shelter and food sources. Many religious

Numerous health care facilities, such as (a) some of the largest medical centers in major cities, and (b) nursing homes, are operated by religious orders, agencies, and denominations.

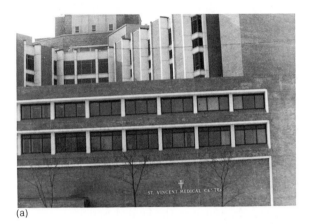

(a)

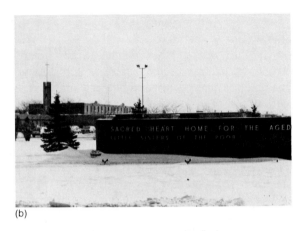

(b)

organizations have developed "soup kitchens" to feed the homeless. These facilities are often the only places where the homeless can come for food and for protection from inclement weather conditions.

Several religious agencies have also been involved in helping refugees relocate in the United States. Usually sponsors—individuals or interested church groups—are found to assist the refugee family upon their arrival in this country.

Many more religion-sponsored programs in the health sector are carried out in countries other than the United States. Health care provision has been a major goal of missionary agencies. The health clinic, nurse, and medical missionary provide health care to many people, particularly in the Third World. In recent years such agencies have become involved in coordinating rural community development projects, including health care, preventive health, and agriculture.

With the increased interest in health promotion in the United States, churches, mosques, synagogues, and other religious facilities provide strong potential as sites for health promotion activities.[12] Several reasons can be given for the effectiveness of churches as agencies in health promotion:

1. Religious organizations are a type of organization that is found in nearly every community.
2. Religious organizations are able to draw on the important role of volunteerism to carry out their program activities.
3. Religious organizations can have an influence on whole families.
4. Religious organizations usually own facilities that have space for use in health programming.[13]

Summary

The private sector plays an important role in community health. With reduced government spending for health and social service programs, the activities sponsored and funded by nongovernmental agencies and organizations have taken on increasing importance. Four private-sector groups are involved in the health field: (1) voluntary health organizations, (2) private philanthropic foundations, (3) business and industry, and (4) religious organizations.

Though voluntary health organizations differ in emphasis, size, and organizational structure, there are some similarities between them. All are funded by nongovernment sources. They are administered by a board of directors with a professional staff that conducts the day-to-day activities of the agency. In addition, volunteer workers provide professional services, supportive services, and fund-raising activities.

The activities of most voluntary health organizations include provision of health services, support for research, both general public and professional educational programs, and service as a lobby agent in the legislative process. Fund-raising efforts include a variety of activities, including media coverage. In addition, many athletic events, charity performances, and community fund-raising campaigns are conducted to raise money.

A number of philanthropic foundations provide funding for the planning and development of health care projects. Support is usually allocated for services to people residing in medically underserved localities. Biomedical research activities and both medical professional and general community health education programs also receive support from the foundations.

The business and industrial community conducts various health programs, most often for the benefit of the employee and his or her family. Increasingly, corporations have been developing health promotion programs.

Though not nearly as extensive nor as well known, various religious organizations play an important role in community health programming. Activities include the operation of health care facilities such as hospitals and nursing homes, assisting in relief and disaster efforts, and organizing refugee placement in the United States.

Discussion Questions

1. Discuss the role that the private sector plays in community health programming in the United States.
2. How does a voluntary health organization differ from an official governmental health organization?
3. What types of health services are provided by the various voluntary health organizations?
4. Identify the advances in medicine and health care made by private-sector-funded research through the years.
5. Discuss the differences and similarities in programming between three voluntary health organizations.
6. In what ways do voluntary agencies work with the legislature in health-related legislation?
7. How are funds raised to support voluntary health organizations?
8. Identify three different foundations with specific interest in health programming.
9. What are some of the differences between a voluntary health organization and a philanthropic foundation?
10. Discuss various ways in which the philanthropic foundations interested in health have become involved in primary health care.
11. Should private industries push their products with the educational promotions they make available to the schools and to the public? Explain your answer.
12. What roles in community health programming do religious agencies play in your community?
13. Why are religious organizations often effective community agencies to provide primary health care?
14. How do religious organizations and the philanthropic foundations work together to improve the health of certain population groups in our communities?

Suggested Readings

Hatch, John, and others. "The Fitness Through Churches Project." *Hygie* 5, no. 3 (1986): 9-12.

Lasater, Thomas M., and others. "The Role of Churches in Disease Prevention Research Studies." *Public Health Reports* 101, no. 2 (March/April, 1986): 125-31.

Shapes, Cecil G. "Review of the National Preventive Dentistry Demonstration Program." *American Journal of Public Health* 76, no. 4 (April, 1986): 434-45.

Tobin, Sheldon S., and others. "Enhancing CMHC and Church Collaboration for the Elderly." *Community Mental Health Journal* 21, no. 1 (Spring, 1985): 58-61.

Westberg, Granger E. "Churches Should Get (Back) into Health Care." *Journal of Holistic Medicine* 2, no. 1 (Spring/Summer, 1980): 40-43.

Endnotes

1. Information provided by the District Office, Muscular Dystrophy Association, Toledo, Ohio.

2. Lyman, R. W. "The President's Review." In *The President's Review and Annual Report, 1980.* New York: The Rockefeller Foundation, 18.

3. Ibid., 24.

4. Ibid., 71.

5. Information provided in correspondence with the Henry J. Kaiser Family Foundation, 525 Middleford Road, Menlo Park, California 94025.

6. Annual Report, Henry J. Kaiser Family Foundation, 1985.

7. Information provided in correspondence with the Robert Wood Johnson Foundation, P.O. Box 2316, Princeton, New Jersey 08540.

8. *W. K. Kellogg Foundation: 1980 Annual Report.* Battle Creek, Michigan, 1981.

9. Information provided in correspondence with the W. K. Kellogg Foundation, Battle Creek, Michigan.

10. Information provided in correspondence with the Metropolitan Life Foundation.

11. Ford Foundation Report.

12. Lasater, Thomas M., and others. "The Role of Churches in Disease Prevention Research Studies." *Public Health Reports* 101, no. 2 (March/April, 1986): 125-31.

13. Ibid., 126.

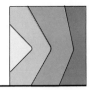

UNIT THREE

Community Health Programming

9

Disease Control: Concern for Both Communicable and Chronic Diseases

Leading Causes of Death, United States

1900	1980s
1. Influenza and Pneumonia	1. Heart Disease
2. Tuberculosis	2. Cancer
3. Diarrhea and Related Diseases	3. Stroke
4. Heart Disease	4. Accidents
5. Stroke	5. Influenza and Pneumonia

Source: Division of Vital Statistics, National Center for Health Statistics, Washington, D.C.

Ten Leading Causes of Death and Related Risk Factors, 1980s

Cause of Death	Risk Factors
1. Heart Disease	Smoking, Diet, Lack of Exercise, Hypertension, Stress
2. Cancer	Smoking, Diet, Environmental Carcinogens
3. Stroke	Smoking, Diet, Hypertension, Stress
4. Accidents (Excluding Motor Vehicle)	Alcohol, Smoking (Fires), Drug Use
5. Influenza and Pneumonia	Smoking, Vaccination Status
6. Accidents (Motor Vehicle)	Alcohol, Speed, Nonuse of Safety Restraints
7. Diabetes	Obesity
8. Cirrhosis of Liver	Alcohol
9. Arteriosclerosis	Diet (Elevated Serum Cholesterol)
10. Suicide	Stress, Alcohol, and Drug Abuse

Source: Department of Health and Human Services, *Report of the Office of Disease Prevention and Health Promotion,* Washington, D.C., 1980.

A significant change in disease patterns in the United States has occurred during the 1900s. At the turn of the century, communicable diseases were the principal health problems, causing serious illness and death. Today many of these once common communicable diseases are no longer a threat. In fact, chronic diseases, not communicable diseases, are now the major health problem faced by millions of people.

Chronic diseases cause long-term problems and are closely related to personal life-style, to environmental hazards, and, in some instances, to inherited biological characteristics. Often the exact cause of a chronic disease is unknown since a specific organism cannot be isolated as is the case with a communicable disease. The risk factors associated with most chronic conditions, however, are identifiable in some, though not all, chronic diseases. Usually the risk factors that are unidentifiable affected the individual's health long before the signs of the disease actually appeared.

An analysis of the leading causes of death proves that chronic diseases now pose a more serious health threat to most Americans than communicable diseases. Today the four leading causes of death are (1) heart disease, (2) cancer, (3) stroke, and (4) accidents. By comparison, the three most life-threatening diseases in 1900 were (1) influenza and pneumonia, (2) tuberculosis, and (3) diarrhea and related diseases.[1] The latter diseases, though still health problems among certain populations, are not a serious concern for most Americans today. Safe drinking water, public water purification systems, and public sanitation systems have effected this change.

Tuberculosis has been reduced significantly in this century. In 1900, it was the second leading cause of death; today it ranks twentieth.[2] Tuberculosis is a little-known ailment to much of American society though the economically disadvantaged, with their poor living conditions, still experience the disease.

Of the three leading causes of death in 1900, only influenza and pneumonia still rank high—fifth—as a cause of death today. For the general population influenza and pneumonia do not pose a serious threat because medication and good personal health care normally counter them. For the elderly whose general health has declined, influenza and pneumonia pose serious threats.

Disease Organisms

Communicable diseases are caused by small living organisms, plant or animal, that are invisible except when viewed through a microscope. These organisms, referred to as microorganisms, or microbes, are found in the body and throughout the environment. Many microorganisms play important roles in the maintenance of good health and in the stability of ecosystems. For example, microbes in the digestive tract aid digestion, and microorganisms in the soil increase fertility by causing decay.

Some microorganisms, known as pathogens, invade the human body and cause disease. This invasion can occur in several different ways. The pathogen may enter the host through a wound or a break in the skin; the microorganism can be transmitted from an infected animal to a human host; or infection can be spread from one person to another.

The major pathogenic microorganisms are bacteria, viruses, fungi, protozoa, rickettsiae, and metazoa. *Bacteria* are small, single-cell microorganisms that are visible only under a microscope and appear in three different shapes: (1) spiral, (2) spherical, and (3) rod. They constitute the most common cause of human disease. Diseases caused by bacteria include cholera, diphtheria, gonorrhea, syphilis, tetanus, typhoid fever, trench mouth, tuberculosis, and yaws. In addition to the many communicable diseases caused by bacteria, infection also results from this pathogenic microorganism.

The *virus* is the smallest pathogen. It can only be seen with an electron microscope and relies upon other living cells to complete its life cycle. Viruses are found in various sizes and shapes. They are known to cause the common cold, influenza, measles, rabies, smallpox, chicken pox, polio, yellow fever, herpes, and Acquired Immune Deficiency Syndrome (AIDS).

Fungi are plantlike organisms that vary in size from a single cell to large multicellular structures such as mushrooms and toadstools. They include yeasts and molds, and, because they contain no chlorophyll, they do not carry on photosynthesis. As a result, the fungus lives on or in another organism. This type of relationship is termed *parasitism*.

Fungal infection results in two types of diseases: (1) superficial skin diseases that affect the skin and hair, such as athlete's foot and ringworm of the scalp, limbs, or trunk, and (2) systemic infections of the respiratory and intestinal tract. Systemic infections can be very serious and occasionally fatal. Histoplasmosis and blastomycosis are systemic fungal infections. Another mycosis, candidiasis, affects the skin and mucous membranes of various parts of the body. Lesions caused by this fungus appear in the mouth, vagina, urinary tract, and in other parts of the body where moisture that favors growth of the fungus is present.

A single-cell microscopic animal form is known as *protozoon.* Though microscopic, the protozoa are larger than bacteria and some forms even feed on bacteria. Pathogenic protozoa in humans cause several diseases, the most common of which is malaria. Dysentery and African sleeping sickness are other communicable diseases caused by protozoa.

Rickettsiae, small microorganisms that resemble bacteria and viruses, are usually transmitted to animals and humans by fleas, lice, or ticks. These microorganisms are smaller than bacteria and grow within the cells of the host. Rocky Mountain Spotted Fever and Q fever are diseases caused by this pathogen.

Typhus is another disease caused by a rickettsia (*Rickettsia Prowazeki*). This disease is spread by the body louse. Lice become infected when they feed on the blood of a person with typhus fever and then transmit the microorganism to another person through their feces. The lice usually defecate at the time of feeding. The individual becomes infected by rubbing the feces and crushed lice into the body through the wounds made by the bites.[3] Treatment requires medical care with administration of appropriate drug therapy. Measures to prevent an outbreak of typhus include improved sanitation, insecticide use to reduce lice, and frequent bathing and washing of clothes. Immunization for typhus is available and recommended for individuals living and traveling in high-risk areas.

Multicellular animals (*metazoa*) that infect humans are parasitic in nature. One example is *helminths.* These pathogens, not considered microorganisms, usually enter the body when the human consumes food and fluids containing them. Tapeworms in beef and pork are examples of this pathogen.

Natural Disease Defense

The human body has several natural defenses against disease-causing organisms. The skin and mucous membrane linings of the body serve as barriers to microorganisms. Thus, a cut or wound that interferes with this barrier can result in an invasion of the body by pathogens. The cilia of the respiratory system help to keep disease-causing organisms from entering the lungs. In the digestive system, the acidity of the stomach is resistant to pathogenic microorganisms. In the bloodstream the leukocytes destroy foreign organisms; and lysozyme, a chemical found in human tears and saliva, dissolves the cell walls of certain bacteria.

When illness and infection are present, the body temperature often rises. This elevated body temperature is also an important protection against pathogens. High body temperature or fever tends to have a negative effect on the pathogen's ability to carry on normal metabolism. As a result, body temperatures above one hundred degrees Farenheit counter the disease-causing ability of pathogens.

A newborn infant is able to resist disease as ably as its mother. This immunity is obtained directly from the mother as maternal antibodies (protein substances) cross through the placental membranes and enter the baby's blood. This protection is potent for only a short period of time. As a result, it is important for infants to begin receiving immunization at about two to three months of age.

Immunity

Resistance to the pathogenic microorganism of a disease is known as immunity. In the presence of specific disease-causing microorganisms, the body produces antibodies. These antibodies neutralize and destroy the pathogens and, as a result, the individual overcomes the illness. This human ability to produce antibodies is referred to as natural acquired immunity, and is often obtained when a person has a given disease. The body produces the antibodies to counter the infection, and when the pathogens for the disease invade the body, the antibodies immediately function and the individual does not develop the signs and symptoms of the disease.

Immunity without contracting the disease is acquired by *immunization.* Immunization involves administering a vaccine containing preparations of killed or weakened strain of the pathogenic microorganism. With the introduction of this vaccine, the body produces antibodies without the observable signs and symptoms of the disease. Toxoids are also used to provide immunity against disease. Toxoids are preparations of altered bacterial poisons or toxins that do not cause the disease.

Immunization is a widely accepted disease-control procedure in the United States. Vaccines have been developed for such diseases as diphtheria, pertussis (whooping cough), polio, mumps, rubella (German measles), rubeola (measles), tetanus, typhus, yellow fever, cholera, plague, and rabies. Some vaccines have also been developed for influenza and pneumococcal pneumonia.

For certain diseases, often referred to as the "childhood diseases," all fifty states require immunization before the child is permitted to enter school. The immunizations most commonly required for school admittance include those for diphtheria, pertussis, tetanus, mumps, polio, measles, and German measles. In the past, smallpox vaccination had been included in this listing, but is no longer a requirement. The worldwide eradication of smallpox led to the recommendation by the World Health Organization and the medical profession that this vaccination was no longer needed.

In 1921 there were more than 200,000 cases of diphtheria—with about 5 percent being fatal—in the United States. The effectiveness of immunization for this disease can be seen by noting that in 1984 there was only one case reported, this being a sixty-six-year-old female.[4] For the past ten years there has been an average of ninety cases of tetanus a year. Two out of every three have been reported among individuals over fifty years of age.[5] The importance of this can be seen when one realizes that the protective levels for tetanus immunizations last for about ten years.

It is important that children begin to receive the immunizations as infants. Most medical doctors recommend that babies be given the first DPT (diphtheria, pertussis, and tetanus) immunization and the first oral polio feeding as early as two to three months of age. Unfortunately, many parents fail to have their children immunized as recommended. This is particularly true among the economically disadvantaged. Because of the cost of the injections, many simply do not have it done. In some poor inner-city areas, the government estimates that the immunization rate is less than half.

Many children, particularly the poor, are immunized at the local health department or community health center. Funding for these programs has been made available through various federal programs. As funding has been reduced for these programs, many are concerned that the national level of immunization of children may become a serious health problem.

It is important that mothers of newborn infants receive instruction about immunization schedules. Education of the public should help to increase the percentage of children who are immunized. Also, school immunization regulations must be enforced. In many communities, children are permitted to enroll and attend school when they have not had the full complement of injections.

Adult Immunization

In 1985 a report of the immunization committee of the American College of Physicians reported the importance of giving attention to the immunization of adults.[6] Most individuals fail to consider the necessity of checking their personal immunization records as they reach adulthood. The Centers for Disease Control reports that many American adults are not protected against communicable diseases for which there are appropriate, effective immunizations. Not only does this include the traditional childhood diseases such as diphtheria, tetanus, measles, mumps, and polio, but also hepatitis and influenza.

Adults should receive ten-year boosters for diphtheria and tetanus. Many adults have not been vaccinated for rubella and rubeola nor have they had the disease. This is particularly important for young adults, as was seen in 1985 when outbreaks of measles occurred on a number of college campuses throughout the nation.

Adult cases account for 86 percent of all instances of Hepatitis B, yet vaccine is available to provide protection. This vaccine should be given to health care workers who are at risk for hepatitis. A series of three doses is assumed to be satisfactory for giving lifetime protection. A major barrier to the use of this vaccine is that it is rather expensive. If an individual is planning to travel abroad to areas where polio is endemic it is necessary to be completely protected for this communicable disease.

Immunizations among the elderly for influenza and pneumonia should also be of concern. Standard procedure is that anyone over sixty-five years of age should be given yearly influenza shots, as should other people with such chronic health conditions as heart disease, lung disorders, and diabetes. These vaccines are usually made available through local health departments, medical care facilities, and individual physicians.

Respiratory Diseases

Respiratory illnesses, especially if acute, are frequently the cause of short-term debilitation and sickness. It is estimated that as many as 250 million people fall victim to acute respiratory diseases each year in the United States.[7] These illnesses account for a minimum of 400 million days in bed, 125 million days lost from work, and 125 million days of absence from school.[8]

Respiratory infections follow a similar pattern. Each begins when the pathogenic microorganism, the virus, or bacteria, invades the host. The period from this time of invasion until the first appearance of symptoms is known as the *incubation period*. The incubation period varies in length from one disease to another. It may last only a day or two, as in the case of the common cold and influenza, or, as with rubella and rubeola, have a much longer incubation period. Because there are no disease symptoms during the incubation period, the individual is unaware of infection. As a result, the person will continue to work or attend school, continuing with an active routine and so spreading infectious organisms to others.

The symptoms of respiratory infections vary. However, the initial symptoms are usually fever, chills, headache, sweating, and general aches and pains. These symptoms occur for only a short period of time, known as the *prodromal period*. This period ends when the specific disease symptoms appear. During the prodromal period the respiratory

infection is very contagious. For effective disease control, individuals experiencing symptoms of a slight cold should be kept away from school, work, and other locations where the disease could spread to others.

As the specific disease signs and symptoms develop to their fullest intensity, the *acme stage* of the disease is reached.[9] The disease is communicable during this stage although the patient is usually not well enough to move in settings where the disease can be easily spread. The individual is either home in bed or hospitalized, and under the care of a physician.

The defense mechanism of the body, the development of antibodies, and various drug therapies reduce the effect of the pathogens. In many instances the sick person also receives treatment for specific symptoms—fever, sore throat, or chills.

The last stage of a respiratory disease is the *convalescence stage*. During this time the disease subsides and the host's body returns to normal. There are times after recovery, however, when the host may still be a reservoir of infection. Even though there is no outward indication of the disease, the host may be a *carrier* of the pathogenic microorganisms and is capable of transmitting the disease to another human host. During this stage the overall body resistance is also weakened. If the person is not particularly careful, a relapse can occur. For this reason, the patient should not return to work or school until certain that the infection is no longer present.

There are numerous respiratory diseases that affect people of all ages, races, and localities. The common cold, influenza, and pneumonia are examples of those infectious respiratory diseases that cause a great deal of illness and debilitation.

Common Cold

Possibly the most prevalent respiratory disease is the common cold, which is caused by a number of different viruses classified as rhinoviruses. The common cold is a highly contagious disease of the upper respiratory tract, affecting particularly the nose and throat. The pathogens involved can be easily transmitted to another individual by coughing, sneezing, talking, and even breathing.

The incubation period of the common cold is from one to three days, and the greatest period of communicability is at the onset of the disease. However, the length of illness varies, often lasting up to two or more weeks.

The principal care and treatment of a person with the common cold involves symptom relief. Bed rest and liquids are usually recommended. Aspirin may be helpful in relief of fever and pain, although there is no drug therapy that will cure the common cold. Antibiotics, such as penicillin, are not effective against the viruses.

Though some measures can be taken to prevent the common cold from developing there is no guarantee of protection. Vaccination is ineffective because of the number of viruses (possibly one hundred or more) that cause colds; protection against one virus does not protect against all others.

Influenza

Another infectious respiratory illness is influenza, which is more severe than the common cold. Four different types of viruses cause influenza. These viruses are spread by direct contact (as by kissing) and by the common use of objects, such as cups, glasses, and towels. The influenza viruses are most likely transmitted by droplets on these objects that have been expelled by coughing, sneezing, and breathing.

The influenza incubation period is from one to two days. The early symptoms include high fever (101 to 104 degrees F), chills, headache, sore throat, aches and pains, and exhaustion. In addition, a dry cough may appear.

Influenza often occurs in epidemic patterns in a specific geographical area. Historically, pandemics (worldwide incidences) of influenza have caused the death of millions of people. It is estimated that the influenza pandemic in 1918 caused the death of more than twenty-one million people. But such widespread epidemics have been reduced with the development of vaccines that are effective in the prevention and control of influenza. Public health policy today is to vaccinate those populations at greatest risk: the aged, those with chronic diseases, and individuals with other respiratory problems.

The normal treatment for influenza includes bed rest, plentiful liquids, regular doses of aspirin, and warmth. As with the common cold, the use of drugs is not effective in combating the influenza viruses.

Pneumonia

The fifth leading cause of death is pneumonia combined with influenza. Approximately 2.4 million cases of pneumonia occur each year, causing an estimated 57,000 deaths.[10]

Pneumonia is an acute inflammation of the lungs caused by bacteria, viruses, or mycoplasmas. It can be an original infection or it can be the result of a complication of some other illness. For example, pneumonia often develops after a person has had the common cold or influenza. Because of lowered body resistance, the pathogenic microorganisms gain control, multiply, and spread; pneumonia develops.

The signs and symptoms of pneumonia include high fever, chills, sweating, and chest pain. In many instances breathing may be difficult and the victim may cough up colored sputum.

Treatment of bacterial and mycoplasma-caused pneumonia includes the use of antibiotics, though there is no antibiotic effective against the viral infection. As with other respiratory diseases, treatment is symptomatic. Measures are taken to lower the high body temperature caused by fever since sustained high body temperature can cause convulsions and severe brain damage. If the person is having difficulty breathing, oxygen intake must be assisted. Relief from coughing is also important, as is rest.

Prevention is extremely important in limiting the spread of the common cold, influenza, and pneumonia. Good health habits are more helpful than the use of vaccines in the prevention of these respiratory diseases. Proper diet, adequate rest, and good hygiene provide resistance to respiratory diseases. Prompt remedial action is also important whenever the initial signs of a respiratory disease appear.

Tuberculosis

One of the most feared of all respiratory diseases has been tuberculosis. At the beginning of the twentieth century tuberculosis was as dreaded as AIDS is today. This disease has caused millions of deaths since the beginning of human history. Despite the fact that tuberculosis is no longer a problem of epidemic proportion in the United States, a little over 20,000 cases are reported annually, and of these, nearly 3,000 victims die.[11] Currently the tuberculosis incidence rate is 9.4 per 100,000 population.[12] The United States government set 8 per 100,000 as the objective for the nation by the year 1990.[13] Worldwide the incidence of tuberculosis is much higher; about three million people die from tuberculosis each year.[14]

The majority of tuberculosis in the United States today is found among the elderly. Most of these individuals were infected years ago and are experiencing a recurrence of old infections. Tuberculosis is also found among recent immigrants to this country, the poor, and the homeless.

The primary cause of tuberculosis is the tubercle baccillus *mycobacterium tuberculosis.* Though this disease primarily affects the lungs, it can spread to other parts of the body, such as the bones, joints, kidneys, and skin.

There are a number of secondary causes of tuberculosis. Throughout history it has been closely associated with poverty. Tuberculosis is frequently found in overcrowded environments, locations having poor hygiene and sanitation, and in settings where there is poor ventilation. It is associated with malnutrition, inadequate sleep, and emotional stress. In the United States, tuberculosis is concentrated among the economically disadvantaged in urban ghettos, in Appalachia, among the Native American population, and in the Southwest among Hispanics.

There are two commonly used measures for detecting tuberculosis in humans: (1) the tuberculin skin test and (2) the chest X ray. The tuberculin skin test indicates the presence of the tuberculosis bacillus in the body. If the reaction is positive, it indicates that the individual has the bacillus. However, this does not indicate whether the case is active or dormant.

The chest X ray ascertains the infection's degree of activity. It is the most accurate procedure for detecting pulmonary tuberculosis as well as the extent of the development and spread of the infection.

Treatment of active tuberculosis often involves hospital inpatient care as well as extended outpatient medical supervision. The need for extended hospital care has been reduced in recent years largely due to drug treatment. The use of drugs to combat and cure tuberculosis has been very successful. Such drugs as isoniazid (INH), streptomycin, and para-aminosalicylic acid (PAS) do not kill the tubercle bacillus, but keep it from multiplying so that the body can more effectively counter the disease organism.

A vaccine, called the BCG (Bacillus-Calmette-Guerin) vaccine, has been developed for tuberculosis. This vaccine provides a degree of active immunity. It also makes the person "TB positive" and thereby destroys the usefulness of the tuberculin skin test as a diagnostic screening device. As a result, the vaccine is only used in the United States among populations at risk for tuberculosis, such as the elderly, the poor, and certain medical care providers. The BCG vaccine has been used extensively in some nations with high incidences of tuberculosis and where a large number of people have already tested positive for the disease.

Tuberculosis is a disease that is best combated by providing better living conditions for the population at risk. Improved housing and living conditions for the poor, better nutrition, and the development of positive health habits can be very effective in reducing tuberculosis incidence. It is felt that the current need is to develop better diagnostic, treatment, and preventive procedures.[15] A need exists for biotechnological development of methods that involve simple, rapid, and low cost tests to diagnose the disease.

Gastrointestinal Diseases

Many communicable diseases are spread through the gastrointestinal tract. The pathogenic microorganisms enter the individual through the digestive system—they are present in the food or water that is ingested—and usually leave the body through the feces or urine.

Worldwide, the principal cause of such diseases is impure, unsanitary water supplies. Millions of people do not have access to a pure water supply. Their basic source of drinking and cooking water is a stream used by cattle, by other members of the community for bathing and washing of clothing, and by other polluters. A number of different diseases affect people as a result of these cleanliness problems.

Dysentery affects millions of people. Unfortunately many young children and infants cannot withstand the rigors of the disease and fall victim to it. Dysentery is not as life threatening to adults as it is to the younger population.

The two most common types of dysentery are caused by bacteria (bacillary dysentery or *Shigellosis*) and protozoa (amebic dysentery or *Amebiasis*). The human serves as the reservoir of infection in both types.

There are several ways that the infection is transmitted, the most obvious of which is the ingestion of contaminated food and water. Transmission can also result by the hands coming in contact with sewage containing the cysts, or by eating uncooked vegetables, berries, and fruits that have grown on soil that was fertilized with human feces.

Some cases of dysentery, particularly bacillary dysentery, are relatively mild. However, amebic dysentery is often prolonged and can be debilitating. This form of dysentery can be exhausting because of the number and frequency of stools and the resultant dehydration. The dysentery patient should drink large amounts of noncontaminated fluids to compensate for this dehydration. Warmth is also important in the treatment of dysentery.

As with tuberculosis, the best prevention against dysentery is a more sanitary living environment including the sanitary removal of human feces. Sanitary pits are being built as part of rural community development projects in Third World nations. Protection of human water supplies against human fecal material is also a necessity. People must be educated about personal hygiene.

Sexually Transmitted Diseases

There are a number of diseases that are transmitted primarily by sexual contact. These are known as *sexually transmitted diseases (STD)* or, as they are referred to in some reports, "sexually transmissible" diseases. In the past, sexually transmitted diseases were referred to as venereal disease.

The term *venereal* comes from Venus, the Roman goddess of love. Venereal diseases were once associated with lovemaking, but since this classification does not necessarily involve lovemaking today it now is felt that the term sexually transmitted better describes this group of diseases.

A number of infections can be classified as sexually transmitted diseases, with the most common being AIDS, chlamydia, genital herpes, gonorrhea, syphilis, and trichomoniasis.

Sexually transmitted diseases cause a number of physical and economical problems for millions of people each year. If left untreated, they can cause serious complications and even debilitation since damaged or destroyed body structures cannot be replaced. Reinfection is possible with new exposure since the body does not build up an immunity to these diseases. Some sexually transmitted diseases are incurable and may affect one with pain and suffering throughout life. The cost for treatment and cure of the sexually transmitted diseases exceeds one billion dollars each year.[16]

The microorganisms that cause most of the sexually transmitted diseases have been identified. For the most part, it is relatively easy to diagnose the diseases and all but herpes are curable. Yet the National Insititute of Allergy and Infectious Disease reports that one in twenty Americans is still affected by sexually transmitted diseases.

In spite of the fact that most sexually transmitted diseases can be identified and treated, the incidences continue to rise. Among teenagers and young adults this problem is viewed as a public health epidemic. There are several reasons for this continued increase in sexually transmitted diseases, but the primary reason is the increased number of sexually active individuals in our society. Sexual activity is particularly important in the fifteen- to thirty-year age group. The sexually active individual runs the risk of becoming infected and spreading the sexually transmitted disease, particularly when sexual behavior is casual—with several different partners. Often one infected person can spread the disease to a multitude of contacts.

In spite of the increased sexual activity, most people do not understand the dangers of sexually transmitted diseases. These diseases are a topic that many people find difficult to discuss because of taboos relating to historically negative attitudes toward sexual activity, particularly intercourse. Victims find their problem demeaning, as does society in general.

Some believe that a discussion of these diseases is unwarranted, particularly in the schools. They reason that any introduction to these diseases necessitates a discussion as to how they are spread, and so is inappropriate for school-age children. As a result of this ignorance, our society continues to have a problem with these diseases.

Surgeon General C. Everett Koop in 1986, recognizing the dangerous lack of information about AIDS among the general population, called for the development of extensive school sex education programs. These programs should include instruction on AIDS. The surgeon general recommended that such instructional programs should begin as early as the primary grades.

When infected, many young people do not seek medical care. This is often due to the stigma placed upon them by their peers and also due to fear of their parents' reactions. They fear that in the eyes of their peers they will be viewed as "pimps," "prostitutes," or other social outcasts. Many do not seek treatment because they do not know the symptoms. The infected individual may attempt to treat the problem with over-the-counter drugs, none of which is effective, or may even ignore the symptoms.

The question of whether the teenager's parents should be informed that their child is being treated at a public health clinic for a sexually transmitted disease is a difficult problem. In some jurisdictions, young people below the age of sixteen or eighteen are not treated in public clinics unless the parents

are informed. But this policy discourages many young people from seeking badly needed help, since they do not wish to have their parents aware of the problem.

Many public health personnel who work with young people having sexually transmitted diseases feel that there should be no parent notification. The likelihood of the individual seeking early treatment is more probable if parents are not notified. Because of the importance of early diagnosis and treatment in protecting against permanent body organ damage the issue is one of medical, legal, and social importance.

Health Effects of STDs

The sexually transmitted diseases cause many health problems. Generally, the initial symptoms are more easily noticed in males than in females, so the male usually seeks treatment earlier in the infectious stage than does the female. The female frequently has neither clinical signs nor other complaints during the first stages of the disease, though lesions and tissue damage may occur within the vagina or the cervix at this time.

One of the most serious problems is pelvic inflammatory disease, which causes sterility in many women. This condition results when microorganisms from the vagina and endocervix ascend to the endometrium, the fallopian tubes, and other reproductive organs. There are numerous ways in which such infection can occur. For example, the intrauterine device is a risk factor for the development of pelvic inflammatory disease. Since there may be different microorganisms involved in the infection, there is no single treatment of choice. Major surgery is sometimes required, often resulting in the removal of the reproductive organs.

Syphilis and Gonorrhea

Gonorrhea and syphilis are caused by bacterial organisms. Syphilis is caused by the spirochete bacterium and gonorrhea by the gonococcus bacterium. Gonorrhea is the most frequently reported communicable disease in the United States with over

The initial indication of syphilis is a chancre. This painless sore is oval-shaped and disappears in time.

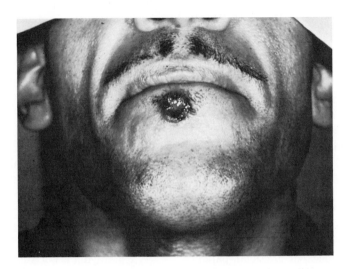

878,000 cases being reported in a recent year, while syphilis is the third most commonly reported infectious disease.[17]

Syphilis

Nearly every organ of the body can be affected by syphilis. Its incubation period ranges from several days to as long as three months, but the normal span is about three weeks. The initial sign of syphilis is the presence of the chancre, a painless sore that develops at the site of the infection. It is oval in shape with hard edges. Within a few weeks the chancre disappears, regardless of whether or not the individual receives treatment. This stage is known as *primary syphilis,* when the disease can be cured by penicillin.

If the patient is not treated, the disease advances to the next stage, known as *secondary syphilis.* The signs and symptoms appear within about six months after the chancre disappears. The indications of secondary syphilis include a rash that covers different parts of the body, patches of hair loss, and the general symptoms of illness—fever, headache, and weakness.

During this stage the disease is highly infectious. This infection begins to damage the various organs and structures of the body. In time, the second stage's symptoms disappear and syphilis enters a *latent stage.* The latent stage may last for a lengthy period of time during which second-stage symptoms disappear, and the individual appears healthy and is noninfectious. However, at some point in the future, possibly as long as ten to twenty years, the defenses of the body break down and the disease is reactivated. During this latent syphilis stage, the disease can still be cured, but whatever organ and tissue damage has occurred is permanent.

Gonorrhea

The incubation period of gonorrhea is normally about three to five days. The first sign of infection in males is a discharge during urination of a thick, yellowish pus. A burning sensation often accompanies urination. These initial indications are usually of such a nature that males will seek some kind of treatment.

The situation is quite different for women. The initial symptoms may be an itching or burning in the genital area with a slight discharge. Often this is not enough indication to cause alarm. Consequently, the female often does not seek proper medical care during the early stage. Left untreated, the disease spreads to the upper organs of the reproductive system. Severe pain, pelvic inflammatory disease, and damage to the fallopian tubes often occur. If treatment is not sought in time, sterility results.

Gonorrhea is particularly dangerous if the woman is pregnant. As the infant passes through the birth canal, the bacteria can get into the baby's eyes and cause blindness. For this reason, drops of chemoprophylactic agents are put into the eyes of newborns.[18]

Genital Herpes

A particularly serious sexually transmitted disease, genital herpes is occurring more and more frequently. In the past two decades physician-patient consultations for this disease have increased fifteen fold.[19] This increase has been about equal between males and females.

The disease is caused by the herpes simplex virus type 2. The initial symptom is the presence of small blisters on the genitalia of females or the glans penis in males. The prime reservoirs of infection are the cervix in females and the semen in males. The blisters of herpes tend to come and go; however, the virus is still present. For this reason one cannot consider that the individual is healed when the blisters go into remission. They are likely to return again.

These fluid-filled sores may burn and itch and are usually quite painful, as is urination. Many people with herpes get the burning, itching, and tingling symptoms just prior to the development of the lesions.

This disease is serious because there is no effective treatment, though some control measures are recommended by physicians. It is important to keep the sores clean and dry and to not scratch them. For an otherwise healthy person genital herpes is usually not dangerous. However, if the virus comes in contact with the eyes and is left untreated it can cause blindness. It can cause many problems during pregnancy such as spontaneous abortion and stillbirth. Pregnant women can transmit the disease to their babies if they have active lesions in the birth canal at the time of delivery. In the female, the infection may locate on the cervix and may cause cervical cancer. Women with genital herpes should get Pap smear tests annually. The frequency of the active disease can be reduced by taking the drug acyclovir.[20]

Chlamydia

The fastest growing sexually transmitted disease is *chlamydia*. This disease is transmitted only by sexual contact or at birth from an infected mother to the infant. The exact number of cases is unknown because many times it is without symptoms and may be overlooked.

Chlamydia is not a fatal disease and is curable. However, there are a number of complications that can be serious. In females, pelvic inflammatory disease sometimes leads to ectopic pregnancy—the fetus growing in a fallopian tube rather than the uterus. Sterility may occur. Symptoms and signs in females include abnormal vaginal discharge, pelvic pain, nausea, fever, and pain upon urination.

Males with chlamydia may experience a number of genital infections. Infection of the tube between the testes and the penis—epididymis—can occur. Some of the symptoms are similar to those of gonorrhea: painful, burning sensation upon urination, and milky discharge from the urethra.

Antibiotics are very effective in halting this infection. Tetracycline and erythromycin are the antibiotics of choice at the present time.

Chlamydia is not a reportable disease. As a result many physicians do not report cases. The Centers for Disease Control recommends that clinics specializing in the treatment of sexually transmitted diseases screen all patients for chlamydia. There are several diagnostic tests. The standard procedure is to culture a sample in tissue culture. This may take as long as a week, during which time the individual can infect others. Thus, the importance of prevention and education can be understood.

Prevention of STDs

Prevention must be emphasized in controlling sexually transmitted diseases. In order to reduce the possibility of contracting or spreading one of these diseases, sexually active males are advised to practice good genital hygiene and to use a condom during intercourse. Proper genital hygiene and medical examinations are precautions the female should take.

The most important preventive measure is immediate treatment after infection. When a case of STDs is reported, it must be investigated. The infected individual must identify all previous sexual contacts for the public health clinic or medical personnel. Only as these sexual partners are identified, contacted, examined, and treated will the epidemic proportions of STDs be reduced.

Ongoing research and development continue to supply more knowledge about the prevention and treatment of all sexually transmitted diseases. For example, attempts have been made to develop a vaccine to treat gonorrhea and to provide prolonged immunity against it. Research also is attempting to identify a satisfactory treatment for genital herpes. But a whole new generation of STDs, such as chlamydia diseases, still needs to be investigated for effective treatment and diagnostic procedures.

Acquired Immune Deficiency Syndrome (AIDS)

Possibly no human communicable disease in the twentieth century has caused as much fear, uncertainty, and emotional concern as has Acquired Immune Deficiency Syndrome (AIDS). This disease is characterized by loss of the immune mechanism which combats certain infections. Its incidence has increased from a few thousand in the early 1980s to over 20,000 by 1986, and projected incidence to reach over 300,000 by the early 1990s. The number of cases of AIDS reported each six-month period continues to increase. Cases have been reported in all fifty states with 90 percent being in the twenty to forty-nine age group. Ninety-three percent of AIDS cases have been among males.[21]

This disease was unknown until 1979 when it was noted in two individuals who died after receiving plasma for hemophilia. So far there is no treatment or cure for AIDS. It is 100 percent fatal with death usually occurring within two to three years from the onset of the symptoms.

When AIDS first surfaced as a health problem, it was found mostly among homosexual males having numerous sexual partners. The greatest number of cases is still found among this population group. A second group at risk for AIDS is intravenous drug abusers using common, unsterile needles. Increasing numbers of AIDS victims can be found among heterosexual persons having multiple sex partners, particularly with male and female prostitutes. A small number of cases are found in infants born to mothers carrying the Human Immunosuppressive Virus (HIV). Some cases have been reported from receiving blood transfusions, particularly hemophiliacs. This population risk is dropping since there is now a test to ascertain whether blood is positive for the virus before it is made available for transfusion.

The etiologic agent that causes AIDS is a virus known as Human Immunosuppressive Virus (HIV). This virus was first identified in 1981 and is believed to have arisen in Africa.

The virus was isolated and identified at about the same time by researchers working separately at the National Cancer Institute in the United States and at the Pasteur Institute in Paris. Research has shown that the virus attacks the T-4 lymphocytes (a subgroup of white blood cells), which help defend the body against certain infections. It is believed that the virus enters the T-cell and incorporates itself into the genetic material (DNA) in the nucleus. The virus reproduces itself and kills the T-cell, which then releases new viruses that invade and kill other T-cells.

The AIDS virus (HIV) is carried in body fluids: blood, semen, and saliva. It is transmitted by blood and semen into the bloodstream of a recipient. There is no proven transmission of the virus by saliva. The virus is very fragile and does not survive outside of the body. For this reason medical authority points out that it cannot be transmitted by casual contact such as touch or kissing.

Symptoms of the AIDS Patient

1. Early influenza-like symptoms (swollen lymph glands, night sweats, diarrhea) with recurrent respiratory and digestive infections
2. Recurrence of fungus infections
3. Development of purplish skin lesions (Kaposi's Sarcoma)
4. Spread of Kaposi's resulting in bleeding from vital organs
5. Development of non-Hodgkins Lymphoma
6. Recurrent infections becoming more severe
7. Forgetfulness, impaired speech, tremors, seizures

Current screening tests cannot diagnose AIDS, but can only detect antibodies in the blood. The tests will not tell whether an individual will develop the disease, it is only an indicator that a person has at one time been infected by the virus, HIV. This means that the person is capable of transmitting the virus to another person by way of the blood and/or semen. The person with a positive HIV test has three possibilities: (1) never developing the disease, (2) developing AIDS Related Complex (ARC), or (3) developing AIDS.

The most commonly used test is an enzyme-linked immunosorbent assay (elisa). This test is easy to conduct, relatively inexpensive, not technically difficult to do, and can be completed in about two or so hours. The elisa test identifies blood that contains antibodies to HIV. A problem with this test is that it sometimes produces false positive readings in blood that does not contain the antibodies, so the elisa test alone is not a valid screening procedure.

Another more expensive, difficult, and complex test, the western blot, or immunoblot, is used to confirm a positive elisa test. This test is currently too expensive to be used as a primary test in large group screening efforts. Research is presently being conducted to develop more accurate, less expensive tests.

AIDS Related Complex (ARC) is the presence of influenza-like symptoms and recurrent infections. It is unknown at this time what the likelihood is of developing AIDS.

Ongoing research is taking place in an effort to find a cure for AIDS. In the meantime education about the disease and an understanding of it are important for everyone. Schools must develop policies on how to cope with AIDS patients. The corporate world is faced with decisions about preemployment screening measures for AIDS.

In 1985 the Public Health Service published several life-style recommendations designed to reduce the risk of contracting AIDS. The recommendations were:[22]

1. Do not have sexual contact with persons known to have or suspected of having AIDS.

2. Do not have sex with multiple partners.

3. Do not use intravenous drugs.

4. Do not have sex with people who are known to inject drugs.

5. Do not use inhalant nitrites. They may play a role in regard to Kaposi's Sarcoma.

6. Avoid anal intercourse.

7. Protect yourself and your partner during sexual intercourse by using condoms, avoiding oral-genital contact and open mouth kissing, and avoiding contact with body fluids (semen, blood, urine, and feces).

Smallpox: Eradication of a Disease

Possibly the most dramatic disease eradication program in history was conducted during the 1970s. Smallpox, a viral disease transmitted from person to person, has been one of the most feared diseases through the centuries. Because it was so threatening, in 1967 the World Health Organization embarked upon a worldwide smallpox eradication program.

Smallpox has caused the deaths of hundreds of millions of people throughout history. Many cities, nations, and cultures have been weakened or destroyed during epidemics of this disease. European explorers introduced smallpox to the Native Americans in both North and South America. Millions of these natives, who had no natural defenses against this disease, contracted smallpox and died. There is little doubt that smallpox contributed to the destruction of the great Inca and Aztec civilizations of South and Central America.

Edward Jenner discovered the vaccination process in the late eighteenth century. Through the years, science and medicine have worked to develop an effective measure to distribute the vaccination to people on mass scales at low cost. It was not until the 1940s that smallpox was eradicated in the developed world—North America and Europe. However, it continued to be a serious health problem in many Third World nations. In 1967, when it was estimated that there were ten to fifteen million cases of smallpox in forty-four countries, the World Health Assembly established a policy of worldwide smallpox eradication.[23]

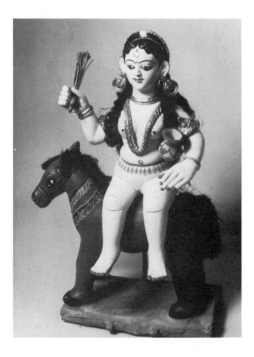

There was a great deal of doubt that such a goal was achievable. Many in the scientific community questioned the validity of such a program. Even the well-known authority René Dubos stated that such an attempt would be ". . . economically and humanly unwise."[24]

The World Health Organization program of smallpox eradication included mass vaccination. This was made possible by the development of a two-tined needle that could be used by trained personnel. The needles could be sterilized and reused, and the training did not require a high level of skill. This had a profound effect on the cost of such a massive program.

An important strategy built into the smallpox eradication program was that of surveillance.[25] The practice of surveillance and containment involved moving directly into areas of smallpox outbreak and

isolating known victims. In addition, everyone in the victims' communities was vaccinated. This procedure required several modes of transportation and the employment of many local people to aid the WHO medical teams.

In addition to mass immunization and surveillance, education and record keeping were employed. The educational efforts were designed to enlighten people about the disease so that they could report any suspected cases to the surveillance teams. Extensive efforts at collecting data about the presence of smallpox and the effect of the vaccine were important parts of the overall campaign.

Within eight years of the start of the program, smallpox had been eradicated from all but five countries. With concentrated efforts in these nations, the incidence of smallpox continued to be identified and eliminated. On October 26, 1979, the Director General of the World Health Organization declared that smallpox had been eradicated in all the world. The last known case was in 1979 in Somalia, in northern East Africa.[26]

As the result of this successful worldwide program of smallpox eradication, routine vaccination is no longer required. In the United States it is even impossible to obtain the vaccine in most communities. Some have questioned the future of a generation of children who have reached maturity without having smallpox vaccination. Is it possible that smallpox could reappear in the future and create serious problems for an unvaccinated civilization? Scientists and medical professionals say this is most unlikely.

Chronic Diseases

Increased surveillance, expanded availability of immunization and vaccination, and continuing research have led to the elimination of many communicable diseases as major causes of death and debilitation in the United States. Of the ten leading causes of death in the mid-1980s, six are chronic diseases. Of the remaining four, one (suicide) results from interpersonal violence, and two are the result of accidents (motorized and nonmotorized), while only one is a communicable disease, influenza and pneumonia. Seventy percent of all deaths in the United States result from chronic diseases.

Chronic diseases are generally considered to not be caused by microorganisms, to be long lasting, and to be the result of a variety of different factors. Some of these causative factors of chronic diseases are unknown. Many chronic diseases have their originations early in life with the development of certain behavioral life-styles that place an individual at risk for the disease.

Of the numerous chronic diseases that affect mankind, four result in the greatest incidences of fatality and debilitation. These are (1) cardiovascular disease, (2) cancer, (3) cirrhosis of the liver, and (4) diabetes. Heart disease, stroke, and cancer account for the three leading causes of death.

Unfortunately, there is no medication that can be given that can "cure" most chronic diseases. It is possible that medication and health care procedures can be provided that will bring relief and a reduction of the specific problem. However, damage to the body caused by the stroke, the malignancy, the diabetic condition, or whatever other problem a person may have, is unlikely to be corrected.

Chronic diseases often cause much debilitation. The various arthritic diseases often result in crippling conditions. A person's ability to use his or her fingers and hands may limit the ability to work or to provide personal care. Advanced stages of arthritic conditions often lead to total incapacity to function alone and the need for permanent, long-term nursing care.

The person with diabetes may also experience various stages of debilitation. From the initial recognition that a person is diabetic major efforts are needed to control his or her diet and insulin levels. Advanced stages of diabetes may result in blindness and other crippling conditions needing long-term care.

Chronic obstructive lung disease, emphysema, and chronic bronchitis result in very difficult breathing, which greatly reduces the ability of the patient to function normally. As chronic obstructive lung diseases progress the individual requires long-term, continuous nursing services and the use of assistive breathing devices.

Cardiovascular Disease

The leading cause of death and debilitation of humans in the United States is cardiovascular disease. Cardiovascular heart disease includes several different specific diseases: coronary heart disease, stroke, and hypertension. These are conditions which affect the body's circulatory system—the heart and the blood vessels.

When circulation of blood in the blood vessels of the heart or throughout the body is obstructed, *coronary heart disease* is the result. Such a situation may occur as the result of a narrowing of the artery reducing blood supply to the muscles of the heart, a saclike bulging of the weakened arterial wall, or a rupture of the artery with loss of blood into the surrounding tissues.

Numerous factors may cause a heart attack. Most cardiovascular heart disease results from atherosclerosis which is the underlying condition in most cardiovascular-related deaths. Atherosclerosis is a slow, progressive hardening of the arteries. Fatty deposits called *plaques* form on the inner layer of the arterial walls. Growth of this plaque over time can reduce or totally block the flow of blood through the arteries.

A *stroke* occurs when there is impairment or blockage of the blood supply to the brain. Such an impairment may be the result of blood clotting or hemorrhaging in one of the blood vessels of the brain. Different parts of the brain control various physical and mental functions. When an individual has a stroke the indications may vary depending upon which part of the brain is affected. In some people it may include paralysis of a limb, in others a loss of speech or balance, and in others difficulty in swallowing or mental functioning. The early symptoms of a stroke may be a massive weakness or numbness of a part of the body. In other instances the symptoms may last only a few seconds or minutes. The increased interest and screening for hypertension in recent years has led to a decline in deaths due to stroke in the United States.

As blood is pumped through the cardiovascular system, pressure is exerted on the walls of the blood vessels. With increased and sustained elevation of this blood pressure, there is a greater risk of damage to the blood vessels and the development of stroke and coronary heart disorder. This condition is known as *hypertension.* Hypertension, if identified early enough, can be kept under control with medical assistance. Prescribed antihypertensive drugs, the reduction of high caloric foods and sodium in the diet, and reduction and control of stress can all be important factors in reducing hypertension.

Extensive research into the causes and treatment of cardiovascular diseases has resulted in increased knowledge and more effective treatment modalities.[27] With increased interest in preventive medicine, it is now known that there are a number of risk factors for cardiovascular disease. An individual can take specific action to help prevent or reduce the likelihood of developing cardiovascular heart disease. Diet plays an important role in the reduction of several factors that have a relation to cardiovascular disease. The reduction of cholesterol and triglycerides, fats normally occurring in the blood, is important. A diet that is low in saturated fats can be important in maintaining a healthy circulatory system.

Sedentary individuals appear to have a significantly higher death rate by heart attack than those who exercise regularly. Not only does exercise strengthen the heart muscle, but it is an important factor in weight control. Obesity is an identified risk factor for cardiovascular heart disease.

There is increasing evidence that cigarette smoking is a major risk factor in the development of cardiovascular diseases. The exact relationship is unknown, but the effects of nicotine and carbon monoxide probably have some relationship.

Though cardiovascular heart disease affects millions of people throughout the United States, there has been an increased awareness of measures an individual can take to reduce the possibility of heart attack. Various changes in individual life-style such as reduced smoking,[28] changes in diet,[29] and increased physical activity have helped to improve cardiovascular health in recent years.

Cancer

The second leading cause of death in America is cancer. This chronic disease has been one of the most dreaded afflictions. However, due to increased research, improved and more effective treatment modalities, and earlier detection, the possibility of cure from cancer has increased in recent years.

Throughout the life cycle of the human being new cell growth continuously occurs, replacing old worn-out tissue. For example, in a case where there has been tissue damage, repair of the injury occurs after a period of time. The body is continually replacing worn-out cells on the skin's surface. Cells sometimes reproduce in such a way that new, undesirable, and nonfunctional masses of cells are noted. This results in the formation of a *tumor.* Unlike cells that adhere to normal body tissues, tumors continue to grow. They lack the adhesiveness that is present in normal cells. Some tumors remain localized, nonspreading, and for the most part are non-life-threatening. These are *benign* tumors. They are usually only dangerous to the individual when the growth harms nearby structures.

On the other hand, some tumors spread into nearby tissue with clawlike protrusions and interfere with the function and nourishment of neighboring organs. These tumors are *malignant* or *cancerous* growths. The process by which a normal cell is changed to an abnormal cell is known as *oncogenesis.*

Cancerous cells have distinctive microscopic appearances. For some unknown reason these cells, unlike normal cells, do not stop growing and reproducing. They proceed to grow and expand in a logarithmic progression. As growth occurs, displacement of normal tissue results. The cancerous cells take over the blood supply of the normal tissue. In time the malignant cells may separate from the mass of tissue and spread to another location in the body. This process is known as *metastasis.* This malignant tissue can implant itself in foreign cellular environments and continue to reproduce, grow, and expand.

Much research has been directed toward identifying what factors initiate the uncontrolled growth of cells. Certain factors that have been identified include exposure to various chemicals or exposure to various physical agents such as sunlight and X rays. There is increasing interest in the role that dietary factors play in the causation of cancer cell development and growth. Research has also focused on the role of viruses in this process. It is known that viruses do cause oncogenesis. However, there is no evidence that any human cancer can be directly linked with a specific virus. Much still remains to be learned about what precipitating factors cause the initial development of cancer cells.

There is scientific agreement that as much as 80 percent of all cancer is linked with individual lifestyles.[30] Smoking, diet, and environmental pollutants are the three factors that presently are receiving the most attention by scientists studying malignancies in the United States. Smoking is directly linked with several different types of cancer—lung cancer in particular as well as cancer of the mouth and trachea. The National Cancer Institute has estimated that as much as 35 percent of all cancer deaths may be associated with dietary influences.[31] Findings of various studies reported by the National Cancer Institute that support this statement include the following:[32]

1. Populations that consume higher amounts of fiber have a lower rate of colon and rectal cancer.
2. Eating too much fat may increase the risk of getting cancer of the colon, breast, and prostate.
3. Obesity is linked with higher risks of developing colon, breast, prostate, gallbladder, and uterine cancer.
4. Heavy drinking of alcoholic beverages increases the risk of cancer of the mouth, throat, and liver.

Early identification of certain signs and indications presents the best way to reduce the possibility of fatality from cancer. There is no single sign, symptom, or test for cancer, but numerous signs and symptoms are considered important by the physicians. An unexplained weight loss is an indication that further examination for cancer is necessary, as is any unexplained bleeding. Anemia in adult males and in postmenopausal females is a strong indicator of cancer unless proven otherwise. Changes in elimination, digestion, or appetite are other indications of cancer. Pain may result from the tumor enlarging or pushing on surrounding organs. Enlarged lymph nodes may be indicative of cancerous growth. The American Cancer Society has identified seven danger signals of cancer with which every person should be familiar:

1. Change in bowel or bladder habits
2. A sore that does not heal
3. Unusual bleeding or discharge
4. Thickening or lump in breast or elsewhere
5. Indigestion or difficulty in swallowing
6. Obvious change in wart or mole
7. Nagging cough or hoarseness

A number of risk factors have been identified that seem to be associated with increased possibility of the development of cancer. For example, excessive exposure to the sun is a risk factor for skin cancer. Cigarette smoking is related to cancer of the lung and the oral cavity. Dietary patterns have been associated with cancer of the stomach and the colon. Other risk factors include age and family history.

Treatment for cancer includes three different procedures: (1) use of surgery, (2) use of chemotherapy, and (3) use of radiation. Surgery is used to remove the malignant tissue. It is a major surgical procedure and is most effective when there is reasonable assurance that the tumor is localized; that is, it has not spread beyond its original site. Surgery is most effective for treating cancer of the colon and rectum. Cancer of the breast is also treated primarily by surgery.

Chemotherapy, the use of drugs, is an effective treatment procedure that is used separately or in conjunction with surgery. There are hundreds of chemotherapeutic agents that are used to treat cancer. The ideal procedure is to identify a drug that is toxic to the cancer cells, but will produce minimal harm to the surrounding normal cell tissue. This is not always easy to accomplish in that often a chemotherapeutic agent that will destroy malignant cells will also damage noncancerous cells.

Chemotherapy may be given intermittently using several different drugs. Drug therapy may also be given on a continuous, daily basis. Exposure to the drugs tends to cause a number of side effects. Many people who are given chemotherapy develop anemia. There can also be a drop in white blood cell count which creates problems with infections. In addition, many individuals being treated with chemotherapy lose body hair. This mode of cancer treatment is most effective with the most serious malignancies.

Radiation treatment, the use of X rays and gamma rays, is effective for treatment of many kinds of cancer. About half of all cancer patients receive radiation either as the sole treatment modality or in combination with other therapy. Some tumors respond temporarily, but are not cured by radiation. This treatment modality slows down the cancer cell growth and is used for cancer of the oral cavity, bone, brain, prostate, testes, skin, and Hodgkin's disease. Radiation has been particularly successful in the treatment of Hodgkin's disease. Cure rates of nearly 90 percent are now being reported.[33]

Extensive technological procedures and research are ongoing in the attempt to improve the chances of long-term cure for cancer. For example, cryosurgical procedures in which a stream of liquid nitrogen is directed into the cancer has been developed. Repeated freezing and thawing kills the malignant cells. Current efforts are being directed toward the development and use of immunotherapy in the treatment of cancer. This approach is designed to activate the body's immune system to destroy the cancer cells. Most use of immunotherapeutic agents is still in the early testing stages with humans.

Means of diagnosing malignancies have improved with highly developed technological procedures in recent years. Ultrasound, a procedure in which machines bounce sound waves off internal organs, is effective in locating tumors. Thermography, use of heat patterns, is also used to locate cancerous tissues. Computerized X rays provide three-dimensional pictures that facilitate cancer screening.

Increased knowledge about cancer has led to significantly improved chances for treatment and recovery. However, as with many other health problems, prevention and early detection are still major factors that all individuals must practice.

Summary

Communicable diseases were once the principal cause of sickness and death in the United States. Today, they are no longer a major threat to life. However, millions of people in America and elsewhere still suffer from one or more of these diseases annually. Communicable disease control, therefore, is still an important responsibility of the public health department.

Small living microorganisms are the causative agents of communicable diseases. The major pathogenic microorganisms are bacteria, viruses, fungi, protozoa, rickettsiae, and the multicellular metazoa. Communicable diseases are the result of these pathogenic microorganisms residing in a host and producing specific symptoms that lead to illness and debilitation.

When the microorganism enters a prospective host, certain defense mechanisms attempt to counter the disease. The human body has the ability to produce antibodies that can neutralize and destroy the pathogens. This ability is known as immunity. Immunity may be obtained through the process of immunization in addition to the naturally acquired immunity.

The various communicable diseases affect many different body systems. A major focus of communicable disease control is directed at diseases of the respiratory system. All respiratory diseases follow a similar pattern. There are a number of different respiratory diseases, with the common cold, influenza, and pneumonia the most widespread in the United States.

Tuberculosis has been the most feared respiratory disease throughout history. This disease, caused by the tubercle bacillus, has led to the death of millions. The incidence of tuberculosis has been greatly reduced in the United States, owing to effective screening procedures and improved hygiene, nutrition, and health care. However, this disease is still a widespread problem in many Third World nations and among the economically disadvantaged in America.

The number of sexually transmitted diseases is increasing in America. Ignorance, social restraints, and an increase in sexual activity have contributed to the upward swing in spite of the availability of diagnostic procedures and treatment measures. The sexually transmitted diseases are a problem particularly among teenagers and young adults in their twenties.

Gonorrhea and syphilis are probably the best known of the sexually transmitted diseases. Genital herpes is of particular concern as there is presently no effective treatment. The most prevalent sexually transmitted disease is chlamydia.

During the 1980s a new disease, Acquired Immune Deficiency Syndrome (AIDS), has caused much concern and fear throughout the United States. This disease, for which there is presently no cure, is caused by the HIV virus. It has been found principally among the homosexual population, intravenous drug users, and those who have received blood transfusions. Extensive research efforts are ongoing in an attempt to find a cure for this serious disease.

The leading causes of death and debilitation among the American population in the 1980s are various chronic diseases. These diseases are not caused by microorganisms, as are the communicable diseases. There are a variety of different causes for chronic diseases.

Chronic diseases include the cardiovascular diseases, cancer, diabetes, chronic pulmonary diseases, arthritic diseases, and numerous others. Many life-style behavioral patterns present risk factors for these various diseases. For example, smoking has been linked with cardiovascular diseases, pulmonary diseases, and cancer. Diet patterns are linked with several of the chronic diseases. In that these diseases are usually long-term in nature and may become debilitating, many problems arise for the caretakers, as well as for the patients.

Discussion Questions

1. What factors have led to the reduction in deaths caused by communicable diseases in the past century?
2. Explain the differences in the various pathogenic organisms that cause a majority of communicable diseases.
3. Describe the ways that pathogenic microorganisms are transmitted from a host reservoir to a new host.
4. Explain what is meant by immunity.
5. What role does the public health department play in immunization programs?
6. How do the common cold, influenza, and pneumonia differ?
7. What are the secondary factors that result in tuberculosis?
8. What are the two most effective measures available in the United States for identifying cases of tuberculosis?
9. Explain why the BCG vaccine is not widely used in the United States.
10. Trace the development of the smallpox eradication program and describe its related activities.

11. Do you believe that it is a good policy to destroy or stop production of all smallpox vaccine? Why or why not?

12. Why is it difficult to control and reduce the incidences of sexually transmitted diseases?

13. Explain the differences between syphilis and gonorrhea.

14. Why is genital herpes such a serious disease?

15. How does AIDS affect the immune system?

16. Discuss the emotional factors surrounding Acquired Immune Deficiency Syndrome.

17. Identify some of tne preventive measures that have been suggested regarding AIDS.

18. Explain how chronic diseases differ from communicable diseases.

19. Discuss the relationships between individual life-style patterns and the development of cardiovascular diseases.

20. What factor does hypertension play in heart disease?

21. Identify some of the possible indications of cancer.

22. What are some of the factors to be decided in the treatment of cancer?

23. Explain how life-style patterns relate to the development of cancer.

Suggested Readings

Anderson, Elizabeth T. "Plague in the Continental United States, 1900–76." *Public Health Reports* 93, no. 3 (May/June, 1978): 297–301.

Benenson, Abram S., ed. *Control of Communicable Diseases in Man,* 12th ed. Washington, D.C.: American Public Health Association, 1979.

Boyd, William. *An Introduction to the Study of Disease.* Philadelphia: Lea and Febiger, 1971.

Bres, P. L. "Could the Great 'Plagues' Recur?" *World Health* (November, 1980): 7–9.

Dowdle, Walter. "The Search for an AIDS Vaccine." *Public Health Reports* 101, no. 3 (May/June, 1986): 232–33.

Francis, Donald P., and Chin, James. "The Prevention of Acquired Immunodeficiency Syndrome in the United States." *Journal of the American Medical Association* 257, no. 10 (March 13, 1987):1357–66.

Guinan, Mary E., and Hardy, Ann. "Epidemiology of AIDS in Women in the United States." *Journal of the American Medical Association* 257, no. 15 (April 17, 1987): 2039–42.

Henderson, Donald A. "Smallpox—Epitaph for a Killer?" *National Geographic Magazine* 154, no. 6 (December, 1978): 797–805.

Henderson, Donald A. "Smallpox Eradication." *Public Health Reports* 95, no. 5 (September/October, 1980): 422–26.

Mason, James O. "Statement on the Development of Guidelines for the Prevention of AIDS Transmission in the Workplace." *Public Health Reports* 101, no. 1 (January/February, 1986): 6–8.

Mason, James O.; Koplan, Jeffrey P.; and Layde, Peter M. "The Prevention and Control of Chronic Diseases: Reducing Unnecessary Deaths and Disability—A Conference Report." *Public Health Reports* 102, no. 1 (January–February, 1987): 17–20.

Mausner, Judith S., and Bahn, Anita K. *Epidemiology: An Introductory Text.* Philadelphia: W. B. Saunders Co., 1974.

Endnotes

1. Public Health Service, *Health, United States, 1980.* Washington, D.C.: U.S. Government Printing Office, 272.

2. Ibid., 273.

3. Benenson, Abram S., ed. *Control of Communicable Diseases in Man,* 12th ed. Washington, D.C.: American Public Health Association, 1979: 354.

4. Centers for Disease Control. Annual Summary 1984: Reported Morbidity and Mortality in the United States. *Morbidity and Mortality Weekly Report* 33, no. 54 (March, 1986): 23.

5. Ibid., 61.

6. Report of Immunization Committee of the American College of Physicians reported in *The Nation's Health* (March, 1985): 6.

7. Department of Health and Human Services. *Promoting Health, Preventing Disease: Objectives for the Nation.* Washington, D.C.: U.S. Government Printing Office, 1980, 57.

8. Ibid., 57.

9. Carroll, Charles, and Miller, Dean F. *Health: The Science of Human Adaptation.* Dubuque, Iowa: Wm. C. Brown, 1982, 363.

10. Department of Health and Human Services, *Promoting Health,* p. 57.

11. Centers for Disease Control. Annual Summary 1984: Reported Morbidity and Mortality in the United States, 66.

12. Ibid., 66.

13. Department of Health and Human Services, *Promoting Health,* 58.

14. "Tuberculosis in Profile." *World Health* (January, 1982): 8–9.

15. Blach, Alan B., and Snider, Dixie E. "How Much Tuberculosis in Children Must We Accept?" *American Journal of Public Health* 76, no. 1 (January, 1986): 14–15.

16. Department of Health and Human Services, *Promoting Health,* p. 25.

17. Centers for Disease Control. Annual Summary 1984: Reported Morbidity and Mortality in the United States, 25.

18. Benenson, Abram S., ed. *Control of Communicable Diseases in Man.* Washington, D.C.: American Public Health Association, 1979, 132.

19. Centers for Disease Control. "Genital Herpes Infection—United States, 1966–1984." *Morbidity and Mortality Weekly Report* 35, no. 24, (June 20, 1986): 402.

20. Centers for Disease Control. "1985 STD Treatment Guidelines." *Morbidity and Mortality Weekly Report Supplement* 34, no. 4S (October 18, 1985): 88S.

21. Centers for Disease Control. "Update Acquired Immunodeficiency Syndrome—United States," 35, no. 2 (January 17, 1986): 17–21.

22. Centers for Disease Control. "Update Acquired Immunodeficiency Syndrome—United States," 34, no. 18 (May 18, 1985): 245–47.

23. Henderson, Donald A. "Smallpox—Epitaph for a Killer?" *National Geographic Magazine* 154, no. 6 (December, 1978): 803.

24. Dubos, Rene. *Man Adapting.* New Haven, Conn.: Yale Press, 1967.

25. Henderson, Donald A. "Smallpox Eradication." *Public Health Reports* 95, no. 5 (September/October, 1980): 425.

26. Henderson, Donald A. "Smallpox—Epitaph for a Killer?" *National Geographic Magazine* 154, no. 6 (December, 1978): 805.

27. Discussion of research relating to cardiovascular disease is discussed in chapter 2.

28. Discussion of cigarette smoking is presented in chapter 17.

29. Discussion of diet and health is presented in chapter 11.

30. National Cancer Institute. *Cancer Facts* (May, 1986): 1.

31. Ibid., 1.

32. Ibid., 2.

33. American Cancer Society. *Facts on Cancer Treatment* pamphlet: 11.

10

The Environment: More than a Search for the Cause of Disease

Selected Federal Environmental Legislation, 1970s

Clean Air Act Amendments of 1970 and 1977
Noise Control Act of 1972
Federal Water Pollution Control Act Amendments of 1972
Federal Insecticide, Fungicide, and Rodenticide Act Amendments of 1972, 1975

Safe Drinking Water Act of 1974, Amendments of 1977 and 1979
Toxic Substances Control Act of 1976
Clean Water Act of 1977 and 1978
Resource Conservation and Recovery Act of 1976

Since the mid-nineteenth century, environmental health has been a vital component of public health programming. Classics in the field of public health literature have focused attention on the importance of improving the sanitary environment.[1] Sanitary concerns as they affect the health of the public have become important aspects of public health programming.

Numerous communicable diseases have resulted from unsanitary conditions throughout recorded history. During much of the nineteenth century, the causes of sickness and ill health were thought to be impure atmospheric and environmental conditions. The germ theory of disease was then unknown. As a result, sanitation programs were developed to create and maintain a clean environment. These were the beginnings of many local public health departments in the United States.

Throughout the first half of the twentieth century, local and state environmental sanitarians focused on such problems as food sanitation, public building sanitation, housing, rodent control, and prevention of air and water pollution. But efforts to improve environmental conditions seem to have peaked in recent years. There have been numerous projects, programs, and activities devoted to providing a better ecosystem for humanity. Concern over the despoiling of the environment was highlighted in April 1970 with the national observance of Earth Day. Hundreds of thousands of people demonstrated throughout the country for improved environmental conditions and effective government environmental policies. Throughout the 1970s citizen involvement in the environmental movement resulted in increased environmental awareness and the subsequent passage of legislation.

In the United States a number of federal legislative acts were passed that provided impetus for environmental health programming. Environmental Protection Agencies were legislated at the national level and in many states. Today the responsibility for managing environmental health programs is found in a number of different agencies although the basic governmental unit having environmental program responsibility is the state health department. Other departments with programming for the environment are the state agricultural department and the departments of water resources, human resources, and natural resources. There are differences from one state to another, yet all have programming that will result in a cleaner environment that is conducive to the health and well-being of citizens.[2]

A Safe Water Supply

How safe is the water we drink, in which we bathe, and which flows in the rivers and streams of North America? Water pollution has become a matter of increasing concern in community health in recent years. Today, once pure sources of water are contaminated by a variety of pollutants. Increased population, additional sewage, growth of industrial wastes, and the dumping of other contaminants have been major contributors to water pollution.

Water pollution is often the result of such industrial processes as energy production. When the water used to generate electricity is returned to its source, it is usually polluted and is often warmer, causing an ecological disruption.

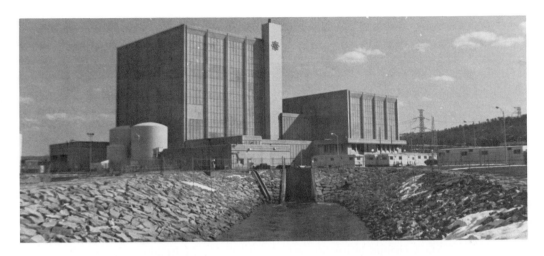

In the United States, citizens assume that the drinking water is pure. Little thought is given to the quality of water from a tap in the office building, the glass of water served in the restaurant, or the water obtained from a park drinking fountain. This complete trust in the purity of drinking water is due to the activities of public health departments.

There is little incidence of waterborne disease today in the United States. Many of the water-related problems common in other parts of the world have been nearly eliminated in our country. For example, such widespread diseases as typhoid and cholera are rarely seen. But illness does result from water contamination and is usually gastrointestinal illness. The Centers for Disease Control has estimated that there are four thousand cases of waterborne illnesses reported every year. It is probable that many more cases of illness associated with the ingestion of contaminated water go unreported or are assumed to be linked to other causes. Waterborne outbreaks are primarily caused by overflow or seepage of sewage from septic tanks, chemical contamination of water supplies, and surface runoff contamination.[3]

In spite of the fact that there is no widespread epidemic of waterborne disease in the United States today, it is important to be concerned about the safety of the water supply of our communities. Episodes of acute illness resulting from water contamination are easily traced, but prolonged exposure at very low levels to contaminants such as cadmium, lead, mercury, and pesticides may have long-term negative health effects. There is speculation that such exposure may eventually cause cancer, heart disease, and other chronic diseases, plus a host of other health problems.

Concern must be expressed over contamination of groundwater. Half of the nation's drinking water—80 percent in rural localities—is groundwater. Contamination can make the water useless for humans and animals as well as for irrigation of crops.

Numerous chemicals have been found in groundwater that have been shown to have adverse effects on human and animal health. Particular concern has been expressed regarding the long-term, low-level exposure to drinking water containing toxic chemicals from waste disposal landfills. Water contamination has been reported to occur by a number of different industries. Even the high tech electronics industry has been responsible for contaminating water resources. Two to three times as high a rate of miscarriages and birth defects has been reported to be related to contamination by the industry's toxic chemicals.[4]

In Congressional testimony it was reported that "no community in the country is free from . . . sources of groundwater contamination."[5] Testimony indicated that there is no data currently available to reveal the true extent of the problem.

Water Pollution Sources

Industrial and agricultural operations are the major users of water and so are responsible for much of the water pollution in our nation. Industry uses water in the manufacturing process to cool equipment and also converts it to steam to provide heat and generate electrical power. Many chemicals are dumped into rivers, streams, and lakes as the result of industrial processes.

Industry

Water is used as a machinery coolant in many industrial settings. Over 80 percent of water used by industry is used for cooling.[6] The water is usually taken from a stream, river, or lake and poured over the heated equipment. When the water is returned to its source, it is warmer than normal, thus raising the temperature of the principal water supply. Warmer water absorbs less oxygen, which results in a retarded decomposition of organic matter. This problem, termed *thermal pollution,* is of particular concern to power-generating plants, especially nuclear power plants.

Fish cannot adjust to abnormal changes in water temperature, though their life cycle is closely related to normal changes in water temperature. Some fish, for example, spawn when water temperature drops in the fall; others spawn when temperatures rise in the spring. Imagine, then, how artificially induced changes in temperature can affect this delicate system. In other instances, fish have adjusted to a higher water temperature caused by a manufacturing process or by a nuclear power plant. But when the plant closes down for repairs or for other reasons, the fish cannot readjust to the cooler water and so die.

Agriculture

Agriculture is the largest user of water in America. Not only is water consumed by cattle and other livestock, but it is necessary for growing all crops. It has been estimated that one bushel of wheat requires fifteen thousand gallons of water from the time the seeds are planted until the wheat is eaten as bread. Water irrigation, which makes agriculture possible on land that would otherwise be useless for growing purposes, requires tremendous amounts of water.

Agriculture's abundant use of water results in water pollution. Besides water, crops require nutrients and so are fertilized. Up to one-fourth of these inorganic fertilizers, however, are lost in surface runoff before the plants can utilize them. They are carried to the stream or river and become part of the downstream town's water supply. Siltation from erosion creates a very similar problem. As the soil is plowed, it is exposed to erosion. Erosion, as well as damaging the terrain and removing badly needed topsoil, carries the nutrients from the eroded areas. The soil and nutrients end up in streams and rivers, polluting the water.

Animal wastes present another water pollution problem. Animal feedlots, where cattle are brought for fattening, have created a particular problem. A feedlot holding ten thousand head of cattle produces as much waste as a community of 160,000 people. Runoff from these feedlots obviously creates serious water pollution problems.

Acid Rain

Not only are lakes, rivers, streams, and underground water tables often polluted, but there is evidence that even rainfall is polluted. This is a condition known as *acid rain* and results when the oxides of sulfur and nitrogen are released into the air from tall industrial smokestacks. These pollutants react with water vapor in the clouds and form acids. The clouds become acidic so when rain and snow fall from them, acid falls to the earth and affects the flora, water, fish, and probably humans and animals.

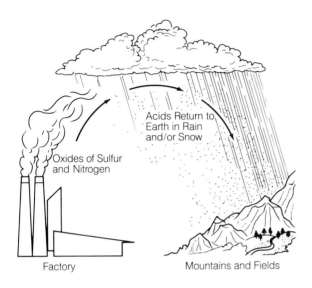

Acid rain results when the oxides of sulfur and nitrogen are poured into the air from tall industrial smokestacks. These pollutants react with water vapor in the clouds and form acids. These acids fall to the earth some distance away in the form of rain or snow.

Acids Return to Earth in Rain and/or Snow

Oxides of Sulfur and Nitrogen

Factory

Mountains and Fields

Acid rain has developed into a significant problem—especially since the early 1970s, when industries began building taller smokestacks. Today many smokestacks are more than five hundred feet high and some are even taller than one thousand feet. These smokestacks emit nitrogen and sulfur oxides high into the atmosphere; as a result, the upper-level winds carry the oxides a great distance from their source, resulting in serious pollution problems several hundred miles downwind.

In the United States, environmentalists have become particularly concerned about fish kills in the Adirondack Lakes region of upstate New York. It is believed that the sources of this lethal acid rain are industrial plants along the Great Lakes.

Acid rain has also become an international problem. In 1981 the Ontario, Canada, government attempted to persuade the United States Environmental Protection Agency to maintain its air pollution standards. Acid rain, a by-product of midwestern industries, was killing fish in Ontario lakes. Since tourism in Ontario depends upon the lakes, this problem has serious economic consequences as well as environmental ramifications.

Although acid rain has proven toxic to fish, its effects on vegetation and wildlife are still uncertain.[7] Although no direct health cause-and-effect relationship with human health has been documented, acid rain must be considered a possible health hazard. It is probable that increased exposure to acid in the environment will in some way be detrimental to human well-being.

Efforts to control acid rain have encountered roadblocks. One Environmental Protection Agency regulation allows each state to regulate its own output of sulfur and nitrogen oxides. Hence the level of acceptable emissions differs from one state to another. As a result of this variance, states with strong emission control regulations may be affected by acid rain originating in distant states having less stringent regulation standards.

The cost of implementing a solution to the acid rain issue has proven to be another stumbling block. It is costly to place scrubbers in the smokestacks of all industries. In spite of this, Japan has proven that not only is such action possible, it can be effective and economical, too.[8] Emissions were decreased by 50 percent in that nation after strong sulfur oxide regulations were implemented in 1968. Today there are six times more scrubbers in Japan than in the United States.[9]

Legislation for Clean Water

In 1914 the first federal drinking water standards were developed.[10] These early standards applied only to water provided by interstate carriers—in those days, trains. Until the 1950s, this and other federal water pollution control programs were designed to prevent the spread of communicable diseases.

The Water Pollution Control Act of 1956, amended in 1965, was the first legislation to establish water quality standards. Other legislation in 1966 and 1970 provided monies to build water treatment plants and prohibited the discharge of harmful waste materials into navigable waters.

In 1972 Congress passed the Federal Water Pollution Control Act, which established a national system of permits aimed at controlling discharges of pollutants by industries, municipalities, and agriculture. Pollution control equipment had to be installed by those agencies and by industries discharging effluents into navigable waters. This legislation also provided large sums of money for building municipal sewage treatment facilities. This legislation was reauthorized in 1987 when Congress overrode the president's veto of it.

Another federal law, the Safe Drinking Water Act of 1974, directed the Environmental Protection Agency to establish drinking water standards. These standards would ensure that drinking water contaminants, such as cadmium, fluoride, mercury, and other elements, did not exceed a specified limit, thus meeting purity standards. Noncommunity settings, such as trailer parks, camping sites, and roadside motels with their own water supplies, also must meet the standards.

The establishment of such standards is no easy task. There are more than three hundred organic chemicals that have been identified in drinking water in the United States. Little or no testing has been done on most of these to ascertain the specific cause-and-effect relationships on health. The Safe Drinking Water Act was strengthened and reauthorized in 1986.

Municipal Water Systems

There are between thirty and forty thousand municipal water supply systems in the United States. With an increasing urban population, water pollution control has focused on the reduction of pollution of these water resources. The Environmental Protection Agency has reported that 28 percent of the larger public water systems and 17 percent of the smaller systems show detectable levels of synthetic chemicals in their water resources.[11]

Municipal water purification systems should contain primary and secondary treatment processes. Primary sewage treatment is the process of screening and sedimentation. Water is placed in a tank where the large impurities, such as sand, trash, and other suspended solids, settle. There is also a filtration process that removes large objects as the water passes through a series of screens. About one-third of the communities in the United States are served by systems providing only this primary treatment of water prior to returning it to the original source. After this treatment the water does not look bad, but it still contains microorganisms and organic nutrients.

The secondary sewage treatment process is important because it is in this stage that microorganisms and organic nutrients are removed. For particles too small to filter, a coagulation process is used. Small particles are made larger through coagulation so that they will settle or can be filtrated.

During this secondary process, the water is sprayed over a bed of stones. While it is trickling around the stones, the nutrients are reduced by bacterial action, thus biologically purifying the water. Aerobic bacteria, air, and sunlight help oxidize and purify the water. The final step in the secondary process involves disinfection of microorganisms by means of chlorination. This process reduces the bacterial content.

Air Pollution

Life on earth cannot exist without oxygen, the most vital component of air. Air is limited and must be reused, and if polluted, it can cause a variety of health problems.

There has always been limited pollution of the air. Fires, wind erosion, and dirt particles have naturally contaminated the air. However, nature solves this problem too: wind, snow, and rainfall clean the air. In environmental settings not disturbed by humans and modern technology, the air is relatively pure and does not contribute to health problems.

Industrialization, the development and growth of the motor vehicle, increased human population, and growth of urban communities have significantly aggravated the problem of air pollution. As a result, the quality of the air today in many parts of the world, including America, is poor. The major sources of air pollution in the United States are the burning of fossil fuels, the internal combustion engine in motor vehicles, fuel furnaces used to generate electricity, and expanding industrial processes.

One of the many sources of air pollution in the United States is factories. Not only is the air quality affected in the immediate vicinity of the factory, but areas downwind must also contend with the pollutants.

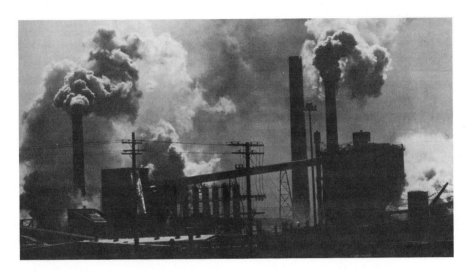

The effect on humans of some types of air pollution is observable. Catastrophic air pollution episodes have caused illness and death of many people on several occasions. For example, in 1948, twenty people in Donora, Pennsylvania, died from respiratory complications, and nearly half the people living in the region had some type of eye, nose, or throat irritation due to a period of severe air contamination. Such an episode in London, England, in 1952 resulted in the death of nearly four thousand people. Again in 1956, a similar occurrence in London caused the deaths of some one thousand people. In many localities (Los Angeles, for example) a continuously contaminated environment exists, endangering the health of residents.

Many indirect, nonobservable effects of air pollution are a concern to scientists, medical professionals, and public health personnel. Long-term exposure to only traces of air contaminants has a very detrimental effect on people's respiratory systems.

Pollutants

Each of the many air pollutants has some known negative effect upon human health or the potential for causing illness and poor health. The Environmental Protection Agency has identified seven pollutants found in large amounts in the air, and has issued regulatory standards designed to control them. These seven are (1) carbon monoxide, (2) hydrocarbons, (3) lead, (4) nitrogen oxide, (5) ozone, (6) particulate matter, and (7) sulfur oxide.

Carbon Monoxide

Produced by the incomplete combustion of organic materials, carbon monoxide's major source is the internal combustion engine of the automobile. This gas is breathed into the lungs and enters the red blood cells where it combines with hemoglobin, which normally carries oxygen to the body cells. Because of the hemoglobin affinity for carbon monoxide, normal oxygen supply is replaced by carbon monoxide. This causes a reduction in oxygen supply to the various body cells.

The action of carbon monoxide in the body can cause death if too much oxygen is replaced, particularly in the brain cells. Exposure to carbon monoxide over a lengthy period of time has a detrimental effect on respiratory functioning, the cardiovascular system, and the mental capacities of alertness and perception.

Hydrocarbons

Compounds containing both carbon and hydrogen, hydrocarbons are the products of incomplete combustion of gasoline and the evaporation of petroleum fuels and industrial solvents. The main sources of hydrocarbons are motor vehicles, refineries, and petroleum-processing facilities.

Hydrocarbons have been shown to have a negative effect on people with upper respiratory problems. Hydrocarbons are also a concern because they are a major factor in the reaction that forms ozone and other photochemical oxidants.

Lead

This substance enters the atmosphere principally from automobile exhaust and from industries that process this metal. Most airborne lead is created by automobiles, so all new automobiles must now use lead-free gasoline. However, many older cars still use leaded gasoline.

Lead is injurious to several body systems since it is absorbed into the blood and accumulates in several locations, principally the bones. Concern has been expressed regarding the effect of lead on young children, who are particularly susceptible to lead poisoning.

Nitrogen Oxides

These are highly toxic gases that are the result of high-temperature combustion of such energy sources as coal, oil, and gasoline. The major outlets of nitrogen oxides are electric utilities, industrial boilers, and motor vehicles.

Exposure to high levels of nitrogen oxides can be fatal. The general public usually is exposed to low levels, which can irritate the lungs, the eyes, and compound the causes of certain lung diseases. Nitrogen dioxide in combination with water vapor in the air produces nitric acid, which can corrode metal surfaces and damage vegetation.

Ozone

Produced by chemical reactions that occur when hydrocarbons and nitrogen oxides are exposed to sunlight, ozone is a photochemical oxidant. Hydrocarbons and nitrogen oxide compounds are broken up and oxygen atoms are released. These oxygen atoms join other oxygen atoms already in the atmosphere to form ozone. Ozone acts as an irritant to the respiratory system and the eyes, and has been shown to damage plants.

Particulate Matter

Airborne particles of solid or liquid substances are particulate matter. Soot, dirt, dust, and fly ash are examples of particulate matter found in the air. Particulate matter is the result of many industrial processes. For example, steel plants, electric generating plants, cement factories, and other similar industrial processes put wastes into the ambient air.

Particulate matter damages the protective cilia of the respiratory system. The damaged or destroyed cilia are likely to be a factor in disease and infection. In addition, toxic chemical substances may be carried into the respiratory system by particulate matter or may cause serious eye irritation.

Sulfur Oxide

The combustion of fuels that contain sulfur results in the production of sulfur oxides. Coal burning accounts for the major portion of sulfur oxides in the air. In addition to coal, the burning of residual oil, paper, rubber, and other solid wastes contributes sulfur dioxide to the air.

The major health effect of the various sulfur oxides is irritation of the respiratory system, so it is especially detrimental to bronchitis, emphysema, and asthma victims. Children and the elderly are particularly susceptible to sulfur oxides. In addition to contributing to respiratory problems, sulfur oxides cause corrosion and damage vegetation.

Legislative Action

The increased awareness of health problems, particularly of respiratory and cardiovascular disease, and the exposure to air pollutants have provoked action to improve the quality of air. This action has taken several different directions. Some actions have been directed at individual behaviors, such as prohibiting the burning of leaves in the fall. Others have been directed at industrial sources of air pollution, requiring emission-control devices on smokestacks. Since the motor vehicle is a major contributor to air pollution, changes in the exhaust system have been mandated by federal government.

Unfortunately, measures designed to clean the air are costly. These costs have been passed on both directly and indirectly to the consumer, to the industrial manufacturer, and to government. All too often the costs to industry and to government are then passed along to the individual. For example, air pollution emission regulations mandate the installation of exhaust devices on all cars, an expense that is passed along to the buyer in the purchase price of the automobile, hence contributing to the higher prices of automobiles.

Many industries, corporations, and individuals feel that current air pollution laws and regulations are inflationary and should be reduced or eliminated. This issue has resulted in one of the major political debates in the 1980s. For instance, the automotive industry would like to see reductions in the regulatory requirements of the Clean Air Act. On the other hand, many environmental groups and public health organizations are opposed to any weakening of such standards.

The federal government took legislative action in 1955[12] and in 1963[13] to deal with the problems of air pollution. These legislative actions provided funds for research and financial assistance to local agencies. In 1970, Congress enlarged the role of the federal government by passing the Clean Air Amendments of 1970 (PL 91–604), legislation that gave the Environmental Protection Agency the responsibility to establish standards for all major air pollutants.

Since 1970, the Environmental Protection Agency has set standards for seven major pollutants. In addition, strict emission standards for the manufacture of new automobiles and the building of power plants and factories were established. Compliance time tables were set, revised, and extended in many instances. Through the 1970s, the Clean Air Act was the principal legislation for improving the quality of air in the United States.

The future of the Clean Air Act is on shaky ground. Officials in industry, business, and government are opposed to the strict standards and compliance time tables. They question the way these federal standards have been established. For most pollutants, there is little clear evidence to indicate the level at which a pollutant can be considered safe, so it has been difficult to develop acceptable threshold levels. For these reasons, those opposed to the Clean Air Act suggest that current standards cannot be justified and therefore must either be compromised or totally eliminated.

Opponents also contend that it is too costly to enforce and to meet standards. Such standards interfere with the concept of free enterprise and create governmental interference.

Environmental and health advocates have argued strongly that the Clean Air Act should not be weakened, but, in fact, should be strengthened. They contend that any action that would extend compliance deadlines into the late 1980s or early 1990s, that would weaken implementation requirements, or that would raise already established standards would only add to the problems of air pollution. These environmentalists also want regulated standards for other pollutants, too. (There are no standards for pollutants such as benzene, arsenic, radioactive emissions, and formaldehyde.) They believe that voluntary compliance will not be effective and that governmental regulations are necessary.

The Bhopal Incident

In December 1984 a lethal cloud of methyl isocyanate (MIC) was released from a Union Carbide storage plant in Bhopal, India. This incident caused the death of some 2,250 people and injuries to over

50,000 individuals, required the evacuation of thousands of other people, and killed many animals. Long-term effects were noted among women such as menstrual bleeding and uncommon vaginal discharges. Methyl isocyanate is used as an insecticide that is important in decreasing insect damage to cotton and vegetables. In spite of laws and regulations designed to prevent such a catastrophe, leakage of gas and chemicals into the atmosphere is an all too common occurrence. Obviously concern must be expressed as to whether a situation such as took place in Bhopal could happen again in the United States.

Solid Wastes

Billions of tons of solid waste are produced annually in the United States. Solid waste includes paper, food stuffs, glass, metals, plastics, pesticide containers, paint cans, tires, batteries, old cars, disposable diapers, and a number of other items found in every household. Permanent disposal of these materials is an ever-increasing problem in the world.

The problem of solid waste removal has been amplified in recent years because of the increased population in the world, the increased manufacture of consumer products, and the manufacture and use of materials that do not burn or decay. For example, the use of plastic containers, which are very difficult to burn and do not decay, has increased extensively in recent years.

Solid waste removal is not just a problem in urban communities. Agricultural wastes, including animal manure and orchard prunings, account for much of the solid wastes produced each year. Two billion metric tons of animal waste are produced annually, half generated by livestock and poultry.

Methods of Disposal

The disposal of solid wastes is achieved in several different ways. Dumping has been a time-honored measure, and sanitary landfills are widely used today. Incineration and recycling, though not as widely used, are also found in many localities.

Dumping

Probably the oldest and most traditional method of solid waste disposal is *dumping*. Waste material is brought to a specified location and thrown away. No effort is made to cover the waste, and it is usually burned to reduce the bulk. In these settings, the wind scatters the paper and other light objects, rodents and other scavengers search for food, and mosquitoes and flies reproduce in the open garbage.

Many dumps are situated where they drain into the groundwater supply. This drainage results in contamination of drinking water and may create many health problems.

Open dumps not only hold a potential for disease but are also an eyesore in any community. They also contribute to environmental problems, such as air pollution, water contamination, and a rodent population. Burning, either purposeful or spontaneous, almost always occurs in dumps. Organic matter that is not consumed by insects, rodents, and other animals is slowly reduced by decomposition.

Today open dumping and burning is prohibited in much of the United States. The sanitary landfill has replaced the open, uncontrolled dumping as the procedure for elimination of solid wastes.

Sanitary Landfill

A much more effective procedure for the removal of solid wastes is an adequate, well-designed, and well-engineered sanitary landfill. At a properly operated sanitary landfill, the waste material is compacted when dumped, then covered with dirt. After a period of time, during which the landfill area is covered with dirt each day, the site is compressed and smoothed by large bulldozers.

A major advantage of a sanitary landfill is that the waste material is buried each day. As a result, burning and blowing of material is kept to a minimum and rodents are few. Land that is of little other use may be reclaimed by the fill and then developed into a park, recreation site, golf course, or a housing area.

Many problems result from an improperly engineered and operated sanitary landfill. Anaerobic decay of the buried wastes may lead to continuous settling of the land for many years. As a result, it becomes difficult to utilize the reclaimed area until the settling is minimized. It is also extremely important that the landfill area is well planned and operated to protect against possible contamination of water supplies. Numerous geological considerations are important in site selection. Water table levels are crucial since areas with high levels are potential runoff sites and so are not satisfactory as landfill locations.

Methane gas is a by-product of the compaction at a sanitary landfill. Landfill methane gas, when mixed with air in a 5 to 15 percent concentration, is flammable.[14] Because of the methane, vegetation has been destroyed, fires have resulted, and on the site of a New Jersey landfill, two individuals were killed by a methane explosion.[15] These dangers can be reduced by proper venting of the sanitary landfill.

It is increasingly difficult to find suitable localities for the sanitary landfills. Residents are usually opposed to a sanitary landfill in their neighborhood. It is also a politically unpopular action to be responsible for a policy decision that establishes a sanitary landfill in a given location.

Incineration

The burning of solid wastes has probably been practiced since the beginning of humanity. Today, incinerators are still operated by municipalities, and in private homes, apartment complexes, and industries. Incineration is useful because it destroys solid substances and in the process reduces the volume of solid waste. However, as a result of burning, soot, smoke, and particulate matter are released into the air.

Incineration is also expensive. Not only is the cost of building an incinerator expensive, but the operation of community incinerators is more than twice as costly as using a sanitary landfill.

Incineration could be used to generate heat and energy if properly developed. This process has had rather limited application in the United States, but some European cities do use the heat and energy generated by incineration. In many cases residences and apartments are heated by garbage-burning facilities. The increased shortages and costs of energy that have been experienced during the past decade make incineration a more viable alternative.

Recycling

Recycling solid waste materials has aroused interest during the past decade. Americans, oriented to throwing away all waste products, have only recently introduced the concepts of conservation and recycling into their life-styles.

In the past it was not economical to recycle, and the availability of resources made recycling unnecessary. Today, however, many products can be recycled. For example, paper is a solid waste product that can be recycled. Old newspapers can be recycled into tar paper for roofing, cardboard cartons, and numerous other items. Metals, including copper, lead, and zinc, are other resources that can be recycled.

Glass, too, can be recycled effectively and completely. One out of every fifteen bottles and jars currently produced in the United States is recycled into new bottles and jars.[16] Through the process of grinding, glass can be reduced to particles that can then be used as soil conditioners in compost or for road surfacing.

Future technology will develop new and more economical uses for recycled solid wastes in our society. It is important that people become conscious of the importance of recycling solid wastes and discontinue their "throw-away" habits.

Toxic Wastes

The disposal of toxic wastes creates many serious problems and concerns. American industry generates an estimated 275 million metric tons of hazardous wastes each year.[17] Included are numerous chemicals—such as dioxin, PCB, PBB, vinyl chloride, mercury, arsenic, and lead—that are potentially hazardous to human health. These threaten to contaminate groundwater supplies; kill vegetation, birds, and animal life; and emit toxic fumes.

Usually chemical wastes are deposited in dumps and sanitary landfills in steel drums. Solid waste disposal sites vary in terms of geological, hydrological, physical, chemical, and ecological nature. For example, clay soils retard leakage and absorb many chemicals, whereas sand and gravel do not provide good containment of chemicals.

(a) This site included several toxic wastes that had seeped into the underground water table. Several small lakes such as this one were in need of cleaning up by the Environmental Protection Agency. (b) Work on this site for over a year resulted in cleaning of the polluted lake and a signficant improvement in the overall environment.

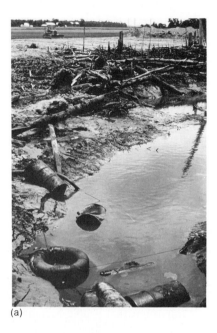

(a)

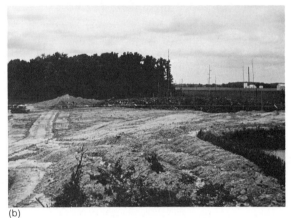

(b)

As time passes and rust develops, poisons seep from the drums into the soil and eventually work their way into the groundwater. Some sixty thousand chemicals in use by industry today may be potentially hazardous to human health.[18] The Environmental Protection Agency estimates that a frightening 90 percent of all industrial wastes are improperly disposed.[19]

In addition to concern over leakage from old and/or improperly managed dumps and landfills, accidental spills and illegal dumping of toxic substances occur all too often. Transportation of toxic wastes is a particularly dangerous action. Spills of highly toxic chemical wastes have occurred on the nation's transportation arteries: roads and expressways, rivers and streams, and railroads.

Often toxic wastes are transported by rail. One of the most serious rail accidents involving chemical wastes occurred in Louisiana in 1982. Freight cars carrying chemicals such as vinyl chloride and phosphoric acid derailed, causing serious explosions and fires. Nearby residents were forced to evacuate their homes for more than a week until the danger had subsided.

Within a month of this text's writing, the news reported three different rail accidents involving chemicals being transported. Each necessitated temporary evacuation of people living in the immediate area, people being hospitalized for emergency care, and in one case a fire that lasted nearly forty-eight hours. Unfortunately, news of additional toxic chemical spills on the rails will continue to be part of daily newscasts.

In 1976, Congress passed the Resources Conservation and Recovery Act, which established safety regulations for landfills. The Environmental Protection Agency was assigned the responsibility of establishing regulatory standards for landfills and of monitoring and enforcing these standards. The law, in spite of its good intentions, provided exemptions for many businesses and industries. For example, any business that produces less than one ton of toxic wastes each month is exempt. Other loopholes in the law have permitted disposal of many toxic wastes without penalty or punishment of any kind.

One of the most toxic chemicals that has received recent attention is dioxin. This chemical has caused the forced evacuation of towns in Missouri and Michigan. In Times Beach, Missouri, more than two thousand people were forced to relocate. In 1972, chemical sludge combined with waste oil was used as a sealant on the roads of this rural community. The sludge contained dioxin. For the next decade there was no concern. However, in 1982, following a widespread flood, residents of the city became aware of the dangerous situation in their town. Following the flood the residents were warned that they should not return due to the toxic danger. Today Times Beach is a vacated town; nearly all of its home owners had to relocate.

Another classic case relating to toxic waste is the case of Love Canal at Niagara Falls, New York. In the latter 1970s residents were suffering from an unusual amount of skin ailments, respiratory problems, headaches, epileptic seizures, and hair loss. It was also noted that the rate of miscarriage and birth defects was higher among residents of this area than for those in surrounding communities. For several years previously a chemical company had deposited some twenty-one thousand tons of hazardous toxic chemicals in an area dumpsite. By 1978 a national emergency was declared at Love Canal and over six hundred families had to be evacuated. Since 1978 scientists have identified over 240 different toxic chemicals in this area, and in 1985 dangerous levels of dioxin were still being reported in the area by the Environmental Protection Agency.

Though much is unknown about the long-term effects of dioxin on human health, it is known that it causes hair and weight loss, headaches, tingling of the extremities, and may well be a cause of cancer. At lowest levels it has been shown to cause birth defects, miscarriage, and death in laboratory animals. It can adversely affect immunosystem response and liver function in humans.[20]

Superfund

Efforts to clean up toxic wastes have been minimal. With as many as ten thousand hazardous waste sites in the United States the cost of cleaning up would possibly run into the hundreds of billions of dollars. Obviously, the expense would be enormous.

In 1980 Congress created a $1.6 billion, five-year program under the authority of the Comprehensive Environmental Response, Compensation and Liability Act, which provided funding and authority for cleaning up hazardous waste sites. This program was established to clean up thousands of dumps that were leaking toxic wastes into underground water sources. Funds for this program came from taxes on petroleum and certain chemicals as well as from general federal appropriations. The program came to be referred to as the Superfund Program.

The Environmental Protection Agency identified some 850 sites as having priority for cleanup. The program became enmeshed in controversy. By 1985 when the law expired the money was gone, and little impact had been made on the problem of solid waste contamination. Only six sites were reported to have been cleaned up.[21] Even then many questions were raised as to whether the cleaning of these sites had been successful. It has been pointed out that the cleaning of these sites has only transported the problem elsewhere. For example, in one case, soil contaminated by PBB, PCB, and DDT was removed from a golf course developed next to an old chemical dump and was deposited at another location.

Much political debate, argument, and controversy between Congress, the president, and the Environmental Protection Agency undercut any chance of effectiveness of this program. The lack of funds to perform these measures, the reduced funding and staff of the Environmental Protection Agency to oversee the corrective measures, and the reluctance of industry and the general public to comply with the orders have all contributed to less than successful cleanup results.

There is difference of opinion as to how much it would cost to effectively clean up priority sites. In 1984 the Environmental Protection Agency estimated that as much as $22.7 billion would be needed to clear up all priority sites. Congress had asked for over $10 billion and finally in 1986 settled on an appropriation of $9 billion for continuation of the Superfund program. Unfortunately, it is still cheaper to dump and only when the dangers of toxic wastes seem to affect the population directly, as at the time of a spill, a fire, or contamination of a water supply, do people become concerned enough to demand action.

Radiation

When atoms are split, energy and radiation are released. This release of radiation is known as *radioactivity*, which has been shown to have a major effect upon the health and well-being of people. Radiation at certain high levels can kill outright or it may linger in the body for years. Exposure to radiation injures human tissue and causes a number of health problems. When a person is exposed to 25–50 roentgens (r) the white blood cells may be affected. Radiation sickness, a condition resulting in nausea, fatigue, anemia, diarrhea, and loss of hair, occurs as the result of exposure to 100 to 200 roentgens of radiation. Exposure to 350 to 500 r will usually be fatal.

More subtle, but just as much of a concern, is the effect of exposure to low levels of radiation over a long period of time. Such exposures often occur in occupational settings, in various community settings, and as has been reported recently in the case of radon, in our own homes. We do not know as much as we would like about long-term effects of continuous or intermittent exposure to low levels of radiation. There is evidence that certain kinds of cancer—skin, bone, skeletal, leukemia, and lung—can be caused by such exposure.

Increasing concern has also been expressed about the damage that may be done to reproductive cells over a long period of time. This exposure may result in damage or alteration of human genes—damage to chromosomes—and the long-term effects may not be revealed until future generations are born. The exact effect of radiation on a person depends upon the body part exposed, the potency of the dose, and the rate at which it is received.

Humans have been exposed to small amounts of radiation in nature since the beginning of time. Radioactive gases are released by soil and rock formations as uranium. Cosmic radiation is given off in outer space and is measurable on earth in small amounts. Radioactive agents in the atmosphere result from sunflares, which give off solar particle beams. People are exposed to an average of 175 millirems a year of natural radiation.[22]

Radon Gas

Radon is an odorless, colorless, tasteless, natural radioactive gas that is produced naturally in the ground. It is the product of underground uranium decay. The Environmental Protection Agency has indicated that as many as 12 percent of American homes may have radon levels above the EPA recommended standard for safe exposure. These radon problems have been reported in some thirty states with the most prevalent concentration being in several states in the eastern United States.

Radon seeping through soil and rock enters homes through cracks in walls, drains, along pipes, and house floors. Radon is also released into the atmosphere when water is heated, as in showering or when washing clothes. Construction of energy conscious homes in the 1980s with increased insulation has played an important factor in keeping radon inside. The radioactive particles become airborne, attach themselves to dust and are breathed in and can cause serious tissue damage. This natural radioactive gas, which decays into four radioactive elements, is thought to be a contributing cause of lung cancer. The Environmental Protection Agency has announced the need for homes in areas with potential for radon gas to have ventilation systems constructed that can help in removing the radon from the interior of the house.

Exactly how many homes are affected and how many related cases of illness and death are due to radon exposure are unknown. Reports of incidence run as high as eight million homes with as many as twenty thousand lung cancer deaths being contributed to radon.[23] These figures are estimates of the Environmental Protection Agency. Even if these data are an overestimation it is important to note that environmental health sanitarians in many locations of the country will be faced with a serious problem for some time in attempting to identify ways to eliminate the threat of this source of radioactivity.

New Sources of Radiation

Since the atom was first split in 1942 at the University of Chicago and ushered in the nuclear age, many new sources of radiation have been introduced into the environment. The development, testing, and use of nuclear weapons have contributed to this increased exposure to radiation. In addition, many domestic uses of radioactive rays have been found. For example, some home appliances emit small amounts of radiation. X rays used in medicine and dentistry account for much of the radiation exposure.

The world's need for and consumption of energy have resulted in the development of nuclear energy power plants. Nuclear energy creates heat that is used for steam-generated electricity. This production of electricity is the most important use of nuclear power today. The nuclear power plant contains a core of nuclear fuel, primarily uranium. The energy potential in uranium, the primary ingredient of nuclear power, is exceptional. One pound of this fuel contains nearly three million times the energy found in a pound of coal.[24] Uranium does not burn like the fossil fuels—oil, coal, and wood. Heat is produced in the nuclear reactor by a process known as *fission*. During this process uranium atoms in the reactor are split and energy in the form of heat is released. The heat from fission turns water into steam and steam spins the turbin generators.

About two decades ago, many people felt that the eventual solution to the world's energy shortage rested in nuclear power. The first nuclear power plant in the United States began operation in 1957 in Shippingport, Pennsylvania, on the Ohio River. This plant was shut down in 1982 and decommissioning of it will be a five-year $100 million project. Since 1957, approximately fifty-five plants have been built and are operational. More than twenty nations in the world have nuclear power, but the United States is the world's greatest producer.

Future of Nuclear Power

The future use and development of nuclear power are clouded in controversy since many oppose both the development and expansion of nuclear energy. These opponents are concerned about the safety of this energy source. For many, their questions have not been satisfactorily answered.

Small amounts of radiation are released from the reactors of nuclear power plants. It is unknown how much of this radiation humans can withstand before health is affected. Although there are claims that the amount released is infinitesimal and of no danger, the long-term risks of exposure are not known.

The disposal of nuclear wastes presents another serious environmental problem. The wastes must be buried in isolated locations and every measure must be taken to assure that the radiation does not escape. Since nuclear wastes are radioactive for years after their burial, opponents are concerned that future contamination could result from an accident, a natural occurrence such as an earthquake, or damage to the burial vaults. In spite of assurances by the nuclear power industry that these disposal procedures are safe, many opponents of nuclear energy remain unconvinced.

Nuclear energy can best be developed near large sources of water, as large amounts of water are needed to cool the reactors. Many nuclear power plants use millions of gallons of water per minute in this cooling process. It is important that the used water be kept in a holding lake or pond before being returned to its original source. Even then, care must be taken not to upset the ecological balance of a lake or river by returning water that is warmer than the natural temperature.

In 1979 the attention of the entire United States was focused upon Three Mile Island near Harrisburg, Pennsylvania. A nuclear accident caused many people to question the safety of nuclear power plants. The accident was kept under control, yet small amounts of radioactivity were measured in the air around the site. Fortunately, dangerous meltdown did not occur.

Meltdown occurs if the water that cools the heat-producing nuclear reactor core is shut down. This action would result in the melting of the nuclear core. The liquefied uranium core would then drop through the protective shielding. Without this shielding, the radioactive uranium would spread radiation into the air and the ground, causing serious consequences to the environment and to human life. The potential for large-scale destruction by nuclear accident was exemplified at Three Mile Island.

The most serious nuclear accident in history occurred in 1986 in Chernobyl, USSR. An explosion followed by fire in one of the four nuclear reactors resulted in the release of a cloud of radiation into the air that spread far beyond the Soviet Union throughout Eastern Europe and into Scandinavia. This incident resulted in the release of the largest quantity of radioactive material ever in an accident. The release measured millions of *curies,* the radioactive decay rate of one gram of radium. By contrast, Three Mile Island is reported to have released fifteen curies.[25]

The radioactive cloud spread northwest over Poland, into the Scandinavian countries, then two days later it spread west–southwest, over Europe, as far as England, Germany, and Holland. Some 300 to 400 million people in fifteen nations were placed at risk.[26] Several hundred people died, and thousands were hospitalized with radiation sickness. Many of the hospitalized victims were treated with bone marrow transplants.

This tragic incident showed that there was no adequate international warning system to alert governments and people of impending nuclear danger. Nor have any international standards for nuclear safety been developed and implemented.[27]

Problems with the design and operation of some nuclear plants have caused shutdowns until repairs or appropriate corrections could be made. The corrosion of the steam generators that carry hot radioactive water has caused several plants to stop operation until repairs could be made. The Nuclear Regulatory Commission has warned a number of nuclear plants that radiation was making the steel shell that surrounds the uranium core susceptible to cracks and possible meltdown.

The future of nuclear energy is dependent on the answers to many questions.The development and construction of new nuclear power plants have been greatly curtailed since the Three Mile Island incident. The accident at Chernobyl only heightened fear and concern of many about the future development and use of nuclear power.

Yet nuclear power is still a major energy producer in many parts of the United States, particularly in New England and the Great Lakes region. If nuclear power is to continue as a viable means of providing energy in the world, it must be proven that radiation can be controlled and the environment kept safe for all humanity.

Military Use of Nuclear Weapons

In spite of concern over radiation and nuclear wastes from nuclear power plants, by far the greatest generation of nuclear wastes has resulted from military nuclear weapons systems programs. The United States weapons programs have generated seven million cubic feet of waste which is seven hundred times more than that generated by nuclear power plants.[28] Concern obviously needs to be directed toward the many problems of nuclear weapons deployment and potential use.

Noise Pollution

Sound moves through the air in waves similar to the movement of water upon an ocean beach. When these waves make contact with the eardrum, sound is heard. These sound waves are then transmitted to and interpreted by the human brain. Human beings communicate by sound, we relax to the sound of music, the sound of an infant's cry tells us that the baby has some need, and most of our contact with the environment takes place by way of sound.

When sound is unwanted, it is termed noise. A sound that is tolerable for one person, however, may be noise to another. For example, the sound of trucks passing in front of a house on the expressway is tolerated by the truck driver because a livelihood is involved. But to the person attempting to sleep, the trucks are making noise. Thus, sound is subject to individual interpretations. It is termed sound or noise depending on the experiences and background of each person.

Sound has three characteristics: (1) pitch, (2) volume, and (3) timbre. Pitch and volume, especially, are of concern to health. Timbre is the quality of sound. Pitch is the height or depth of the sound, and is measured in units based upon the cycles per second (c.p.s.). The human ear can detect sound as low as sixteen c.p.s. and as high as sixteen thousand c.p.s.[29] Volume is recorded in units called decibels (dbs.). Zero decibel is the weakest sound level that can be detected by the human ear.

Decibels are logarithmic, not linear, units of measurement. For this reason, there is a sharp increase in the loudness of sound with each decibel increase. For example, ten decibels of sound is ten times more intense than one decibel. However, twenty decibels is one hundred times more intense than one decibel. Thirty decibels is one thousand times as intense as one decibel. Continuing this progression, one hundred decibels is ten billion times as intense as one decibel of sound.

Most sound that the human being encounters ranges between fifty and ninety decibels. The level at which most people begin to feel pain is about 120 decibels. The sound level of a two-person conversation is usually around sixty decibels, and traffic noise in a city ranges from seventy to over ninety decibels. If you have ever been on the ground near a jet airplane when it is taxiing for takeoff, you will recall the ear-shattering noise. The sound level being generated by that plane is near 140 decibels.

The principal and most obvious health-related problem of noise pollution is the loss of hearing. It has been estimated that over twenty million Americans are exposed daily to noise that may permanently damage their hearing.[30] In addition to this hearing loss, exposure to noise causes a number of other physiological effects. Noise causes an increase in adrenaline output, dilation of blood vessels in the brain, an increase in heart rate, and a rise in blood pressure. All of these physiological reactions are related to cardiovascular disease. Though there has been no proof of a direct relationship between noise pollution and heart disease, it is a possibility, considering the physiological changes that result from exposure to noise.

Noise also contributes to the level of stress in people. The physiological effects of noise on the human body create the same problems associated with other stress-related problems: headaches, tension, and sleep disruption.

Table 10.1	Permissible Noise Exposures
Duration per day, Hours	**Sound level (dbs.)**
8	90
6	92
4	95
3	97
2	100
1½	102
1	105
½	110
¼ or less	115

Source: Table G-16, Occupational Health and Safety Administration General Industry Standards.

Noise pollution is found in many environmental settings. All forms of transportation and construction equipment are the major sources of noise pollution in our society. Though primarily an urban problem, machinery in rural localities is also a source of noise. Studies have shown that farmers and other agricultural workers use equipment that generates noise levels between eighty and ninety decibels.

In the home, appliances produce high noise levels. Garbage disposals, blenders, dishwashers, power tools, and stereos cause noise levels that have been found to exceed ninety to one hundred decibels.

Some people are exposed daily to high sound levels at their place of employment. There is little doubt that this exposure to both continuous and intermittent sound levels is injurious to hearing over an extended period of time.

Since many industrial processes in the workplace produce noise levels above one hundred decibels, the Occupational Safety and Health Act required the establishment of standards for noise exposure in the occupational setting. The standards that have been established by the Occupational Safety and Health Administration allow up to ninety decibels of exposure for an eight-hour day. Higher decibel levels are acceptable for shorter periods of time. Industry is then required by law to reduce the sound levels at the source of the noise generation or to provide protective equipment for all employees.

Summary

Efforts to provide a safe and healthful environment have been a major focus of community health programming. Activities in the latter part of the 1800s were designed to control communicable diseases. Today, however, a greater number of environmental problems necessitates a wider range of environmental program emphasis.

The provision of a safe water supply and the presence of pure air are two important emphases of an environmental health program. In spite of the fact that waterborne diseases do not reach epidemic proportions in the United States today, water pollution remains a problem. Many municipal water systems are not providing the purest water for residents. Various chemicals dumped into the lakes and rivers, industrial processing measures, and agriculture are major sources of water pollution.

Likewise there are many sources of air pollution. Most air pollution in this country is the result of emissions from the internal combustion engine of motor vehicles, the burning of fossil fuels, and other industrial processes. These produce many different pollutants. The Environmental Protection Agency has established standards to control several of these pollutants, including carbon monoxide, hydrocarbons, lead, nitrogen oxide, ozone, particulate matter, and sulfur oxide.

The disposal of toxic chemical wastes has created a number of serious problems. Presence of toxic chemicals in groundwater is an increasing concern in many localities. The presence of chemical dumps and the use of chemical agents for a variety of uses have led to the necessity to evacuate two cities in the United States. The long-term effects of toxic wastes are not totally known.

Increasing concern about radiation has been noted in recent years. The nuclear power plant accidents at Three Mile Island and Chernobyl have caused concern about the potential for catastrophic dangers of nuclear power. Humans are exposed to radiation in a variety of different localities: radon in their homes, radiation from natural sources, and radiation emitted from scientific and military uses.

Discussion Questions

1. In what ways has emphasis in environmental programming changed since the last century?
2. What is thermal pollution?
3. In what ways is groundwater being affected by chemical dumping today?
4. Identify the provisions of federal legislation passed in the 1970s to control water pollution.
5. What is acid rain and what are its effects on humans, animals, and vegetation?
6. How does carbon monoxide physiologically affect the human body?
7. Do you feel that the Clean Air Act should be changed, modified, or rescinded? Explain your answer.
8. What is the difference between a dump and a sanitary landfill?
9. Why have the problems associated with toxic wastes become a serious concern in the United States?
10. Discuss the significance of the incidents at Love Canal, N.Y., and Times Beach, Missouri.
11. What is the Superfund?
12. Identify some of the controversy surrounding the Superfund program.
13. What is radiation?
14. Explain some of the concerns about nuclear power plants in the United States.
15. What is the significance of Chernobyl and Three Mile Island?

16. Do you support further development of nuclear power? If so, why? If not, why not?

17. Explain concerns being expressed about radon in homes.

18. Identify some of the health problems associated with noise pollution.

Suggested Readings

Bacon, J. Maichle, and Gleckno, William A. "Groundwater Contamination: A National Problem with Implications for State and Local Environmental Health Personnel." *Journal of Environmental Health* 48, no. 3 (November/December, 1985): 116–21.

Bowander, B., and others. "Avoiding Future Bhopals." *Environment* 27, no. 7 (September, 1985): 6–13, 31–37.

Craun, Gunther F. "A Summary of Waterborne Illness Transmitted Through Contaminated Groundwater." *Journal of Environmental Health* 48, no. 3 (November/December, 1985): 122–27.

Dowling, Michael. "Defining and Classifying Hazardous Wastes." *Environment* 27, no. 3 (April, 1985): 18–20, 36–41.

Gerusky, Thomas M. "The Pennsylvania Radon Story." *Journal of Environmental Health* 49, no. 4 (January/February, 1987): 197–200.

"Health Aspects of Hazardous Waste Disposal." *Environment* 28, no. 3 (April, 1986): 38–45.

Heil, Jeffrey, and Van Blarcom, James. "Superfund: The Search for Consistency." *Environment* 28, no. 3 (April, 1986): 6–9.

Hesse, John L., and others. "Problems and Responsibilities Associated With Hazardous Waste at the State Level." *Journal of Environmental Health* 48, no. 4 (January/February, 1986); 186–89.

Hileman, Bette. "Acid Rain Perspectives: A Tale of Two Countries." *Environmental Science and Technology* 18, no. 11 (November/December, 1984): 341A–44A.

Hohenemser, C. "Chernobyl: An Early Report." *Environment* 28, no. 5 (June, 1986): 6–13, 30–43.

"Indoor Air Pollution." *Consumer Reports* (October, 1985): 600.

Johnson, Arthur H. "Acid Deposition: Trends, Relationships, and Effects." *Environment* 28, no. 4 (May, 1986): 6–11, 34–39.

Kawata, Kazuyoshi. "Evolution of Drinking Water Regulations in the United States." *Journal of Environmental Health* 48, no. 4 (January/February, 1986): 206–9.

LaVeen, E. Phillip. "Protecting the Nation's Groundwater From Contamination." *Environment* 27, no. 4 (May, 1985): 25–27.

National Geographic Society. *Energy: A Special Report in the Public Interest.* Washington, D.C.: The Society (February, 1981).

Neufeld, William P. "Five Potential Crises: The Greenhouse Effect." *The Futurist* 18, no. 2 (April, 1984): 9–10.

Popkin, Roy. "Hazardous Waste Cleanup and Disaster Management." *Environment* 28, no. 3 (April, 1986): 2–5.

Regenstein, Lewis. "The Toxics Boomerang." *Environment* 25, no. 10 (December, 1983): 36–38, 43–44.

White, Irvin L., and Spath, John P. "Low-Level Radioactive Waste Disposal: How Are the States Setting Their Sites?" *Environment* 26, no. 8 (October, 1984): 16–20, 36–41.

Young, John, and others. "A Survey of State Asbestos Programs." *Journal of Environmental Health* 48, no. 6 (May/June, 1986): 332–35.

Endnotes

1. Carson, Rachael. *Silent Spring.* Boston: Houghton-Mifflin, 1962. Dubos, Rene. *Man Adapting.* New Haven: Yale University Press, 1965. Ehrlich, Paul R. *The Population Bomb.* New York: Ballantine Books, 1971.

2. El-Araf, Amer, and Baca, Thomas E. "The Administration of State and Local Environmental Health Programs: Who is Responsible?" *Journal of Environmental Health* 43, no. 2 (September/October, 1980): 86–100.

3. Craun, Gunther. "A Summary of Waterborne Illness Transmitted Through Contaminated Groundwater." *Journal of Environmental Health* 48, no. 3 (November/December, 1985): 122–27.

4. Reported in the *Wall Street Journal,* January 17, 1985.

5. LaVeen, E. Phillip. "Protecting the Nation's Groundwater From Contamination." *Environment* 27, no. 4 (May, 1985): 26.

6. Wagner, Richard H. *Environment and Man.* New York: W. W. Norton and Company, 1971: 133.

7. La Bastille, Anne. "Acid Rain, How Great a Menace?" *National Geographic* 160, no. 5 (November, 1981): 673.

8. Ibid., 680.

9. Ibid., 680.

10. Oleckno, William A. "The National Interim Primary Drinking Water Regulations." *Journal of Environmental Health* 44, no. 5 (March/April, 1982): 236.

11. USEPA. "National Primary Drinking Regulations, Volatile Organic Chemicals." *Federal Register* (1984): 49:24331–55.

12. Public Law 84–159, passed July 15, 1955.

13. Public Law 88–206, the Clean Air Act, passed December 17, 1963.

14. White, Peter T. "The Fascinating World of Trash." *National Geographic* 163, no. 4 (April, 1983): 440.

15. Ibid.

16. Ibid., 450.

17. Regenstein, Lewis. "The Toxic Boomerang." *Environment* 25, no. 10 (December, 1983): 36.

18. "A Problem That Cannot Be Buried." *Newsweek* (October 14, 1985): 84.

19. "The Toxic Waste Crisis." *Newsweek* (March 7, 1983): 20.

20. News release, American Medical Association, April 17, 1986.

21. "A Problem That Cannot Be Buried." *Newsweek* (October 14, 1985): 77.

22. Plant, Robert. "The Dangerous Atom." *World Health* (January, 1969): 17.

23. "Radon Gas: A Deadly Threat." *Newsweek* (August 18, 1986): 6.

24. National Geographic Society. *Energy: A Special Report in the Public Interest* (Washington, D.C.: The Society, 1981): 67.

25. Hohenemser, C. "Chernobyl: An Early Report." *Environment* 28, no. 5 (June, 1986): 6.

26. Ibid., 39.

27. Ibid., 40.

28. "Nuclear Power: Answers to Your Questions." Edison Electric Institute, Publication No. 78–24, 24.

29. Hammond, Eva. "Hearing Defects of School Age Children." *Journal of School Health* 60 (1970): 405.

30. *You Make the Difference.* Washington, D.C.: U.S. Government Printing Office: VII–10.

11

Community Nutrition: Developing Healthy Eating Patterns

Health problems related to nutrition are prevalent throughout the world, though they vary significantly from person to person, from community to community, and from culture to culture. The problems of hunger, starvation, and malnutrition are grave concerns worldwide. These conditions, affecting millions of people, occur principally in the poorest of the Third World nations and in those localities where political and natural tragedies have uprooted large populations.

Hunger and starvation, for the most part, are not characteristic of the developed world. In fact, a major health problem in the United States and many other industrial nations is *overconsumption* of food. Excessive intake of food, accompanied by a relatively sedentary life-style, results in obesity and an increased risk for major health problems.

Medical science has recorded an association between eating patterns and many of the chronic degenerative diseases. Hypertension, heart disease, and other chronic conditions are related to excessive intake of certain nutrients.

In recent years people have responded to these findings and have altered their life-styles so that weight loss and good nutrition are priorities. This is evident in the array of diet books, the increasing number of natural food stores, and the interest in enrollment in fitness programs. This concern about obesity, fat, and food overconsumption has led to controversial positions concerning the subject of diet and weight control.

Though food overconsumption and limited activity is the principal nutrition problem in America today, malnutrition does exist. It is found in varying degrees among certain segments of the American population. A physicians' task force studying hunger in America in 1984 found evidence of hunger and malnutrition.[1] The task force estimated that twenty million people are hungry at some time each month. This condition was found to be present basically among the economically disadvantaged, who encounter numerous health problems that are caused by malnutrition.

This population group includes many single-parent women, jobless minorities, unemployed blue-collar workers in depressed economic conditions, poor elderly, Native Americans, and migrants. In comparison to the relationships between chronic diseases and overconsumption, a different set of factors is associated with malnutrition. These factors are communicable diseases, developmental retardation, and reduced nutrient intake.

Poor nutrition is a problem for many pregnant teenagers, infants and school children, and the elderly. Local, state, and federal community health programs have been developed to meet the nutrition problems of these individuals.

Community nutrition programs have to account for both malnutrition and overconsumption. Not only must programs be designed to provide foodstuffs, calories, and nutrients for the hungry and malnourished, but some guidance about eating patterns for weight reduction must also be available.

What to Believe?

The American consumer makes decisions about what to eat based upon a variety of information. This information is often confusing and conflicting. Not only are the food advertisements that are developed by marketing specialists biased, misleading, and sometimes difficult to understand, but the recommendations of national boards and commissions often differ.

Standardization of nutrient and energy requirements is an inexact science. These standards, established by committees of experts, are published for public information. These are estimates of the proper nutrient intake for the good health of the average consumer.

Recommended Dietary Allowances (RDAs)

In the United States, the Recommended Dietary Allowances (RDAs), published by the Food and Nutrition Board of the National Research Council, are the standards by which many dietitians, nutritionists, and physicians identify adequate nutritional intake. The Food and Nutrition Board published its first listing of RDAs in 1943 and has updated the chart periodically. The RDAs update is based on newly acquired nutritional knowledge and research findings.

The tenth edition of the Recommended Dietary Allowances (RDAs) was scheduled to be released in 1985. However, controversy kept these guidelines from being accepted and published. The basic conflict centered around RDA values for vitamins A and C.

The committee that was appointed to submit the 1985 RDAs recommended reducing RDA values for Vitamin A and Vitamin C by about one-third. The National Academy of Science rejected these recommendations. They wanted these RDA values retained at the same levels as in the 1980 values. Agreement could not be reached and, as a result, the Academy rejected the entire report.

It is important to understand that RDAs are not standards of minimum requirements, but indications of nutrient and caloric levels that should provide adequate nourishment for most consumers.[2] They establish guidelines for planning diets for public assistance programs, for nutrition education programs, and for other community nutrition activities.[3] The RDA listings as defined by the Food and Nutrition Board are ". . . levels of intake of essential nutrients considered . . . to be adequate to meet the known needs of practically all healthy persons."[4]

Dietary Food Guide

Another set of guidelines, the Dietary Food Guide, is published by the U.S. Department of Agriculture and Harvard University's Department of Nutrition. These guidelines are supported by the American Medical Association.[5] They identify four different food groups: (1) milk and milk products; (2) meats, fish, poultry, dry beans, and other protein sources; (3) vegetables and fruits; and (4) breads and cereals. The guidelines recommend a moderate daily consumption of foods from each of the four food groups.

Dietary Goals for the United States

In 1977, the Senate Select Committee on Nutrition and Human Needs prepared a report that has received widespread attention.[6] The principal outcome of this report was the identification of six basic nutritional goals for the United States.

In addition to establishing the dietary goals, the committee recommended a number of buying guides for the American consumer. It was believed that by following these guides, the dietary goals could be met.

The buying guides recommended an increased consumption of fruits, vegetables, poultry, fish, and whole grains. These foods are important sources of vitamins and minerals yet are relatively low in fats, particularly saturated fat and cholesterol. Foods high in cholesterol, sugars, salt, and alcohol are directly related to six of the ten leading causes of death in America—heart disease, cancer, cerebrovascular disease, arteriosclerosis, diabetes, and cirrhosis of the liver.[7]

The subcommittee reported that the average American consumes 125 pounds of fat and one hundred pounds of sugar per year. Together, these two comprise 60 percent of the average diet.[8] Since two dietary goals call for the reduction of saturated fat and consumption of cholesterol, it was recommended that the American consumer decrease the amount of meat and other foods high in fat content. Americans were also advised to lower their intake of butterfat and eggs, and to substitute nonfat milk for whole milk.

The committee also strongly recommended a decrease in the consumption of sugar and salt. Soft drinks are a major source of sugar in the diet. In 1960, the average American consumed 13.6 gallons of soft drinks per year. By 1976, at the time of the

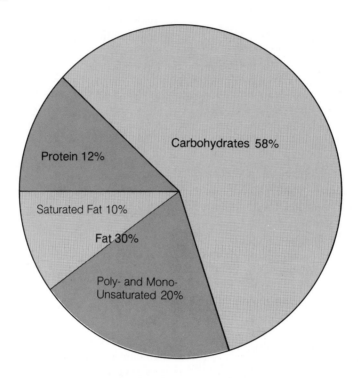

Dietary Goals for the United States

1. Increase carbohydrate consumption to account for 55 to 60 percent of caloric intake
2. Reduce fat consumption from 40 to 30 percent of caloric intake
3. Reduce saturated fat consumption to account for about 10 percent of caloric intake
4. Reduce cholesterol consumption to about three hundred milligrams a day
5. Reduce sugar consumption by about 40 percent
6. Reduce salt consumption by about 50 to 85 percent to approximately three grams per day

Source: Select Committee on Nutrition and Human Needs, U.S. Senate, *Dietary Goals for the United States*. Washington, D.C.: U.S. Government Printing Office, (1977).

The need for decreasing sodium, fat, and sugar in the diet is
noted in an educational display at a community health fair exhibit.

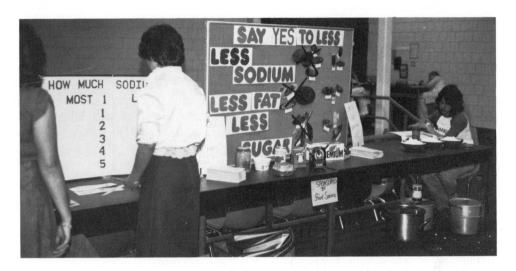

subcommittee report, this amount had more than doubled to 27.6 gallons per year.[9] Not only has this directly contributed to a number of health problems because the sugar replaces necessary complex carbohydrates, but it has also indirectly influenced milk consumption, an excellent source of nutrition.

The American public uses salt, which is primarily sodium, for many purposes, including food preservation, food preparation, and general seasoning.The human body needs about one gram of salt a day to maintain body homeostasis, but the average American consumes between ten and twenty grams per day. Obviously, this is far too much.

Too much sodium in the diet increases the risk of high blood pressure. It has been shown that individuals who live in areas where salt intake is high are much more likely to have hypertension than those who reside in localities with little sodium in the diet. Thus, a reduction in salt intake lowers the probability of hypertension.

Some difference of opinion exists as to what is an appropriate level of sodium consumption. Scientific and medical recommendations suggest a range of from three to eight grams per day.[10] However, an intake of three grams per day means that the individual will be eating a salt-restricted diet,

which is often recommended for those who have hypertension or who are at risk for this condition.

Most people have little idea of how much sodium they ingest each day. In an effort to educate the public about the potential health danger of sodium, it seems reasonable to have warning labels on food products. Individuals who are at risk for hypertension could then avoid purchasing these foods. This would have not only a preventive effect but also would be useful educationally and could result in a long-range economic benefit. In congressional testimony in 1981, it was reported that the benefits of sodium labeling on all processed foods would lower the incidence of high blood pressure and save over one billion dollars because of reduced sodium intake.

The Senate subcommittee, in addition to identifying dietary goals, advised that nutrition education programs be presented in the schools. It also recommended that improved food-processing methods be developed. The importance of food labeling for all foods was addressed in this report. Realizing that there are many questions yet unanswered regarding human nutrition, the subcommittee also called for increased research.

The dietary goals have received widespread attention. As a result, they have encountered opposition from various groups. A frequently expressed concern is that the goals were set by political personnel after hearing hand-selected testimony. The food industry, such as the United Egg Producers, strongly oppose the recommendations that Americans cut back egg and meat consumption. They argue instead that their products contribute to good health.

Toward Healthful Diets

A report by the Food and Nutrition Board of the National Research Council, "Toward Healthful Diets," issued in May 1980, suggested that individuals who are not at risk for atherosclerosis should not be concerned about fat and cholesterol in their diets. They could find no reason to recommend that adults decrease their intake of cholesterol.

This council is an organization of the National Academy of Science, which studies scientific questions for the government. The conclusions reached by this prestigious scientific board raised a great deal of concern and opposition by medical and public health agencies who have long worked for a reduction in the fat intake and cholesterol level in the American diet. This finding contradicted many nutritional guidelines established by these agencies and scientific nutritional organizations.

Dietary Guidelines for Americans

In early 1980 the federal departments of Agriculture, and Health and Human Services issued the report *Dietary Guidelines for Americans*. This report, like the Food and Nutrition Board report, recommended that Americans eat a variety of foods, avoid excess sodium, take alcohol only moderately, and maintain an ideal body weight. However, these two reports differed significantly on the role of fat, cholesterol, and carbohydrates in the diet.

The Department of Agriculture (USDA) and Health and Human Services (HHS) guidelines recommend that Americans avoid excessive fat, cholesterol, and sugar in the diet. It suggests that most

Americans should increase the consumption of complex carbohydrates. On the other hand, the Food and Nutrition Board report suggested that only people at risk for heart disease need to be concerned about cholesterol intake, and only obese individuals and those at risk for heart disease need to be concerned about too much fat.

In 1985 the United States Department of Agriculture and the Department of Health and Human Services issued a Second Edition of the federal dietary guidelines. The original guidelines were slightly modified. The 1985 document stated that the diet of most Americans is adequate. It recommended that large dose nutrient supplements should be avoided. This report noted the usefulness of salt as a food preservative and stated that sodium is but one factor known to affect hypertension. The guidelines included a strong caution warning of the dangers of drinking alcoholic beverages and driving. The public was instructed that if they drink, they should not drive.

These findings and recommendations by such prestigious groups have raised questions in the minds of many Americans about proper nutrition. Who is correct? Is fat a danger? How does cholesterol relate to health problems? If such reputable reports do not agree, where do we turn for accurate nutrition guidance? It is the responsibility of those involved in community nutrition to provide accurate information without bias. Currently, much nutrition information is false or misleading, and the average individual must sort this out in order to develop a healthy diet.

Community nutrition has an important goal: the improved health of all people within the society. In a society where the average life-style results in obesity, heart disease risk, and numerous other diet-related health problems, this goal is most important. Not only is it difficult to cope with measures to control weight problems, but there are many conflicting opinions about what is good nutrition, adequate diet, and appropriate governmental responsibility in nutritional programming.

Nutrition Programs

Child Nutrition

Nutrition affects the health and well-being of all age groups, races, and populations. Special concern should be focused on the problems of malnutrition in infant and child development. Malnutrition increases the likelihood that exposure to infection will lead to disease. Also, it encourages retarded cognitive and social development. Malnutrition has been shown to impair brain development in the early years of life, whereas good nutrition among pregnant and lactating women has an important influence on the health of newborn babies.

Because of the significant problems caused by malnutrition in infants and pregnant women, a number of child nutrition programs have been established in the United States. Child-care food programs provide meals and food supplements for children in day-care centers and other similar facilities. The Head Start Program supplies food for economically disadvantaged children enrolled in the program. Another important program that provides food supplements to mothers and children is the Supplemental Food Program for Women, Infants, and Children (WIC). Many children receive at least one-third of the recommended daily allowance (RDA) for nutrition through the School Lunch Program.[11]

Head Start

Though not designed primarily for nutrition, the federal Head Start Program has an important nutrition component. The basic purpose of Head Start is to provide children from low-income families with services that will enhance their personal development. Since many are physically, socially, and emotionally disadvantaged, this program provides opportunities and services that will help the young children to function adequately once they enter school.

Another important component of Head Start is the health program, in which the physical and mental health of each child are developed. Assessment activities include medical examinations and screening. Immunizations for common childhood diseases are provided by the Head Start Program. Improvement of the children's nutrition is an important aspect of the overall health program.

Meals are served to children enrolled in the Head Start Program. Breakfasts, lunches, dinners, and snacks are provided. The specific meals that each child receives are determined by the child's individual needs and the length of time the child is in the Head Start facility each day.

Not only do children enrolled in the Head Start Program receive nutritious meals, but parents are sometimes included in aspects of the programming. The parents become involved in the planning and preparation of the meals. This part of the program educates the parents. As they become involved in the process of creating good, nutritious meals for their children in the program, they are, in turn, learning to do the same at home for their families.

Special Supplemental Food Program for Women, Infants, and Children (WIC)

A major federal program designed to improve the nutrition of women and children is the WIC program. This program, known officially as the Special Supplemental Food Program for Women, Infants, and Children, was started in 1972 as a pilot program. Throughout the 1970s it was expanded both in focus and emphasis. The WIC Program provides nutritional assessment, counseling, and supplemental foods to certain high-risk population groups in terms of nutrition-related health problems. Four groups were designated as recipients of the aid: (1) pregnant women, (2) new mothers, (3) infants, and (4) children under five years of age.

In order to qualify for the WIC program, the individual must be certified as "low income" by the state, a physician must indicate that there is a nutritional risk to the individual's health, and the individual must live in the geographical area in which the WIC program is located. State and local agencies do not always use the same criteria to establish risk. Only one risk factor is necessary for eligibility. The most common nutritional risks by participant category are:[12]

Infants
    Mother on WIC during pregnancy
    Inadequate nutrition intake
    History or presence of anemia
Children
    Inadequate nutrition intake
    History or presence of anemia
    Low height for age
    Low weight for height
    High weight for height
Pregnant Women
    Inadequate pregnancy weight gain
    History or presence of anemia
    Teenage pregnancy
    Inadequate nutrient intake
    Excessive pregnancy weight gain
Postpartum Women
    Inadequate nutrient intake
    Teenage mother
    History of anemia
    High weight for height

The supplemental food received under this program contains nutrients that are often lacking in the diets of the populations at risk. The foods are high in protein, calcium, iron, and vitamins A and C. Infant formula, milk, juice, and other nutritious foodstuffs are made available through the program.

Those who participate in the WIC program do not have to pay for the food because the program is funded by the United States Department of Agriculture. Funds are channeled through local agencies who certify the eligibility of participants. Local agencies providing direct services for WIC programs are city and/or county health departments, hospitals, and nonprofit organizations serving health and welfare needs. The state health department is

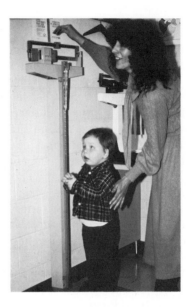

Participation in the WIC Program includes record keeping of the children's growth patterns. Each child weighs in to ascertain the growth that has taken place.

the state agency responsible for this program; funds are channeled through this agency from the federal government. The state agency manages the program and sets standards for its operation.

A component built into the WIC Program is nutrition education. Not only are food supplements available, but participants in the program receive instruction in nutrition. They are taught to read and understand food labels as well as how to prepare nutritious meals. The purpose of this is to improve the eating patterns of the participants. Nutrition education is also seen as an important preventive health measure.

The WIC Program has been a very effective nutritional program because it affects the health status of many women and children.[13] Studies have reported that WIC participants eat more nutritious food than non-WIC, low-income individuals. Nutrient quality of the diet continues to be better for WIC participants.[14] Not only does it have the positive effect of providing needed nutrients, but other health-related benefits have been identified. For example, WIC participants have increased their use

The Special Supplemental Food Program for Women, Infants, and Children (WIC) includes education. Here, "Fred*wick*" discusses good foods with the children to encourage proper eating patterns.

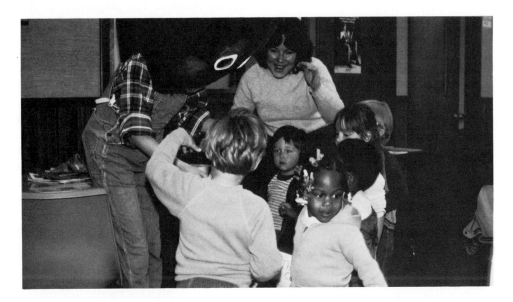

of medical services in the community.[15] It is estimated that for every dollar spent on WIC, three dollars are saved in future health care costs.[16]

The federal government has exempted the WIC Program from inclusion into the block-grant funding programs. Federal support for this program has remained constant while reductions have occurred in other child nutrition programs. Because of increased needs and the relative stability of funding, there has been a reduction in the number of individuals being served in this program. In some localities, this has meant that many women and infants in need of nutritional assistance cannot obtain that help any longer. Often those who are just above the poverty level may not be eligible for involvement in the WIC program. Hopefully this very effective program will continue to be operational in the years ahead.

Infant Formula

Breast-feeding versus bottle-feeding has become a nutritional issue in many parts of the world, including the United States. Throughout many parts of the world, as economic development occurs,

modern procedures are adopted. This has been the case in the way that mothers feed their infants.

Of course the natural way for an infant to be fed is from the mother's breast. Nutrient absorption, particularly of fat and iron, is greater in breast milk. Also, there are immunologic advantages to breast-feeding. The American Medical Association supports breast-feeding unless there are medical reasons for not doing so.[17] The only disadvantage of breast-feeding is in those few cases where insufficient milk can deprive the infant of necessary nutrients.

As countries develop and as mothers become more involved in working outside the home, infants are more often fed infant formula from the bottle, replacing breast-feeding. Unfortunately, a number of health problems have been identified with formula-feeding, particularly in the Third World. These problems include increased diarrhea, sickness, respiratory illness, allergic reactions to the formula, and stomach ailments. Without any question, breast milk is more nutritional and is a major contribution to the improved health and survival of infants.

All too often in Third World settings there are inadequate facilities to wash a used bottle before it is reused. Also, because of low economic status and a lack of knowledge, many mothers dilute the amount of formula with larger than required amounts of water. Usually this water has not been purified and, as a result, many water-borne illnesses are contracted by the infant.

The issue of breast-feeding is a concern not only in developing nations, but also among lower socioeconomic populations in the United States. For example, it has been reported that black mothers are one-third as likely to breast-feed as are white mothers. Breast-feeding by Hispanic mothers dropped nearly one-half in the United States during the 1970s. In the case of Indochinese refugees, the incidence of breast-feeding drops to 25 percent from nearly 100 percent within six months of arrival in America.[18]

In 1981 the United Nations passed a nonbinding code—a statement of principle, which has no enforcement mechanism—restricting the marketing of infant formula in the world. One hundred and nineteen nations supported this action; only the United States opposed it. The American government stated that the code unfairly restricted commerce.

The pressures of corporate industry were more influential than the health of children throughout the world. This unfortunate presidential administration action was soundly opposed by most public health personnel, agencies, and organizations. Interestingly, both houses of Congress passed resolutions that condemned the stand taken by the United States government.

An action as important to the overall health of children as breast-feeding must not be negatively affected by political determinates. Nutrition education programs need to be designed to encourage all mothers to breast-feed their infants. Only as people understand the long-term health values and benefits to children will there be an improvement in the health status of children.

Food Stamp Program

A federal program that has helped to meet the nutrition needs of many American citizens is the Food Stamp Program. This program, in its present form, was started in 1961 as a pilot project in several selected localities. With the passage of the Food Stamp Act of 1964, the program was established nationwide.[19]

The basic purpose of the Food Stamp Program is to provide the means for the economically disadvantaged to obtain needed foodstuffs. The population served by food stamps includes households with incomes below the federal poverty level, with eligibility based upon income and other financial resources. The head of the household must make application to receive food stamps, and then local offices evaluate the application to approve eligibility for involvement in the program.

Those who are qualified and registered to receive food stamps receive them on a regular basis through the mail. The stamps are used to purchase groceries through the normal food-marketing channels, and food stores redeem the stamps at face value. An individual may purchase any food item with the stamps. Nonfood items, such as paper products, alcoholic beverages, pet food, soap, and cleaning products, cannot be purchased with the stamps.

The Food Stamp Program was established principally to improve the nutrition of the poor in America. Malnutrition and hunger affect the elderly, infants and children of the poor, Native Americans, migrants, and pregnant teenagers. It is these populations that have benefited the most from this federal program. Unemployment, as seen in the early 1980s, has resulted in an increase in the number and a distortion of the stereotyped image of those who use food stamps.

Another purpose of the Food Stamp Program, as noted by Congress, is to strengthen the agricultural economy.[20] When people are able to purchase more foodstuffs, the demand for these foodstuffs increases and the agricultural industry is able to sell more products, thus stimulating the agricultural economy.

The effectiveness of the Food Stamp Program is questionable because of the numerous problems associated with it. One problem has been nonparticipation by many who are qualified.[21] Many people who are qualified to receive food stamps do not do so because they do not understand the program, because of bureaucratic problems associated with registering and qualifying, or because of personal pride. On the other hand, a significant problem is involvement in the Food Stamp Program by individuals who do not qualify or for whom the program was not principally designed.

In spite of the problems associated with the Food Stamp Program, it must be recognized that over twenty million people a year benefit who otherwise would not have been able to obtain adequate nutrition. The importance of good nutrition for infants, children, and the elderly, in particular, makes this program seem most worthwhile, despite its abuses.

As with all federal programs, the future of the Food Stamp Program is in question. Since 1981, governmental regulations have reduced the number of people who are eligible to receive food stamps. These regulations have placed greater financial responsibility for this program on the individual states. Certain population groups who could receive food stamps in the past are no longer eligible. Unfortunately, many people who need the assistance, especially borderline poor, may not qualify.

Food Information Labeling

What we eat has a direct relationship to disease and to the quality of our personal health. Failure to obtain certain essential nutrients can result in specific diseases or health problems. In addition, excessive intake of certain nutrients contributes to adverse health problems.

In order to be able to make intelligent food selections, people should have information about the nutrients found in food. Therefore, the public should be provided with as much information about the food they eat as is possible. This means that nutritional labeling should be a part of the marketing of all foods. This labeling must be informative and meaningful to the average consumer.

Food information labeling was introduced in the mid-1970s. Three federal agencies are responsible for governing food labeling in the United States. The labeling of all foods except meat, poultry, and egg products is administered by the Food and Drug Administration. The United States Department of Agriculture (USDA) regulates meat, poultry, and egg products. Food advertising is governed by the Federal Trade Commission.

The Food and Drug Administration requires that all packaged foods display the name of the product and the manufacturer. Any food to which a nutrient has been added or that makes a nutritional claim must have a label. The list of ingredients included in the food must also be indicated.

In 1987 the United States Department of Agriculture began enforcing stricter labeling requirements of meat and poultry products. Under these stricter policies the fat content of these foods must be presented on the labels.

Food labeling is helpful in the selection of foods. It is helpful to those individuals who are counting calories or for people on special diets recommended by their physicians. Reading labels is also helpful in comparing the costs of two similar products.

The data on food labels must be accurate, with information listed about calories, sugars, sodium, fats, carbohydrates, protein, and other important nutrients. All packaged food should have information labels, and where nonpackaged foods are sold, the information should be displayed prominently for the consumer to read. The federal government, in its objectives for the nation, recommended that by 1990 all packaged foods should have labels to inform consumers about calorie and nutrient levels.[22] Since the mid-1980s there has been an increased demand for explicit health-related or disease-prevention claims on food labels. A major problem associated with such labeling centers on the difficulty of agreeing on what kind of scientific evidence is necessary in order to substantiate the claims.

Not everyone is in agreement that nutrition labeling, required by both federal and state governments, is needed. As is expected, many in the food industry are opposed to the regulations; they do not

Reading Food Labels

Nutrition labels taken from two different cereal boxes are shown on these two pages.

1. Indicated initially is the average serving size and the number of servings the package will accomodate.

2. Upper portion of the label
   Number of calories
   Amount of protein, carbohydrate and fat, in grams (1 ounce = 28 grams)
   Amount of cholesterol, in grams
   Amount of sodium and potassium, in grams

```
┌─────────────────────────────────┐
│  EACH SERVING CONTAINS          │
│  3 GRAMS OF DIETARY FIBER       │
└─────────────────────────────────┘
```

NUTRITION INFORMATION

SERVING SIZE: 1 OZ. (28.4 g, ABOUT 4 BISCUITS) FROSTED MINI-WHEATS ALONE OR WITH ½ CUP VITAMINS A AND D SKIM MILK.
SERVINGS PER PACKAGE: 20

	CEREAL	WITH SKIM MILK
CALORIES	100	140*
PROTEIN	3 g	7 g
CARBOHYDRATE	24 g	30 g
FAT	0 g	0 g*
CHOLESTEROL	0 mg	0 mg*
SODIUM	5 mg	65 mg
POTASSIUM	80 mg	280 mg

PERCENTAGE OF U.S. RECOMMENDED DAILY ALLOWANCES (U.S. RDA)

	CEREAL	WITH SKIM MILK
PROTEIN	4	15
VITAMIN A	25	30
VITAMIN C	25	25
THIAMIN	25	30
RIBOFLAVIN	25	35
NIACIN	25	25
CALCIUM	**	15
IRON	10	10
VITAMIN D	10	25
VITAMIN B_6	25	25
FOLIC ACID	25	25
PHOSPHORUS	8	20
MAGNESIUM	8	10
ZINC	10	15
COPPER	4	6

*WHOLE MILK SUPPLIES AN ADDITIONAL 30 CALORIES, 4 g FAT, AND 15 mg CHOLESTEROL.
**CONTAINS LESS THAN 2% OF THE U.S. RDA OF THIS NUTRIENT.

INGREDIENTS: WHOLE WHEAT, SUGAR, SORBITOL, GELATIN,

VITAMINS AND MINERALS: VITAMIN C (SODIUM ASCORBATE AND ASCORBIC ACID), VITAMIN B_3 (NIACINAMIDE), ZINC (ZINC OXIDE), IRON, VITAMIN A (PALMITATE; PROTECTED WITH BHT), VITAMIN B_6 (PYRIDOXINE HYDROCHLORIDE), VITAMIN B_2 (RIBOFLAVIN), VITAMIN B_1 (THIAMIN HYDROCHLORIDE), FOLIC ACID AND VITAMIN D.

**MADE BY KELLOGG COMPANY
BATTLE CREEK, MICH. 49016, U.S.A.
©1982 BY KELLOGG COMPANY
® KELLOGG COMPANY**

CARBOHYDRATE INFORMATION

	CEREAL	WITH MILK
COMPLEX CARBOHYDRATES	15 g	15 g
SUCROSE & OTHER SUGARS	6 g	12 g
DIETARY FIBER	3 g	3 g
TOTAL CARBOHYDRATES	24 g	30 g

3. Lower portion of the label
   Percentage of RDAs for several nutrients provided in one serving
4. The last part of the label contains a listing of other ingredients that have been added.

5. Both labels contain special information concerning carbohydrates in these products.

Upon examination of these two labels what factors do you note that are significant? Which cereal would you choose to not eat because of information obtained from reading the labels? Explain.

NUTRITION INFORMATION

SERVING SIZE: 1 OZ. (28.4 g, ABOUT ¾ CUP) FROSTED FLAKES ALONE OR WITH ½ CUP VITAMINS A AND D SKIM MILK.

SERVINGS PER PACKAGE: 20

	CEREAL	WITH SKIM MILK
CALORIES	110	150*
PROTEIN	1 g	5 g
CARBOHYDRATE	26 g	32 g
FAT	0 g	0 g*
CHOLESTEROL	0 mg	0 mg*
SODIUM	200 mg	260 mg
POTASSIUM	25 mg	230 mg

PERCENTAGE OF U.S. RECOMMENDED DAILY ALLOWANCES (U.S. RDA)

	CEREAL	WITH SKIM MILK
PROTEIN	2	10
VITAMIN A	25	30
VITAMIN C	25	25
THIAMIN	25	30
RIBOFLAVIN	25	35
NIACIN	25	25
CALCIUM	**	15
IRON	10	10
VITAMIN D	10	25
VITAMIN B₆	25	25
FOLIC ACID	25	25
PHOSPHORUS	**	15

*WHOLE MILK SUPPLIES AN ADDITIONAL 30 CALORIES, 4 g FAT, AND 15 mg CHOLESTEROL.
**CONTAINS LESS THAN 2% OF THE U.S. RDA OF THIS NUTRIENT.

INGREDIENTS: CORN, SUGAR, SALT, MALT FLAVORING, CORN SYRUP,

VITAMINS AND IRON: VITAMIN C (SODIUM ASCORBATE AND ASCORBIC ACID), VITAMIN B₃ (NIACINAMIDE), IRON, VITAMIN A (PALMITATE; PROTECTED WITH BHT), VITAMIN B₆ (PYRIDOXINE HYDROCHLORIDE), VITAMIN B₂ (RIBOFLAVIN), VITAMIN B₁ (THIAMIN HYDROCHLORIDE), FOLIC ACID, AND VITAMIN D.

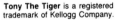

MADE BY KELLOGG CO.
BATTLE CREEK, MICH. 49016, U.S.A.
©1981 BY KELLOGG CO.
®KELLOGG COMPANY

Tony The Tiger is a registered trademark of Kellogg Company.

CARBOHYDRATE INFORMATION

	CEREAL	WITH SKIM MILK
COMPLEX CARBOHYDRATES	15 g	15 g
SUCROSE & OTHER SUGARS	11 g	17 g
TOTAL CARBOHYDRATES	26 g	32 g

believe the government should regulate private enterprise. In addition, they point out that food labeling increases production costs, which are then passed on to the consumers.

Still other opponents suggest that most Americans would neither read nor understand the warning labels. There is some evidence, particularly from experience with selected foods and cigarette sales, that warning labels on products have little effect on the behavior patterns of most American consumers.

Food Additives

Much of the food and drink Americans ingest contains added chemicals. Over thirteen hundred additives have been approved by the Food and Drug Administration (FDA) for use in foods for human consumption. Only about a third of these are actually used as food additives, and these are used for a variety of purposes.

Additives, used as preservatives and food thickeners, for flavor, coloring, and as an emulsifier to improve food texture, have a long and varied history. For centuries people have added substances to their food. Before the advent of refrigeration, meat was salted, smoked, and sun dried in order to preserve it. Some food additives serve other useful purposes. Without preservatives to prevent the formation of mold and bacteria, many foods could not be shipped great distances, which would lead to geographical limitations on the availability of foods. In particular, the vast assortment of foods in urban areas would be greatly reduced.

Concern has been expressed in recent years over the increased use of food additives. These concerns have developed over the uncertainty of the amounts that are safe for human consumption, the quality of testing by the Food and Drug Administration, and the possible connection between certain additives and cancer, cardiovascular diseases, and hyperactivity.

Having food additives in our diet is a topic of great debate. Some additives are felt to be useful only as marketing ploys. For example, artificial coloring and flavoring have no nutritive value. Their sole purpose is to make food appear more appealing to the consumer. Artificial flavoring is used in a variety of foods, particularly in soft drinks.

Artificial coloring gives the consumer the impression that the product has a greater content of a given ingredient than is really present. For example, artificial coloring is used in flavored ice cream to give the impression that there is more lime, raspberry, or cherry than is really in the product. Artificial coloring, the most controversial of food additives, is suspected of being carcinogenic. But little is actually known about the effects of using these chemicals over a long period of time.

It must be noted that most chemicals used as food additives are safe. However, the Food and Drug Administration has banned over twenty-five food additives known to be toxic to humans or animals. Over half have been coal tar dyes known as "artificial colors."[23]

When combined in the digestive system with other chemicals, certain food additives may be dangerous. For example, nitrites that are used in meat to make it look fresh and attractive have been associated with cancer. Research has shown that nitrite, even by itself, might cause cancer.[24] Approved since 1925, it has been used for years as a meat preservative because it inhibits the growth of bacterial spores that cause botulism. In the 1960s, scientists discovered that, in combination with other substances, nitrite produces a family of chemicals called nitrosamines. Some of these chemicals have caused cancer in laboratory animals. This has caused great concern in the meat industry because one-tenth of the nation's food supply is dependent upon this single food additive.[25]

How strict should federal regulations be in controlling the amount of additives in food that is sold in our stores? Should food additives that contain even a small portion of a possible cancer-causing agent be banned? These questions and similar issues have caused serious debate, differences of opinion, and legislative action.

Under provisions of the food and drug laws, known as the Delaney Amendment,[26] any substance found to be carcinogenic in either animals or humans cannot be approved as a food additive. This legislation has been the source of much controversy. Critics say it is inflexible and confusing. For example, the law does not apply to many additives introduced before 1958, the year it became effective.

They also argue that in some situations, additives in trace amounts are essential for human nutrition, but in large doses may be carcinogenic. Advocates of the Delaney Clause suggest that to permit the use of certain additives that may be carcinogenic will "open the door" for other cancer-causing agents.

Several food additives have been declared unsafe for human consumption. In some instances, particularly in the case of saccharin, many people have questioned the efficacy of such a ruling. Under the Delaney Clause, saccharin would have been banned; however, Congress ruled that this could not occur.

It is the position of many, particularly the food marketing industry, that no food additive can be declared absolutely safe. They argue that food additives should be allowed if the risk to humans is not significant.

The quality of additive testing by the Food and Drug Administration has been questioned by consumer groups. A time lapse of as much as five years may occur between the declaration that a substance is dangerous and the actual outlawing of that additive. Consumer groups maintain that the Food and Drug Administration acts too slowly in warning the public, all the time permitting the public to consume the substance in question.

As can be seen, there are many questions about the use of food additives in the American diet. Admittedly, some additives are necessary and there are potential dangers in others. A definitive response to this issue will not appear in the immediate future. In the meantime, the consumer should learn to eat food that does not contain excessive amounts of additives. Eating fresh fruit and vegetables, fresh meat, and whole grain products is most important in order to protect ourselves from additives. Learning to read the labels on foods will also be useful in reducing the amount of nonnutritious food additive intake.

Mass Media Influence

Much of the public's knowledge and information about foods is obtained through the mass media. Advertisements on radio, television, and in newspapers, books, and journals entice the consumer to eat a range of appetizingly packaged foods. Little is said about the nutrient values of these products. Many times marketing and sales of the food—not the product's health value to individuals—are the prime goals.

Children are encouraged by entertaining advertisements to eat sugar-coated cereals, creamy candy bars, and other foods high in sugar content. Numerous sales approaches are used to interest growing children in eating these foods that contain little or no nutrient value. Adults are presented with similar advertisements for soft drinks and other foods high in sugar, salt, and saturated fat.

It is doubtful that society can expect the corporate food industry to highlight the inherent dangers of excessive sugars, high levels of sodium, and increased fat and cholesterol in their marketing promotions. Some consumer and nutrition groups have advocated federal regulations to control media advertising, particularly in television. It is unlikely, though, in a time of increased opposition to federal regulatory activities, that such restrictions will become a reality.

It is increasingly important that public nutrition education programs focus upon these dangers so that the consumer is better prepared to buy intelligently. Food product advertising in the mass media should be countered by effective and accurate nutrition messages informing the population of healthful diets. This would probably be more effective than the regulation of advertising in the mass media.

Eating Behavior

Dietary Factors

The American public displays a significant interest in diet. What we eat, how much we eat, and other factors in our life-style associated with eating are of great importance to many people. Some people spend a lot of time reading food labels, listening to those selling special diets, talking about eating, and taking classes in diet control.

Every year a number of new diets with various claims and promises gain attention. Some diets promise to solve a particular problem, while others indicate that the diet will contribute to weight control and good health. The weight loss diets seem to be the most popular. Anything that promises quick weight loss has much appeal to many people. Other diets, particularly high fiber diets, promise protection against certain diseases.

Certainly how and what we eat does contribute to health and wellness. For example, certain relationships between diet and headache have been established. It has been shown that certain foods which contain tyramine, cheeses for example, can dilate and constrict blood vessels and bring on headaches. Chemical imbalance resulting from diet also contributes to headaches.

In recent years there has been an increased consciousness regarding what we eat and how it affects one's health. Concern over meats that are rich in fat, such as pork, lamb, and beef, has led to a reduction in consumption of these products in the 1980s. In 1976 beef consumption was a little over 94 pounds per person; by the mid-1980s it had dropped to 79 pounds per person.[27] In contrast, the per capita consumption of chicken rose from 43 to 58 pounds in this same time period.

The meat-growing industry is changing its product to address these new concerns of the American public. Both pigs (pork) and cattle (beef) are being bred leaner. Pork is now allowed about half the amount of fat it had twenty-five years ago and the meat-packing industry is making certain efforts to trim fat from the product in the marketplace. Cattle are spending less time in feedlots where they are fattened for market. Leaner cattle from abroad have been imported for mating in an effort to produce a less-fattened product.[28]

Restaurants are providing options on their menus for people wishing diets low in fatty foods and in calories. Today one finds more salad bars and more fish and chicken dishes available on the menus of most restaurants. Margarine, which contains less saturated fat than butter and little cholesterol, is found in many restaurants. In 1986 the McDonald Corporation announced that Chicken McNuggets and Filet of Fish will only be cooked in 100 percent vegetable oil. This popular fast-food chain also indicated that they will no longer serve whole milk; only 2% milk or nonfat milk will be available.

The American Heart Association, working in cooperation with restaurants throughout the nation, has developed menus that are low in cholesterol and other nutrients that contribute as risk factors for cardiovascular disease. The association has set certain guidelines and criteria that the restaurant must meet in order to advertise that their menu is acceptable for positive cardiovascular health. Any restaurant or restaurant chain that wishes to indicate to their customers that items on their menu meet American Heart Association guidelines may do so. This program is known as the "Creative Cuisine" program.

Combined with this increased concern about how and what we eat has been interest in a number of other factors related to weight control and good health. The emphasis of physical activity along with diet in disease prevention has also become an interest of thousands. In addition, the relationships of food intake and chronic diseases and the role of genetics in obesity are receiving increasing research by those involved in community nutrition programs.

Eating Disorders

Two eating disorders have received increased attention in recent years: (1) *anorexia nervosa* and (2) *bulimia*. These two different but interrelated disorders are increasing dramatically in our society, particularly among young women in their teens and early twenties.

Anorexia nervosa is not a new disorder. Documented cases can be traced back to at least the thirteenth century; however, it was about a hundred years ago in England when the disorder was given the description we know today as anorexia nervosa.[29] This disorder is characterized by a refusal to eat and a fear of weight gain.

Concern about weight gain reaches such magnitude that the individual develops an obsession with weight loss, actually resulting in a fear of weight

Diagnostic Criteria for Anorexia Nervosa

1. Intense fear of becoming obese
2. Disturbance of body image; claiming to "feel fat"
3. Weight loss of at least 24 percent of original body weight
4. Refusal to maintain body weight over a minimal normal weight for age and height
5. No known physical illness that would account for weight loss

Source: Northwest Ohio Center for Eating Disorders, St. Vincent Hospital, Toledo, Ohio.

Diagnostic Criteria for Bulimia

1. Recurrent episodes of binge eating
2. At least three of the following:
   A. Consumption of high-caloric, easily ingested food
   B. Unconspicuous eating during a binge
   C. Termination of eating episode by abdominal pain, sleep, or self-induced vomiting
   D. Repeated attempts to lose weight
   E. Frequent weight fluctuations greater than ten pounds
3. Awareness that eating pattern is abnormal
4. Fear of not being able to stop eating voluntarily
5. Depressed mood and self-deprecating thoughts following binges
6. Bulimic episodes not due to any known physical disorder

Source: Northwest Ohio Center for Eating Disorders, St. Vincent Hospital, Toledo, Ohio.

gain. Excessive dieting reaching starvation levels produces a number of serious physiological and psychological problems. There is usually a desired body image of extreme thinness. The individual seems to enjoy losing weight. The refusal to eat is a pleasurable indulgence.

A second eating disorder is bulimia. The term means "ox hunger" or "voracius appetite." In this disorder the individual may stuff oneself with food, then take laxatives or force oneself to vomit in order to eliminate the food. This practice, often referred to as the "binge-purge" syndrome, leads to dehydration, possible damage to the esophagus, and dental decay. Laxative abuse may result in damage to certain digestive organs.

Bulimia is not an incapacitating condition. However, the individual tends to spend time eating alone. After eating the individual feels fat and fears getting fatter; this results in the purging.

Treatment centers have been established in a number of medical facilities throughout the nation. Hospital inpatient care is one part of the program.

During this phase of the treatment program a nutritional assessment is usually conducted. Therapy is provided to help the individual recover lost nutrients. Supplementary feedings and other nutrient disturbances accompany the return to normal eating patterns. While hospitalized the person participates in a number of activities designed to help him or her overcome the psychological problems associated with the eating disorder.

Relaxation therapy designed to teach body awareness, physiotherapy, individual psychotherapy, and group therapy are all procedures that have been used to treat those with eating disorders. Behavior modification strategies have also been used.[30]

Both eating disorders require several years of active treatment once the person is released from the hospital. This requires involvement of family, friends, and others who are important in the lives of the patient. Self-help groups have been established in many communities to provide supportive assistance. The goal of all treatment programs, both inpatient and outpatient, is to positively influence eating patterns and to develop a more appropriate and positive self-image.

Summary

A variety of health problems that involve nutritional patterns afflict humanity. In the United States overconsumption of food results in obesity and an increased risk for a number of different chronic diseases. On the other end of the spectrum, malnutrition is found among certain segments of the American population, particularly the economically disadvantaged.

A wealth of nutritional information, recommendations, and guidelines is available to the American consumer. This information is often confusing and conflicting. For years the Recommended Daily Allowances (RDAs) have served as guidelines for adequate nutrition. More recently, the Senate Subcommittee on Nutrition and Health identified six dietary goals for the country. Some guidelines recommend less sugar, salt, saturated fats, and cholesterol in the diet. Other reports conclude that the concern over fat and cholesterol consumption is unfounded. Increased research is necessary to ascertain the proper human dietary intake.

Even though nutritional status affects the health of people in all age groups, several federal programs have been developed with the goal of improving the diets of pregnant women, newborn infants, and children. The Head Start Program provides meals for economically disadvantaged children. The Supplemental Food Program for Women, Infants and Children (WIC) provides food supplements for mothers and children. These programs, along with others, have been effective in improving the nutritional status of women, infants, and children. However, government funding cutbacks in the 1980s have resulted in reductions in many of these programs.

Another federal program, the Food Stamp Program, allows the economically disadvantaged to obtain needed foodstuffs. The food stamps are used to purchase groceries and so improve the nutritional status of many poor people in America.

In order to make intelligent decisions in food selection, people need information about the nutrients in the food that is purchased. In order to be better informed, people need labeling on all packaged foods. Labeling should inform the consumer of the nutrients and additives in the food. Many foods contain additives that are not nutritious and some may even be harmful.

There is an increasing interest in weight control and disease prevention as it relates to eating patterns among many Americans. This has led to greater intake of such products as chicken and fish, and less consumption of beef, pork, and lamb. Restaurants, the food marketing industry, and agriculture have all been influenced by these changing American eating patterns.

Two eating disorders are noted among many people of high school and college age, particularly women. These eating disorders are anorexia nervosa and bulimia. Anorexia is a condition wherein the individual develops an unrealistic body image and fails to eat adequate amounts of food. As a result there is not only a resultant weight loss, but also serious nutrient depletions. Bulimia is a situation where the individual overeats, then purges the food by vomiting. Both eating disorders usually require the help of medical personnel and self-help therapies to overcome the problems.

Discussion Questions

1. Which is the greater problem in America, overconsumption of food or malnutrition? Explain your answer.
2. What are the Recommended Dietary Allowances (RDAs)?
3. What factors led to the failure to release an updated report of RDAs in the mid-1980s?
4. Discuss the dietary goals for the United States as published by the Senate Select Committee on Nutrition and Human Needs.
5. Do you support the dietary goals of the Senate Subcommittee? Why or why not?
6. Explain which health problems are caused by excessive intake of sodium.
7. What controversy was generated by the report "Toward Healthful Diets"?
8. What provisions for improved nutrition are part of the Head Start Program?
9. Explain the various components and objectives of the Special Supplemental Food Program for Women, Infants, and Children (WIC).
10. In what ways has the WIC Program been successful?
11. What issues were involved in the United States' position taken in 1981 at the United Nations regarding infant formula?
12. Explain the various components of the Food Stamp Program.
13. Do you believe that all foods should have complete information labeling? Defend your answer.
14. What information is included on the labels found on certain foods?
15. What are some of the purposes of food additives?
16. Should food additives that contain a small portion of a carcinogenic agent be marketed for human consumption?
17. Should press and mass media food advertisements be regulated? Defend your answer.
18. How have the diets of most Americans been affected by federal government funding reductions in the 1980s?
19. Discuss some of the measures being taken by the food marketing industry and restaurants to accomodate the concern of many people over diet and health.
20. Explain some of the differences between bulimia and anorexia nervosa.
21. Discuss some of the diagnostic criteria for anorexia and bulimia.
22. What are some of the treatment modalities followed in care for those with eating disorders?

Suggested Readings

Allen, Lindsay A. "Calcium and Osteoporosis." *Nutrition Today* 21, no. 3 (May/June, 1986): 6–10.

Bailey, Sue. "Diagnosing Bulimia." *American Family Physician* 29, no. 5 (May, 1984): 161–64.

Benedick, M.; Campbell, I. H.; Bowden, D. S.; and Jones, M. *Towards Efficiency and Effectiveness in the WIC Delivery Service.* Washington, D.C.: The Urban Institute, 1976.

Caliendo, Mary Alice. *Nutrition and Preventive Health Care.* New York: Macmillan Publishing Co., 1981.

Darby, William J. "Nutrition: Gastronomy, Mythology or Science?" *Nutrition Today* 21, no. 5 (September/October, 1986): 4–11.

Executive Summary. "Review of the Scientific Community's Views on Progress in Attaining the Public Health Service National Nutrition Goals for 1990." *Nutrition Today* 21, no. 3 (May/June, 1986): 30–36.

Gietzen, Dorothy, and Vermeersch, Joyce A. "Health Status and School Achievement of Children From Head Start and Free School Lunch Programs." *Public Health Reports* 95, no. 4 (July/August, 1980): 362–68.

McSherry, James A. "The Diagnostic Challenge of Anorexia Nervosa." *American Family Physician* 29, no. 2 (February, 1984): 141–45.

Miller, Virginia; Swaney, Sheldon; and Deinard, Amos. "Impact of the WIC Program on the Iron Status of Infants." *Pediatrics* 75 (1985): 100–105.

Olson, James Allen. "Vitamins A and C—Proposed Allowances." *Nutrition Today* 21, no. 5 (September/October, 1986): 26–30.

Potts, Nicki Lee. "Eating Disorders: The Secret Pattern of Binge/Purge." *American Journal of Nursing* 84, no. 1 (January, 1984): 32–35.

Rush, David. "National WIC Evaluation." *Public Health Currents* (1986): 17–20.

Select Committee on Nutrition and Human Needs, U.S. Senate, *Dietary Goals for the United States.* Washington, D.C.: Government Printing Office, 1977.

Slattery, Marty. "Developing a Community-Based Program." *The Community Nutritionist* 1, no. 1 (January/February, 1982): 9–11.

Vaden, Allene G. "Child Nutrition Programs: Past, Present, Future." *Nutritionist* 13, no. 1 (Winter, 1981): 7–10.

White, Philip L. "Setting New Diet and Health Directions." *Nutrition Today* 21, no. 4 (July/August, 1986): 4–6.

Endnotes

1. American Public Health Association. *The Nation's Health* (April, 1985): 20.

2. Council on Scientific Affairs. "American Medical Association Concepts of Nutrition and Health." *Journal of the American Medical Association* 242, no. 21 (November 23, 1979): 2335.

3. "Recommended Dietary Allowances Revised 1980." *Dairy Council Digest* 51, no. 2 (March/April, 1980): 10.

4. Food and Nutrition Board. *Recommended Dietary Allowances, 9th Ed.* Washington, D.C.: National Academy of Sciences, National Research Council, 1980.

5. Council on Scientific Affairs. "Concepts of Nutrition and Health," 2335.

6. Select Committee on Nutrition and Human Needs, U.S. Senate, *Dietary Goals For the United States.* Washington, D.C.: U.S. Government Printing Office, 1977.

7. Ibid.

8. Ibid., 9.

9. Ibid., 46.

10. *Promoting Health, Preventing Disease: Objectives for the Nation.* Washington, D.C.: U.S. Government Printing Office, 1980, 75.

11. The School Lunch Program is discussed in chapter 13.

12. U.S. Department of Agriculture, Food and Nutrition Service. *Study of WIC Participant and Program Characteristics* (1986): xxiii.

13. Testimony before U.S. Senate Subcommittee on Agriculture, Nutrition, and Forestry. Washington, D.C.: U.S. Government Printing Office, April 12, 1978.

14. Rush, David. "National WIC Evaluation." *Public Health Currents* (1986): 19–20.

15. Benedick, M.; Campbell, I. H.; Bowden, D. S.; and Jones, M. *Towards Efficiency and Effectiveness in the WIC Delivery Service.* Washington, D.C.: The Urban Institute, 1976.

16. "Child Nutrition Programs Update." *Dairy Council Digest* 53, no. 6 (November/December, 1982): 35.

17. Council on Scientific Affairs. "Concepts of Nutrition and Health," 2336.

18. "Infant Formula Promotion A Domestic Threat, Too." *Nutrition Action* (August, 1981).

19. Food Stamp Act of 1964, P. L. 88–525, August 31, 1964.

20. Ibid.

21. Caliendo, Mary Alice. *Nutrition and Preventive Health Care.* New York: Macmillan Publishing Co., 1981, 594.

22. *Promoting Health, Preventing Disease,* 75.

23. Hausman, Patricia. "The Cancers of Affluence." *Nutrition Action* (December, 1981), 7–11.

24. Select Committee on Nutrition and Human Needs, *Dietary Goals,* 46.

25. *FDA and the 96th Congress.* Washington, D.C.: U.S. Government Printing Office, 1981, 86.

26. Food Additives Amendment, P. L. 85–929, passed by Congress, 1958.

27. Mayer, Jean, and Goldberg, Jeanne. "Nutrition." Syndicated column, December 23, 1986.

28. Ibid.

29. National Dairy Council. "Eating Disorders." *Dairy Council Digest* 56, no. 1 (January/February, 1985): 1.

30. Chng, Chwee Lye. "Anorexia Nervosa: Why Do Some People Starve Themselves?" *Journal of School Health* 53, no. 1 (January, 1983): 22–26.

12

Community Mental Health: From Sad Past Toward a Dynamic Future

> " . . . even at its best state hospital care is bad for many patients; . . . mental hospitals can be valuable social institutions only if they are restricted to caring for patients they do not harm . . . alternatives to hospital care and methods of redistributing patients must be devised—and quickly."[1]

As recently as two decades ago this statement might have summarized the major mental health need in the United States. By the mid-twentieth century, people should have developed more effective, positive outlooks regarding the care, treatment, and rehabilitation of mental health. Yet in spite of significant programs, government funding, community mental health centers, public education, and extensive research on the dynamics of mental illness, this statement is still relevant in the latter part of the twentieth century.

The extent and nature of mental health problems are difficult to ascertain. In some measure, this is due to the fact that there is little agreement on what constitutes a mental disorder. Some people have the idea that mental illness involves only such matters as severe depression, schizophrenia, and suicide. Yet there are many factors that result in mental retardation that must be considered in discussing community mental health. Many people find it difficult to recognize mental illness in their own families or in a member of the community.

Mental illness should be considered a community concern because of the number of people affected by it. One family in three is affected by mental illness and one person in ten is hospitalized for mental or emotional disorders at some point in life. However, instead of focusing primarily upon mental illness as was the case in the past, there has been an increased emphasis on maintaining and restoring mental and emotional well-being. Efforts to prevent mental illness and emotional problems are receiving increasing attention. In spite of these new directions in understanding mental health, there are still many misunderstandings and misconceptions about mental health.

Learning to cope with mental problems is a significant community health concern. People who experience emotional and mental disorders must receive care. This care is time-consuming and costly in terms of both money and stress on the family. As a result, mental illness does not involve only the patient, but also the family and, in turn, the community at large. Because the community often misunderstands those individuals experiencing mental problems, these people are often denied a very vital support framework.

As a result of this misunderstanding a major goal of any mental health program is to educate the public about mental illness and positive mental health. With such educational efforts, mental health and mental illness can be better understood and a healthier emotional climate will result.

History of Mental Health Care

Care of the world's mentally ill has not been a "bright" chapter in the history of humanity. The mentally ill were often neglected or were the recipients of cold, harsh, impersonal care. They were kept in jails or poorhouses, known as almshouses, along with convicted criminals. They were placed in these environments because, like the criminals, they had behaved in a manner considered improper by the community. In most almshouses no medical care was provided, no effort was made to rehabilitate the patient, and only basic sustenance was provided.

Inhumane treatment of the mentally ill was common in the past. Stories of torture and brutality are frequent and disgustingly true. The mentally ill were often kept in iron cages with no heat and little or no light. In many parts of Europe in the seventeenth and eighteenth centuries, the mentally ill were shackled with irons and chains. There were times these individuals were exhibited in towns, fairs, and circuses for the amusement of the general population.

The mentally ill were also considered to be possessed by evil spirits. They were tortured in order to exorcise the evil spirits from individuals and the community. These patients were burned, flogged, and forced to endure other inhumane treatment in efforts to "purify" the community.

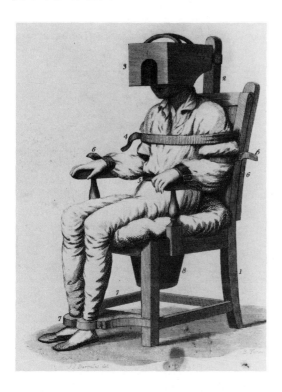

In the 1700s, a mentally ill individual might have been tied to a chair, with feet locked and head tightly restrained. Such inhumane action left no opportunity for treatment, rehabilitation, or improvement in conditions.

Historically, the care of the mentally ill in the United States has not reflected any great enlightenment either. Adequate care was never provided for these unfortunate people. Often those in need of care for mental and emotional problems were placed in large, impersonal, public institutions. The type, quality, and effectiveness of care in these settings left much to be desired. Usually, however, patient care was primarily custodial and little effort was made to rehabilitate the patient.

By the end of the eighteenth century, reforms in the treatment and care of the mentally ill occurred in parts of Europe. During the 1790s, Philippe Pinel worked for the reform of the treatment of the mentally ill in France. Pinel felt that these patients should not be kept in chains, but should be cared for in hospitals. He worked for the placement of patients in dry, sunlit rooms rather than in dungeons. He also did away with violent treatment, bleeding, and purging. Pinel encouraged talking with patients and listening to their problems. He began to use case histories by keeping records of patients. Pinel's theories and practices were highly unpopular among the public, who had no understanding of the true nature of mental illness and emotional disorders. Even Pinel's fellow physicians opposed his ideas.

During the nineteenth century, care of the mentally ill in the United States gradually became the responsibility of the individual states. The work of Dorothea Lynde Dix in the mid-1800s established the insane as "wards of the state." Thus, it became the state government's responsibility to care for the mentally ill. This resulted in state-operated mental hospitals. However, care received in these institutions was still custodial in nature and only a few treatment programs were made available. The consensus in the late 1800s and early 1900s was that the mental patient needed to be isolated from society and the family. As a result, many government mental hospitals were located some distance from cities.

The poor condition of state mental hospitals concerned many people in the early twentieth century. Clifford Beers's 1906 book, *A Mind That Found Itself*, has become a classic of the sad state of affairs in mental hospitals.[2] Beers told of his experiences during the three years he was a patient in several mental health institutions. His experiences convinced him of the need for change in the nation's mental health system and he called for reform of care for the mentally ill. He also emphasized the need for better understanding of the nature of mental health and mental illness. As an outgrowth of this book and other efforts led by Beers, the Connecticut Society for Mental Hygiene was founded in May 1908. This organization was the first state association in the United States established for mental health.

Other individuals worked to improve the condition of mental health care during the early twentieth century. Though well-meaning and effective in some settings, none of these efforts had a major national impact.[3]

Later efforts were designed to cure the mentally ill. Insulin shock treatment and electric shock therapy were introduced during the 1930s. Psychosurgery was also performed on some mental patients during these years. These and other procedures created some controversy.

Until World War II little substantive change occurred in the care and treatment of the mentally ill. The war, however, amplified the serious state of mental health in the United States, especially the lack of effective treatment and rehabilitative services. Over a million men were rejected for military duty because of neuropsychiatric disorders.[4] Three out of every five beds in Veterans Administration hospitals following the war were occupied by individuals with mental disorders.[5]

Many military personnel returned from combat in need of psychological care and treatment. The sheer numbers of those needing treatment encouraged the improvement of mental health programs. In spite of the need, mental health personnel were still inadequately trained and treatment facilities remained overcrowded.

This state of affairs, despite good intentions, generated some discussion about the inhumane care of those isolated in state mental health institutions. A well-received book written in 1948 proved that, indeed, there were tragic problems in the state institutions. Albert Deutsch, in *The Shame of the States,* enlightened readers of the plight of the institutions patients.[6]

Change was accelerated by the passage of federal legislation designed to improve the care and treatment of mental health patients. In 1943, vocational rehabilitation legislation (the Barden-LaFollette Act) was amended so that mental as well as physical rehabilitation was funded. For the first time, vocational counseling and training for the mentally ill were made possible.

Another major breakthrough occurred in 1946 with the passage of the National Mental Health Act. This established the National Institute of Mental Health and supported programs to train professionals for work in the mental health fields. It also made monies available to states for development of community mental health clinics. Even more significantly, the act funded research into the cause, diagnosis, and treatment of mental disorders. The National Institute of Mental Health was also charged with developing demonstration projects, experiments, and studies to find improved and effective ways to rehabilitate the mentally ill.

Mental Health Facilities

The mentally ill and emotionally disturbed are cared for in a number of different facilities. Historically, the mental health movement existed within the confines of the institutional setting. Today, services are provided outside the institutional walls.

Most mental health care and treatment is provided in one of the following types of facilities:

1. State mental hospitals—Inpatient care and treatment of the mentally ill are provided. Not all mental hospitals are state-operated; some are private psychiatric facilities. State mental hospitals are often referred to as psychiatric centers.

2. Veterans Administration psychiatric services—One hundred and twenty-nine VA medical centers have psychiatric bed services.[7] In addition, drug dependence treatment programs and mental hygiene clinics are available for individuals qualified for veterans' benefits.

3. Community hospital psychiatric services—Usually a separate psychiatric unit operates within the general hospital setting.

4. Community mental health centers—Centers are established in many localities to provide a broad range of mental health care within the community setting.

5. Residential treatment centers—Treatment is available to those who are diagnosed as moderately disturbed. The patient usually resides in these settings under supervision.

6. Outpatient psychiatric clinics—The patient receives care and treatment on an outpatient basis within the community.

7. Psychiatric day/night facilities—The patient spends part of the twenty-four hour day in these settings. Planned therapy and treatment are provided during this period. For the remainder of the day the patient returns to the community.

State Mental Hospitals

The first hospital in the United States specifically for the mentally ill was established in Williamsburg, Virginia, in 1773.[8] Since then, psychiatric care has been considered a responsibility of the state.[9] Large state-operated mental hospitals have been the states' response to this onus. The individual in need of mental health professional services went, or was taken, there to receive proper care. Although the state mental hospitals vary in size, organization, and program effectiveness, their basic function is and has been to provide custodial care for the mentally ill.

The quality of care given to a mental patient varies. There have been questions raised about the adequacy of care and attention given in state mental institutions. Reports have called attention to inadequate diets, poor living conditions, overuse and improper use of drugs, and personal abuse of the patients.

In many states, the professional personnel are inadequate. Often the available staff members are ill-prepared to meet the needs of the patients. Overcrowding of facilities and budget deficiencies have also led to serious problems.

As a result of these conditions, long-term placement in mental institutions often does not help the psychiatric patient. Such placement can further contribute to stress and related problems. Nor are many rehabilitative measures followed in mental hospitals. An institutionalized patient is usually isolated from family and familiar surroundings, lacks exposure to normal role models, and is unable to develop meaningful personal relationships. This traditional approach to the treatment and institutionalization of the mentally ill has recently received negative publicity.

Little change occurred in the mental health care provided in mental hospitals until the end of World War II. In 1955, a congressional committee on mental health studied the national mental health problems. A number of recommendations that served as the foundation for governmental support in the 1960s were made by this commission.

The resident population in state mental hospitals increased annually until 1955, when it reached a total of 558,922 in the United States.[10] In 1956, the number of patients declined and has since continued to drop annually. In twenty years the number of patients decreased 61 percent.[11]

Whereas, in 1955, one-half of all mental health care was provided in state mental hospitals, today less than 10 percent takes place in these facilities. Three-fourths of all mental health care today is provided by outpatient psychiatric services or in community mental health centers, whereas in 1955, less than one-fourth of all care was of an outpatient basis. Today more people are seeking help for emotional disorders but are less reliant upon the mental hospitals.

According to the federal government data there are slightly less than three hundred state mental hospitals currently in operation with a little more than 128,000 beds. This is some fifty hospitals less than were in operation in the mid-1970s, with a reduction in state mental hospital beds of over 150,000 since the beginning of deinstitutionalization.[12] Today state mental hospitals are focusing their services on long-term care for the chronically ill, such as schizophrenics, and on care for the criminally insane.

A number of major changes in the operation of the state mental health hospitals have taken place. In addition to the reduction of inpatient services since 1954, different types of services are often available. Many state facilities provide acute short-term care. Outpatient care, day-care programs, and special service programs for the elderly and children are also available.

The opportunity to obtain professional help on an outpatient basis, in nursing homes, in community mental health centers, or in halfway houses, rather than in the institutional setting, has resulted in major changes in mental health care. A number of factors have contributed to this development. During the latter part of the 1950s, psychotropic drugs for treating the mentally ill were introduced. These drugs and tranquilizers were used to help control two major psychoses that led to many cases of institutionalization: depression and schizophrenia.

In 1954, New York became the first state to enact a community mental health services act.[13] Within the next decade, nineteen other states passed similar legislation. Most states now have legislation that encourages the use of community services in the care of mental patients.

Another factor in the reduction of admissions to state mental hospitals is the change in the basic care of the elderly. There has been an increase in elderly placement in nursing homes. Prior to the mid-1960s these patients were often sent to the state mental hospitals. This change, however, now permits the elderly patient to be near family and familiar surroundings.

Political and economic considerations have also influenced the reduction of state mental hospital use. Maintaining such large and crowded facilities became costly. Long-term hospital care is also very expensive. Many state governments encourage the community mental health service concept to reduce the financial burden of maintaining the hospital system.

Several pieces of federal legislation passed in the 1960s contributed to the decreased patient number in state hospitals. In 1963 Congress passed the Community Mental Health Services Act. This provided funds to local communities for the construction and staffing of mental health facilities. The Mental Retardation Facilities and Community Mental Health Centers Construction Act, also passed in 1963, supported the development of programs in which care of the mentally ill has moved from state hospitals to community facilities. The passage of Medicare and Medicaid also provided funding for mental health services within local communities.

The future of the state mental hospital is open to discussion. Some feel the concept of state hospitals is obsolete.[14] This is amplified by the fact that in many states, the hospital facilities are antiquated, in need of repair or new construction, and are often isolated from population centers. The cost of repairing, upgrading, and constructing new hospital facilities makes alternative programs very attractive.

In several states there has been discussion of possibly discontinuing operation of the state mental hospital system. However, there are still many questions as to whether such a system could be replaced completely. Can an entire population of a locality or state be serviced by community mental health centers? Can the needs of all patients be satisfactorily met by community centers? These are just two of many questions that must be addressed before state facilities can be eliminated. It is doubtful if such a development will occur.

Deinstitutionalization

In order for deinstitutionalization of the chronically mentally ill patient to work there must be appropriate living arrangements for the individual upon returning to the community. There must also be adequate support services. Unfortunately the growth of facilities in the community has not kept up with the need. As a result many chronically mentally ill individuals are now being placed in facilities such as nursing homes or boarding homes, which cannot provide appropriate services to meet their needs. Numerous problems have resulted, homelessness is one of the most apparent.

Has deinstitutionalizing the mental patient been effective? Some view it as a failure. Patients have been removed from mental hospitals and placed in the community where they often cannot find employment. Many times they commit crimes, are imprisoned, or simply live on the streets of the big cities. These individuals find it most difficult to adjust to and be accepted by society. All too often, the patient enters the "revolving door"; unable to adjust to the community, the patient returns to the facility. But the facility fails to rehabilitate and prepare these people for reentering community life.

Many others feel that deinstitutionalization has been successful. They hold that it is a better alternative to keeping the mental patient in an isolated state hospital removed from family, friends, and familiar surroundings. Treatment and rehabilitation near family and friends are felt to be more effective.

General Hospital Psychiatric Services

An important factor in the treatment of mental illness in recent years has been the expanded role of general hospital psychiatry. Both inpatient and outpatient psychiatric services are offered in this setting. The inpatient psychiatric treatment, for those in need of twenty-four-hour services, is the most expensive mode of care in the hospital.

The general hospitals have become involved in psychiatric care in an effort to "deinstitutionalize" the mentally ill and because of the recent emphasis on community-based care. The general hospital is geographically accessible to the majority of the population in any given community. In addition, the general hospital offers comprehensive, collaborating medical services for treatment of the psychiatric patient.

The general hospital has an accessible psychiatric emergency care facility. When a person needs immediate care, as during a breakdown or when under stress, effectively trained personnel are usually available to treat the person. Round-the-clock emergency psychiatric services extended by the general hospital include walk-in clinics, suicide prevention centers, home visitation programs, crisis intervention centers, as well as psychiatric emergency-room care.

Both public and private general hospitals have psychiatric departments. However, the type of patient usually admitted differs between the two. Private hospitals admit a greater number of patients with depressive disorders while public general hospitals admit the more severely disabled who have schizophrenic disorders.[15]

With the continuing phase-out of state mental institutions, there will be a corresponding increase in the use of general hospital psychiatric services. In the years ahead, the general hospital will become the focus for mental health care in communities throughout the United States.[16]

Community Mental Health Centers

Legislation in the 1960s and subsequent developments in community mental health focused upon the involvement of the community in care of the mentally ill. The typical community mental health center is staffed by a multidisciplinary team of mental health workers. The Community Mental Health Services Act identified several priority populations at whom the community health program must be directed. The first group includes the chronically mentally ill who leave the state mental institution and return to the local community. Once back in that community, they need adequate and effective support services.

A second priority population includes disturbed children and adolescents. Many stressful and emotional events occur in the formative years. Communities need to establish and strengthen community services, outreach, and education that assist children with emotional problems. Such programs can be conducted by schools, churches, and families, as well as by other community agencies. Children at high risk for emotional disorders are those who experience family separation, conflict between parents, the loss of parents through death or divorce, difficulty in school, or those with teenage parents. Other children who are more likely to have mental problems are those having multiple stressors in life or whose parents are mentally ill or drug or alcohol abusers.[17]

The elderly constitute the third priority group. For some people emotional problems develop with age, retirement, and the loss of loved ones and close friends. Adjustment to such circumstances merits emphasis. Supportive measures, treatment, and care need to be provided in the community setting. Recently mental health services have been available to the mentally impaired and emotionally distressed senior citizens in nursing homes.

Because the community mental health center developed as an alternative to the state mental hospital, a number of changes have occurred in program direction:[18]

1. Increased emphasis upon community-based services
2. Emphasis upon prevention of mental illness
3. Emphasis upon a mental health "system" with effective community planning
4. Emphasis upon short-term therapeutic approach to mental health
5. Emphasis upon indirect services (educational, consultative)
6. Emphasis upon an expanded use of nonprofessionals in the provision of mental health services

Since passage of the Community Mental Health Services Act in 1963, over seven hundred community mental health centers have been funded. The first such center began operating in 1966. Federal funding supported the construction of the center and its staffing and operation. As the result of federal assistance, community mental health centers were established in all fifty states. Federal funding of community mental health centers was discontinued in 1981 when the block-grant funding programs were established. This resulted in funding decisions relating to mental health being transferred to the states. Between 1981 and the mid-1980s federal funding for community mental health centers was reduced more than one-third.

The National Institute of Mental Health estimates that only about 55 percent of the national population lives within reasonable distance to such services. Since these facilities are basically located in urban population centers, people living in rural areas are usually underserved.

Since the passage of the original legislation supporting these centers, there have been several important amendments. The 1968 amendment included coverage for alcoholics and narcotics addicts. Services for drug abuse were added in 1970. A significant change occurred in 1981 with the passage of the Omnibus Budget Reconciliation Act. This legislation consolidated all federal programs related to mental health, alcoholism, alcohol abuse, and drug abuse into a block grant. This action in effect repealed the original 1963 Community Mental Health Centers Act.

Services are provided in the community mental health centers on both an inpatient and outpatient basis. Community mental health centers provide inpatient care in one of three different administrative patterns.[19] (1) Some operate their own inpatient units. In these the patient is not hospitalized, but kept at the center. (2) Other community mental health centers develop affiliate relationships with a hospital in order for their patients to have access to inpatient facilities. These centers contract with a hospital for use of beds when needed. (3) The third pattern is one in which the community mental health center is based at the hospital. The hospital operates the center in these situations.

The duration of treatment varies from several weeks to a few months on an inpatient basis. Short-term accommodations are available for those who need help for a relatively short period of time. Numerous outpatient services are provided, including group therapy, which has been found to be very effective.

Day-care services, sometimes referred to as Day Hospital, Day Treatment Center, or Day/Night Program, are furnished for those who do not need twenty-four-hour hospitalization, yet for whom normal outpatient care is inadequate. For example, a child might receive schooling in a therapeutic setting, but still be able to live at home with the family. Thus family participation is very important to the success of this program.[20]

The community mental health center also provides emergency care. These services are needed in situations of panic, personal disorganization, destructive outburst, or in times of stress. For instance, personnel are trained to assist potential suicide victims. They frequently operate telephone crisis and other forms of emergency intervention centers.

Both education and consultation are available at these centers. The educational objective is to inform the patient, the family, and the public about mental illness and to encourage measures to cope with such a condition. These activities are also intended to stimulate principles of good mental health. Consultation is provided for a variety of emotional problems.

Residential Treatment Services

In the past decade the community residential treatment approach has expanded to become an effective alternative to institutionalization. A variety of approaches can be used to help rehabilitate the patient in such settings.

The most common community residential treatment program is the halfway house. The halfway house serves as a bridge between hospitalization and the community. While living in a halfway house, the patient continues to receive treatment but is also mobile in the community. The resident may be on medication, but this is often unsupervised; the patient is responsible for this aspect of rehabilitation. There is usually twenty-four-hour staff support, and some halfway houses even hire a live-in staff.

The cooperative apartment type of community residential treatment differs from the halfway house in that there are fewer residents. The staff is available "on-call." A reasonable amount of independent living is permitted, and the residents determine many of the programming activities.

Another approach to community residential treatment involves family homes and foster homes. This approach places the patient in a private home where activities are family-oriented. The patient becomes involved in shopping, house maintenance, gardening, and socializing. Of great importance in the rehabilitative process is the support given by the host family and close neighbors.

There are several other variations of community residential treatment services. Boarding houses, group homes, foster communities, and nursing homes offer these services, too.[21]

Mental Health Personnel

In recent years there has been increased need for professional personnel in the mental health field. This need has resulted in an increase in the number of psychiatrists, psychologists, psychiatric social workers, and psychiatric nurses. These are the "core" professionals who service those in need of mental health care. These professionals work in all of the community settings previously discussed.

The difference in training, skills, and role in the treatment of the mentally ill and those with emotional problems by psychiatrists and psychologists is often misunderstood by the general public. The psychiatrist is a medical doctor whose specialty training lies in the prevention, diagnosis, treatment, and care of individuals with mental disorders. The psychiatrist usually needs three years of training beyond basic medical education in the treatment of the mentally ill in order to become certified. Psychiatrists use a variety of skills. In addition to talking (counseling) with the patient, the psychiatrist can prescribe drug treatment and other medical therapy modalities.

On the other hand, the psychologist studies the nonmedical science of human behavior for the purpose of diagnosing, treating, and preventing mental illness. These individuals are unable to use drug therapy. They use the techniques of case study, experimental research, surveys, and observation in their work. The emphasis of psychology is upon human behavior.

Paraprofessionals have become increasingly involved in mental health services. People with varying degrees of training now work in crisis centers, suicide prevention centers, and rap groups. They have been very effective in dealing with such groups as drug addicts, alcoholics, and the economically disadvantaged.[22] The paraprofessional offers a number of skills in mental health patient care including diagnosis, counseling, and supervision of medication. In addition, patient support, education, referral, admission, and case recording are paraprofessional tasks. They also staff halfway houses and provide child care.

Training of community mental health para-professionals varies. Sometimes this involves a pre-service orientation followed by in-service continuing education sessions including group discussions, seminars, and sensitivity training. More recently, college preparation for such positions has become the norm. The two-year Associate Degree program for the paraprofessional mental health worker is now offered. Some ten thousand students a year graduate from over two hundred such programs.[23]

Several different tasks performed by the para-professional have been identified:[24]

1. Intervene in critical treatment situations
2. Provide psychiatric help for those who could not otherwise receive such assistance
3. Provide needed care where a shortage of mental health professionals exists
4. Mobilize community resources
5. Interpret client needs to a professional
6. Serve as a role model

These tasks, combined with the many services provided by mental health "core" professionals, are significant parts of mental health treatment and rehabilitation. Each person, professional and para-professional, has an important, specific role to play in caring for the mentally ill, assisting the emotionally distraught individual, and setting goals and conducting programs for preventive mental health.

Presidential Commission on Mental Health (1978)

In spite of the movement to a community-based program of mental health services, the increase in the size of the mental health workforce, and greater awareness of mental illness and mental health, many persons' needs for mental health care, support, and prevention are still not met. In 1978, President Carter appointed a national commission to review the status of mental health in the United States and to make recommendations for future direction, legislation, and national goals. The Presidential Commission on Mental Health (1978) concluded in its report that " . . . there are millions who remain unserved, underserved, or inappropriately served."[25]

Many people with chronic mental disabilities are unable to obtain the basic necessities of life, such as food, clothing, and shelter, when they are released from the mental hospital. Because there is no effective follow-up, at least half of those released from mental hospitals are readmitted within a year.[26]

Among the Commission's many recommendations to the president was the suggestion that a major effort should be made to provide personal and community support mechanisms for the individual having mental health problems. Three community groups were singled out to participate in this effort: (1) the public school system, (2) the civil and criminal justice system, and (3) primary health care providers.[27] Most of the Commission's recommendations were based on the premise that people with mental problems are best cared for within their own communities.

The Commission recognized that many people were unable to obtain mental health care services. They advised that measures be taken to implement services in underserved geographical areas. Furthermore, those who were unable to obtain care because of economic or cultural barriers should also have access to the care. In an effort to overcome the economic barrier, the Commission suggested that health insurance include outpatient mental health benefits. Not only should private health programs expand existing coverage, but any future national health insurance proposals should include mental health care coverage for outpatient care, inpatient services, and emergency mental health services.

In an effort to surmount the cultural barriers, it was recommended that minorities be encouraged to enter the various mental health professions. Thus, mental health personnel could communicate with and relate to minorities.

The Commission on Mental Health concluded that an emphasis must be placed on promoting mental health. Efforts must be made to reduce the effects of such stressful life experiences as unemployment, marital disruption, and retirement.[28] Of interest is the fact that the Commission concluded that treatment of children should be a priority. With this in mind, good prenatal care, child health care, and the development of day-care programs were deemed necessary for the prevention of mental health disorders.

As we have already noted, care for the mentally ill in the past two decades has moved from mental hospitals to such community-based facilities as community health centers, halfway houses, and cooperative residences. It is important to emphasize the need of coordinating mental health services and other health services within our states and communities. Such coordination must occur in order to improve the accessibility of mental health services. One approach is to provide mental health services in primary medical care settings as recommended in the report from the president's commission.

National Institute of Mental Health

The federal agency concerned with mental health program development is the National Institute of Mental Health (NIMH), one of the institutes of the Alcohol, Drug Abuse, and Mental Health Administration of the Public Health Services. NIMH was founded in 1946 with the passage of the National Mental Health Act by Congress. Through the years, the National Institute of Mental Health has developed, conducted, and supported programs directed at mental illness and emotional disturbance. Among the most visible has been NIMH's role in mental health research.

NIMH Research

Research has played an important role in improving the status of care, treatment, and understanding of the mentally ill. The National Institute of Mental Health has supported research into the causes, treatment, and prevention of a number of mental and emotional disorders, including schizophrenia, severe depression, anxiety disorders, and manic depressive illnesses. Specific problem areas such as the mental health of children, minorities, the aging, criminals, delinquents, and the elderly have been important research areas.

Although the primary purpose of mental health research is the improvement of treatment for individuals with mental illness and emotional problems, there are other specific goals, too. Extensive efforts have been directed at learning more about the underlying causes of mental illness. Such efforts involve learning more about how the mind works, about the relationship between the body and the brain, and the adjustment into society of the emotionally troubled individual. The biological basis of memory and learning and various physiological and chemical influences on human behavior are also researched.

An important discovery made by biomedical researchers was that information is transmitted through the central nervous system by chemicals in the brain called *neurotransmitters*. Neurotransmitters are essential for normal mental functioning. One of the neurotransmitters, norepinephrine, is considered crucial in the areas of the brain that govern emotions.

Research in recent years has shown that heredity is a factor in schizophrenia. The specific relationship and the measures that would reduce the individual's susceptibility are current areas of research. Other evidence of the role heredity plays in mental illness is under investigation.

Drug therapy for mental illness has resulted in the study and development of many drugs that affect human behavior. For example, tranquilizers and antidepressive medication are effective in helping hospitalized mental patients. Tranquilizers are useful in treatment of patients with schizophrenia. Antidepressive drugs can improve the condition of individuals experiencing various states of depression.

Behavioral research has investigated behavior in a variety of situations. This includes individual behavior as well as interactions in group settings. Studies of sociocultural influences on behaviors that result in emotional disturbances or in alcohol and drug abuse, as well as studies into child development, have led to better understanding of how to care for the patient. The issue of hyperactive behavior among children has been an important research initiative of NIMH.

(a) The rehabilitation medicine program at St. Elizabeth's Hospital in Washington, D.C., considers both physical and mental aspects of recovery for psychiatric patients. (b) Occupational therapy is also helpful in restoring patients' usefulness and productivity, as is (c) recreation therapy.

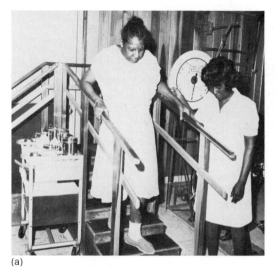
(a)

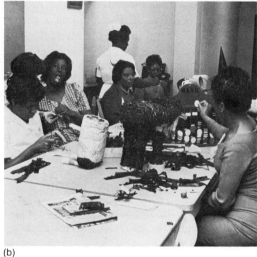
(b)

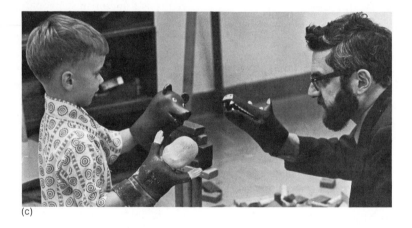
(c)

Epidemiological research looks at the extent of mental illness, stress, and emotional disability in the country. This data, however, is often hard to obtain since many families are reluctant to report that a family member is experiencing a problem. Often the data available is based only on those who are treated in public facilities. However, accurate data is needed in order to ascertain the extent of specific mental health problems in a given community and to assist in appropriate program planning.

National Institute of Mental Health research has been looking at problems related to stress. Not only has such research attempted to learn more about the dynamics of stress on human lives, but also how to encourage health-promoting behaviors.

Numerous community agencies provide meals for the homeless. For most homeless individuals, this is the major source of nutrition they obtain each day.

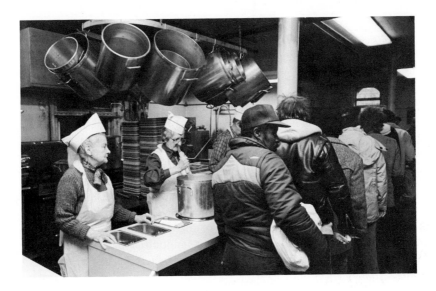

Related NIMH Tasks

Though research is important and consumes a major portion of the efforts and financial support of the National Institute of Mental Health, this federal agency also conducts a number of other activities designed to improve the mental health of the country as a whole. A demand for professional and para-professional personnel in the mental health field has necessitated educational programs. Many training programs, in-service sessions, and financial fellowship programs are funded by NIMH.

A number of mental health services are either provided by NIMH or coordinated by this agency. The national institute supports innovative mental health services in community settings, such as day-care centers, schools, hospitals, and the community mental health facilities. The National Institute of Mental Health operates the St. Elizabeth Hospital in Maryland, where staff members provide treatment and rehabilitation for psychiatric patients. A model community mental health center is operated within this hospital.

The Institute also distributes public and professional literature and information about mental health and related concerns. Monographs, pamphlets, and other publications update the general public and the mental health professionals about effective programs and techniques for the treatment of mental illness and emotional disturbances.

Homelessness

There have always been people who live on the streets, in the parks, and in slum buildings of America's cities. The "tramp," the "wino," or the "bum" has been a part of the landscape of many urban communities. However, in recent years there has been an increasing number of homeless people. The homeless population has become younger, many having a history of psychiatric hospitalization. Whereas the homeless have traditionally been males, there is an increasing number of women and children and families who are found on the streets of our cities. This has been caused by economic setbacks and unemployment.

One Day in the Life of the Homeless in America

"In Dallas . . . shelter . . . use is up 50 percent."

"In Kansas City, Missouri . . . two homeless men froze to death Tuesday."

"In Detroit, shelters . . . forced to turn away a record number of people."

"In New York City, a record 10,000 are in shelters."

"In Milwaukee . . . former cab driver . . . 'will I make it through the night or will I just freeze to death?' "

Quotes taken from: *U.S.A. Today,* November 13, 1986.

The numbers of such people have risen quite dramatically in recent years. It is difficult to define, or to obtain an accurate count of, the homeless in America today. The Department of Housing and Urban Development estimates the number to be between 250,000 and 350,000. Other estimates range as high as two to three million.[29]

The homeless tend to fall into one of three different categories. (1) Some are individuals who have had recent economic setbacks. (2) Others are persons who have had severe personal crises. (3) A large number of the homeless are the chronically mentally ill.

During the early 1980s many people found themselves unemployed. For many this came about as a result of economic recession and increased high level technology in the industrial world. Inability to find work or being released from one's employment after years of seniority with a company often causes extreme psychological frustration. Anxiety and depression manifested by various physical symptoms are often seen among these individuals.[30]

Deinstitutionalization has resulted in neglect of the chronically mentally ill. Many of the social welfare, housing, and other support system needs of these individuals have not been provided.

The original concept of deinstitutionalization was that services would be made available outside of the mental health hospital back into one's community. This concept in theory was good in that

people would be cared for in community mental health centers. In reality this is not what has happened. During the early 1980s, funding cutbacks reduced community mental health services. Many communities are now without community mental health facilities and personnel. Needed ambulatory care is not available in many localities. As a result thousands of chronically mentally ill people have been left on the streets to make their own way without the emotional, financial, and physical resources to do so. Therefore, they are homeless or are living in substandard living conditions. Homelessness has resulted from an absence of follow-up, rehabilitative services, and help outside the hospital within the community. These individuals have shifted from one place to another.

Numerous health problems are found among the homeless. Much untreated illness and disease is noted. Respiratory infections are much more common than among the average nontransient population. Numerous skin problems and nerve disorders have been observed among the homeless.

Trauma is an all too prevalent occurrence among the street people. Muggings, fights, and rape often occur, resulting in lacerations, skin injuries, and fractures.

A variety of different nutritional disorders are found among these individuals. Lack of funds usually prohibits the purchasing of adequate nutritious meals. An increase in the risk of malnutrition is often noted.

Health Problems: Comparison of Homeless with the National Average

	Homeless	National Average
Trauma	30.7%	17.5%
Colds	27.8%	6.3%
Lungs	20.6%	3.6%
Limb Disorders	18.8%	1.3%
Skin	14.7%	4.8%
Nerve Disorders	11.9%	1.9%
Eyes	7.8%	3.7%
Nutritional Disorders	6.0%	1.4%
Infectious Diseases	3.8%	1.4%

The homeless often find a place to sleep in fields, yards, under bridges, or in vacant buildings.

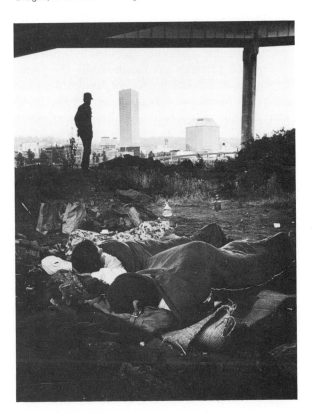

Hypothermia is another health problem found among the homeless. During cold winters in many big cities the street people will often have no place to get out of the extremely cold temperatures and weather elements. Once they lie down to rest or to sleep they either freeze to death or suffer extreme cold and reduction of body temperature.

Alcohol use is common among the homeless. Whether alcohol is a cause of the problems that lead to one's homelessness or a result of the homelessness is a subject of debate and discussion. In all probability, it is a combination of both. Alcohol abuse impacts most of the health problems of the street people. It is a major cause of malnutrition. Drunkenness results in violent behavior and related trauma injuries.

The homeless usually experience a lack of access to needed health care. Many have no health insurance. Without a permanent address it is difficult to obtain Medicaid. People will usually go to a public hospital or a free clinic, or will not seek medical attention when needed. All too often they fail to seek care until the specific health problem is serious, painful, or debilitating. Medically speaking, the problem of establishing continuity of care is always a concern due to the transient nature of the homeless.

The National Institute of Mental Health has established several areas of research activities to cope with problems of homelessness.[31] Epidemiological studies are being conducted to reach agreement as to the way homelessness can be defined, focusing on the nature and extent of the homeless, and on factors relating to how chronic mental illness results in homelessness. The National Institute of Mental Health is working to help health professionals effectively help the chronically mentally ill, homeless person.

Summary

The mentally ill have been treated inhumanely in the past. Mental patients were treated little better than animals: they were chained, imprisoned, tortured, given only subsistence food supplies, and exhibited as human "freaks." Little effort was made to treat or rehabilitate the mentally ill. Isolated attempts in parts of Europe to improve mental health care met with little acceptance, but in the early twentieth century, the work of Clifford Beers initiated a more positive approach to mental health.

Mental patients seeking treatment were institutionalized in state hospitals in the early part of this century. The quality of care they received here was often poor as no major developments in better understanding of the patients or in rehabilitation had occurred.

Since 1955 the number of patients in state mental hospitals has been reduced by about 60 percent. This is due to a number of reasons. The development of drug therapy meant that many mental patients could often be treated on an outpatient basis. Another new concept in the treatment of the mentally ill was the care of the patient in the community—not in an isolated, impersonal state hospital. This led to the Community Mental Health Services Act, legislation that created a community mental health center system. Today over 50 percent of the American population seeking mental health services contact such facilities.

Other community-based facilities provide both outpatient and inpatient mental health services along with emergency care. These facilities include general community hospitals, residential therapy services, and private psychiatric services.

In 1978, with the support of President Carter's administration, a national commission was appointed to make recommendations for national goals and future mental health programs. This commission made a number of recommendations for expanded community services. Several barriers that prohibit many people from obtaining mental health care were identified: geography, economics, and culture. Not only did the commission recommend steps to improve the availability of mental health services, but it emphasized the need for prevention.

The National Institute of Mental Health was established by federal legislation in the 1940s. It has supported major research efforts to learn more about mental illness and the emotionally disturbed. Biomedical research has focused upon the physiological and chemical aspects of mental disorders. Research has also investigated the hereditary, socioeconomic, and epidemiologic dynamics of mental health.

In addition to research, NIMH supports mental health education and training programs, publishes both public and professional material about mental health, and supports and coordinates the mental health services in local communities.

Deinstitutionalization of the state mental hospitals has been a major contributing factor to increased homelessness in the United States. Other factors that have contributed to this development have been unemployment, economic setbacks, and personal crises in the lives of individuals. A number of health needs and concerns are present among those who are found to be homeless in the urban areas of this country.

Discussion Questions

1. Describe some of the abuses that have been reported in the history of treatment of the mentally ill.
2. Identify and compare some of the contributions to the mental health movement made by Pinel, Clifford Beers, and Dorothy Lynde Dix.
3. Following the Second World War, what role did the federal government play in improving mental health care in the United States?
4. What are some of the contributing factors in the reduction of the number of patients in state mental hospitals since 1956?
5. In your state, how many state mental psychiatric hospitals are in operation and what services do they provide?
6. How does a general hospital psychiatric department differ from a state mental hospital?
7. What has been the influence of the 1963 federal legislation that established community mental health centers?
8. Discuss the question: has deinstitutionalization been as successful as hoped in the 1960s and 1970s?
9. Discuss the influence the Omnibus Budget Reconciliation Act has had on mental health programming.
10. What is meant by day-care services in the field of mental illness?
11. Explain the organization and services of residential treatment centers.
12. Discuss some of the recommendations made by the Presidential Commission on Mental Health in 1978.
13. What is the significance of neurotransmitters in mental illness?
14. How has drug therapy changed the care and treatment of the mentally ill?
15. Identify some of the functions of the National Institute of Mental Health.
16. Identify some of the factors that have contributed to the increase in homeless individuals in the 1980s.
17. In what ways has deinstitutionalization impacted the problems of homelessness?
18. What are some of the health problems associated with the homeless?

Suggested Readings

Bachrach, Leona L. "The Effects of Deinstitutionalization on General Hospital Psychiatry." *Hospital and Community Psychiatry* 32, no. 11 (November, 1981): 786–90.

Bachrach, Leona L. "General Hospital Psychiatry: Overview From a Sociological Perspective." *American Journal of Psychiatry* 138, no. 7, (July, 1981): 879–89.

Bachrach, Leona L. "Research on Services for the Homeless Mentally Ill." *Hospital and Community Psychiatry* 35, (September, 1984): 910–13.

Bassuk, Ellen L.; Rubin, Lenore; and Lavriat, Alison S. "Characteristics of Sheltered Homeless Families." *American Journal of Public Health* 76, no. 9 (September, 1986): 1097–1101.

Beers, Clifford W. *A Mind That Found Itself.* New York: Doubleday and Company, Inc., 1906.

Bloom, Bernard L. *Community Mental Health: A General Introduction.* Monterey, Calif.: Brooks/Cole Publishing Co. (1984) 432 pp.

Clarke, Gary J. "In Defense of Deinstitutionalization." *Milbank Memorial Fund Quarterly, Health and Society* 57, no. 4 (1979): 461–79.

Colton, Sterling I. "Community Residential Treatment Strategies." *Community Mental Health Review* 3, no. 5/6 (September/December, 1978): 1, 16–21.

Eisenberg, Leon. "A Research Framework for Evaluating the Promotion of Mental Health and Prevention of Mental Illness." *Public Health Reports* 96, no. 1 (January/February, 1981): 3–19.

Ewalt, Jack R. "The Mental Health Movement, 1949–1979." *Milbank Memorial Fund Quarterly, Health and Society* 57, no. 4 (1979): 507–15.

Feldman, Saul. "Community Mental Health Centers: A Decade Later." *International Journal of Mental Health* 3, no. 2–3: 19–34.

Fisher, Pamela J., and others. "Mental Health and Social Characteristics of the Homeless: A Survey of Mission Users." *American Journal of Public Health* 76, no. 5 (May, 1986): 519–24.

Frazier, Shervert H. "Responding to the Needs of the Homeless Mentally Ill." *Public Health Reports* 100, no. 5 (September/October, 1985): 462–69.

Friedman, Emily. "Hospital Psychiatric Services Begin a Changing of the Guard." *Hospitals* 55, no. 9 (May 1, 1981): 52–55.

Goldman, Howard H., and Morrissey, Joseph P. "The Alchemy of Mental Health Policy: Homelessness and the Fourth Cycle of Reform." *American Journal of Public Health* 75, no. 7 (July, 1985): 727–31.

Keill, Stuart L. "The General Hospital as the Core of the Mental Health Services System." *Hospital and Community Psychiatry* 32, no. 11 (November, 1981): 776–78.

Keill, Stuart L. "Psychiatric Care: A New Role For Hospitals?" *Hospitals* 54 (October 1, 1982).

Lamb, H. R. *The Homeless Mentally Ill.* Washington, D.C.: American Psychiatric Press, 1984.

Leaf, Philip J., and others. "Federally Funded CMHS: The Effects of Period of Initial Funding and Hospital Affiliation." *Community Mental Health Journal* 21, no. 3 (Fall, 1985): 145–55.

Linn, Margaret W., and others. "Effects of Unemployment on Mental and Physical Health." *American Journal of Public Health* 75, no. 5 (May, 1985): 502–06.

Moffic H. Steve, et al. "Training in Community Mental Health." *Community Mental Health Review* 4, no. 3 (1979): 1–11.

Nash, Kermit B., et al. "Paraprofessionals and Community Mental Health." *Community Mental Health Review* 3, no. 2 (March/April, 1978): 1–8.

National Institute of Mental Health. *National Leadership Workshop on the Homeless Mentally Ill: Proceedings of the Workshop.* Rockville, Md.: NIMH (1985).

Neighbors, Harold W. "Seeking Professional Help for Personal Problems: Black Americans' Use of Health and Mental Health Services." *Community Mental Health Journal* 21, no. 3 (Fall, 1985): 156–66.

Parker, Zoe H. "The Chronically Mental Ill, Will the Community Accept Them?" *Hygie* V, no. 3 (1986): 13–16.

President's Commission on Mental Health. *Report to the President.* Washington, D.C.: U.S. Government Printing Office (1978): 1–8.

Ridenour, Nina. *Mental Health in the United States: A Fifty-Year History.* Cambridge, Mass.: Harvard University Press, 1961.

Robertson, Marjorie J., and Cousineau, Michael R. "Health Status and Access to Health Services among the Urban Homeless." *American Journal of Public Health* 76, no. 5 (May, 1986): 561–65.

Tableman, Betty. "Overview of Programs to Prevent Mental Health Problems of Children." *Public Health Reports* 96, no. 1 (January/February, 1981): 38–44.

Thomas, Claudewell S., and Lindenthal, Jacob J. "Issues in Community Mental Health." *Administration in Mental Health* (Winter, 1975): 66–70.

Willer, Barry, et al. "Deinstitutionalization and Mentally Retarded Persons." *Community Mental Health Review* 3, no. 4 (July/August, 1978): 1–12.

York, David R. "The Private Sector: Revenue Source of the 80's." *Community Mental Health Journal* 21, no. 4 (Winter, 1985): 252–63.

Zusman, Jack. "What is Community Mental Health?" *International Journal of Mental Health* 3, no. 2–3: 5–18.

Zusman, Jack, and Bertsch, Elmer F. *The Future Role of the State Hospital.* Lexington, Mass.: Lexington Books, 1975.

Endnotes

1. Ridenour, Nina. *Mental Health in the United States: A Fifty-Year History.* Cambridge, Mass.: Harvard University Press, 1961, 134.

2. Beers, Clifford W. *A Mind That Found Itself.* New York: Doubleday and Co., Inc., 1906.

3. Ridenour. *Mental Health.* 13–15.

4. Brown, Bertrams. *Trends in Mental Health.* Washington, D.C.: U.S. Government Printing Office, (DHEW) Pub. No. (ADM) 76-406, 1976, 2.

5. Ibid.

6. Deutsch, Albert. *The Shame of the States.* Salem, New York: Ayer Company, 1948.

7. Veterans Administration. *1980 Annual Report.* Washington, D.C.: U.S. Government Printing Office, 17.

8. National Institute of Mental Health. *Financing Mental Health Care in the United States.* Washington, D.C.: U.S. Government Printing Office, (DHEW) Pub. No. 73-9117, 1973, 7.

9. Friedman, Emily. "Hospital Psychiatric Services Begin a Changing of the Guard." *Hospitals* 55, no. 9 (May 1, 1981): 53.

10. National Institute of Mental Health. *State and County Hospitals, U.S. 1973–1974.* Washington, D.C.: U.S. Government Printing Office, (DHEW) Pub. No. (ADM) 76-301, 1975, 1.

11. Ibid., 1.

12. *Statistical Abstracts of the United States, 1986.* U.S. Department of Commerce. Washington, D.C.: U.S. Government Printing Office, 106.

13. National Institute of Mental Health. *Financing Mental Health Care.* 9.

14. Ibid., 12.

15. Bachrach, Leona L. "The Effects of Deinstitutionalization on General Hospital Psychiatry." *Hospital and Community Psychiatry* 32, no. 11 (November, 1981): 786.

16. Keill, Stuart L. "The General Hospital as the Core of the Mental Health Services System." *Hospital and Community Psychiatry* 32, no. 11 (November, 1981): 776–78.

17. Tableman, Betty. "Overview of Programs to Prevent Mental Health Problems of Children." *Public Health Reports* 96, no. 1, (January/February, 1981): 38.

18. Bloom, B. L. *Community Mental Health: A General Introduction.* Monterey, Calif.: Brooks Cole, 1977.

19. Leaf, Philip J., and others. "Federally Funded CMHS: The Effects of Period of Initial Funding and Hospital Affiliation." *Community Mental Health Journal* 21, no. 3 (Fall, 1985): 145.

20. Maxey, Joseph T. "Partial Hospitalization: A Review of Growth and Development in the United States." *Community Mental Health Review* 4, no. 4, 1979, 1–8.

21. Colton, Sterling I. "Community Residential Treatment Strategies." *Community Mental Health Review* 3, no. 5/6 (September/December, 1978): 1, 16–21.

22. Nash, Kermit B., et al. "Paraprofessionals and Community Mental Health." *Community Mental Health Review* 3, no. 2 (March/April, 1978): 1–8.

23. President's Commission on Mental Health. *Report to the President.* Washington, D.C.: U.S. Government Printing Office, 1978, 40.

24. Nash. "Paraprofessionals and Community Mental Health," 3.

25. President's Commission on Mental Health. *Report to the President.* 2.

26. Ibid., 5.

27. Ibid., 15.

28. Ibid., 51.

29. Frazier, Shervert H. "Responding to the Needs of the Homeless Mentally Ill." *Public Health Reports* 100, no. 5 (September/October, 1985): 462–69.

30. Linn, Margaret W., and others. "Effects of Unemployment on Mental and Physical Health." *American Journal of Public Health* 75, no. 5 (May, 1985): 502–06.

31. National Institute of Mental Health. *National Leadership Workshop on the Homeless Mentally Ill: Proceedings of the Workshop.* Rockville, Md: National Institute of Mental Health, (1985).

13

Schools: Comprehensive Programs for Better Health

Within nearly every community throughout the United States, the local school is a natural setting for health promotion and disease prevention activities. For at least nine months of each year, millions of young children spend a major part of each day in school. Education is compulsory in all fifty states for children in the age range of six to sixteen. Specific age requirements differ slightly from one state to another, but children's school experiences can have a major effect on their health behavior patterns and personal well-being.

The school health program has historically been an important part of the total school program in this country. It encompasses all school activities directed at the development of healthier individuals. This program has traditionally been divided into three components: (1) *health instruction,* (2) *health services,* and (3) *healthful environment.*

There are many who believe that the health and well-being of the child during school hours are the responsibility of the school. Community health programming works closely with the school health program by screening vision and hearing, instituting dental health programs, and directing drug education and various other related activities. Through these cooperative efforts, both groups can best utilize their capabilities, and the result should be a healthier child.

Comprehensive School Health Program

The concept of a comprehensive school health program has been frequently discussed, although the idea has different meanings for different people. Some people, in discussing the need for comprehensive school health, are referring solely to the systematic planning of a K–12 health instruction program. Other individuals view comprehensive school health as a broader coverage of health services. Programming in this second model uses school facilities, but local health community personnel provide the screening and medical services. Physicians, nurses, dentists, and paraprofessionals are frequently involved in such programming.[1]

Comprehensive school health programs must account for all three components of the traditional school health definition. A successful program is also dependent upon the cooperative efforts of the educational community, the medical community, and the community health department.

Children are products of their environments: their families, cultures, neighborhoods, and communities. In order to respond to the health problem of a school child, it is necessary to involve elements from the community as well as the family. No school health program can be effective without the inclusion of all three areas of influence: school, community, and family.

Health Instruction

The instructional phase of a comprehensive school program imparts information about positive health behaviors. Children are given the background they need to make good decisions about their personal health behaviors. Statements of support for school health instruction have been developed by many professional organizations.

Health instruction in the schools is tailored to the learning capabilities of each specific age group. Regularly scheduled class periods devoted to health instruction are the most effective health education approach, particularly in secondary schools.

In the elementary school, health is usually taught by the classroom teacher. This teacher, trained in elementary education and certified to teach most subjects, often has minimal background and education in the health field. Most elementary education majors have taken only one health course, often in combination with a physical education methods course. At many colleges this health requirement can be met by taking a personal health course, which does not focus on the health of the elementary school-age child. As a result, the elementary school teacher usually lacks broad, current knowledge of health.

The preparation of junior (middle school) and senior high school health teachers is slightly better. In most states, secondary school teachers must fulfill state certification requirements to teach each specific subject. Though requirements vary, a prospective teacher must have as a minimum an academic minor in a subject in order to be certified to teach it. In many states, certification is granted simultaneously for health and physical education, but usually the emphasis in preparation is on physical education rather than health education. Some states, however, have developed separate certification standards for health education.[2]

In order to upgrade the caliber of health teachers, in-service training and continuing education programs in health are often provided. Such educational efforts enlarge and update the teacher's basic knowledge of health concepts and provide exposure to current curricular developments and materials.

Usually the amount of teaching time devoted to health is determined by the state department of education. This time allotment is most often presented in terms of minutes per week. How this instruction occurs, who teaches the class, and what content is covered is decided by the local school district. In the secondary school, the health class is usually a separate class taught over one semester.

Health concepts are also taught in an informal class setting. This is incidental learning through experiences at school. Health discussions may be integrated into other subjects as well, such as science, home economics, and physical education.

A number of questions are often raised about the health instructional program. One concern is whether it is ethical for public schools to include educational experiences that attempt to change personal health practices. Whose values, practices, and beliefs are the standards that are taught? At times these standards for health practices may be contrary to family values, beliefs, and morality. How does the school cope with this matter in developing a health curriculum? All too often these difficult questions are not considered when setting goals and establishing learning experiences for the school health program.

In spite of the fact that there are many approaches to health instruction in the schools, the health education curriculum must still be redesigned. Such an effort should focus upon the total entity of health: the *social,* the *emotional,* and the *physical.* Each component must be presented in light of the most current developments and information.

Curriculum Development

The educational curriculum in the United States is determined and controlled locally. According to the Constitution, education is a state responsibility. It is at the community level that decisions are made regarding school funding, curriculum, and other educational matters.

As a result, curriculum development throughout the United States varies significantly from one school district to another. Though there are state education department guidelines and regulations for many subjects in the curriculum, the actual development of what is taught, and how, is usually a local matter.

The process of curriculum design also varies. During the development phase, curriculum specialists, school administrators, teachers, sometimes parents and students, and occasionally others with specific expertise are often consulted. Such an approach to curriculum development leads to a large variance in curriculum organization, topics, methods, and goals.

Health education has seldom been coordinated in a comprehensive K–12 curriculum. All too often school districts do not coordinate the health learning experiences from one grade level to another. The subject matter may be determined by the knowledge and expertise of the teacher or as outlined by the textbook being used. This unplanned scheme of curriculum development often results in overlap, duplication, and repetition. It is not unusual to hear elementary school students complain that the subject being covered this year is the same as that which was studied the previous year. This problem must and can be solved by offering a sequential curriculum. Though other topics can be added, a well-designed school health program should include at least ten major topics.

National Curriculum Efforts

At times a national curriculum for certain subject areas has been proposed. However, local control of education in America has forestalled any such development. Despite this opposition proponents of a national curriculum, particularly for health, continue to argue for its inception.

School Health Education Study

In the mid-1960s, a nationally developed curriculum project known as the School Health Education Study (SHES) was designed and produced. The development of this curricular project was the outgrowth of a nationwide survey that indicated a serious weakness in school instruction of health. In this study, it was found that little coordination of teaching existed between school levels. Students seriously lacked knowledge of basic health. The overall conclusion was that the level and quality of health instruction programs in the schools were poor.[3]

Ten Content Areas Considered Minimal for a Comprehensive School Health Program
1. Personal health
2. Mental and emotional health
3. Prevention and control of disease
4. Nutrition
5. Substance use and abuse
6. Accident prevention and safety
7. Community health
8. Consumer health
9. Environmental health
10. Family life education
Source: Education Commission of the States, *Recommendations for School Health Education, Report No. 130* (Denver, Colorado, 1981), 31–32.

As a consequence of this national study, a curriculum project was initiated. Its goal was to improve health instruction with a nationally recognized curriculum. This project, known as the *SHES Project,* used a conceptual model of curriculum development. It was a well-designed curriculum effort, in which additional concepts were built onto the previous year's conceptual base. Through the latter part of the 1960s and the early 1970s, a number of school districts throughout the country adopted all or parts of this curriculum. However, it never gained widespread use and the enthusiasm for this curriculum waned by the mid-1970s. One major reason for the lack of interest by many school districts was the cost. In order to use the curriculum on an integrated K–12 basis, the district was forced to spend more money than was usually appropriated for health education.

Health Education Curriculum Models

There is still a need for a carefully planned health curriculum for kindergarten through high school students. This need has led to a number of national efforts for the implementation of such a curriculum. These activities have involved various community health organizations, agencies, and foundations,

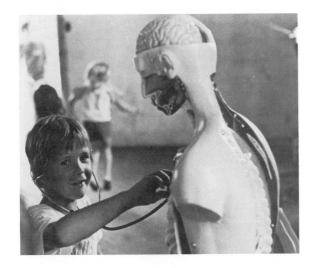

"Feelin' Good" is a cardiovascular fitness curriculum used by school districts in several states. Through education and exercise, health knowledge and values that will last a lifetime are developed.

along with curriculum development specialists and health education personnel.

In recent years, more than 120 school health education curriculum models have been developed.[4] These have been received with varying degrees of attention and acceptance. Some have been designed specifically as health education curriculums, others as cardiovascular health, fitness, nutritional, dental health, and emotional health programs. Though it is impossible to identify all of the health education curriculum models and resources now available, several are noted in this chapter.[5]

Some of these curriculum models are designed for elementary grades (Health Education Curriculum Guide, Know Your Body, Feelin' Good, Health Skills for Life, Learning for Life), while others are designed for secondary school children (Family and Community Health through Caregiving, Skills for Living—Project Quest, Teenage Health Teaching Modules). Some focus primarily on cardiovascular health (Feelin' Good), others on nutrition (Nutrition Education and Training Program), dental health (School Dental Health Education Curriculum— Tampa), or substance abuse. Most tend to focus on

student behavior objectives. They use a variety of values-clarification strategies. Discovery activities, decision-making skills, and student-centered materials for self-learning are primary methodologies in most of these programs. Several of the programs involve the home and the community, in addition to the school. Such programs usually involve workshops and the involvement of family members in activities along with the students.

These programs rely heavily on audiovisual material. Thus it is important for teachers to be trained not only in teaching strategies, but also in the use of such equipment and materials. For example, before using the Self-Discovery Program, teachers receive five days of training. Training workshops for teachers who use Skills for Living—Project Quest are held regularly.

Some financial support for the development, teacher training, and dissemination of several of these health education curriculum models has originated with various philanthropical foundations. The Kellogg Foundation has provided grants for the Learning for Life Program, the Feelin' Good Curriculum, and the Family and Community Health through Caregiving Program. The Zellerback Family Fund financed the development and piloting in San Francisco of the Growing Healthy Curriculum. The Health Education Curriculum Guide was developed with the support of the United Way Health Foundation in Canton, Ohio.

Evaluation studies have been conducted on most of these curriculum models. One three-year comparative study was the School Health Education Evaluation.[6] This study evaluated four projects: the Growing Healthy Curriculum Project, the Health Education Curriculum Guide, Project Prevention of Dalles, Oregon, and the 3Rs and High Blood Pressure Project. More than thirty thousand students in grades 4–7 in one thousand classrooms in twenty states were a part of this study.

In general this study showed that health education instruction in schools is effective. Students in these programs showed improved attitudes toward maintaining a healthy body. Increased knowledge regarding growth and development, human sexuality, and substance abuse was recorded. Also, students in these programs had improved decision-making skills, and less smoking was reported by students in these programs.[7]

The School Health Education Evaluation emphasized the need for administrative support, good teacher training, and the importance of continuity across grade levels.

Growing Healthy Curriculum Project The curriculum project that has received the greatest national exposure has been the Growing Healthy Curriculum Project. This project, formerly known as the School Health Curriculum and the Primary Grades Curriculum Project, is designed to help students understand how the body functions. It has been used in close to six hundred school districts in forty-one states.[8] Various dimensions that affect the body are studied—both environmental and microorganismic. Students are educated to make appropriate personal health behavioral choices throughout their lives. The goal of this project is to "help the child realize that the body is each person's greatest natural resource in life, that the body is uniquely one's own, that it is exquisitely beautiful and complex in its structure and functions, that it is influenced by one's own choices made throughout life and that it has the potential of bringing experiences in life more exciting than anything imaginable because they will be one's own experiences."[9]

The Growing Healthy Curriculum Project has materials for instruction of grades K–7. The units designed for grades 4–7 focus on the body's systems, while the K–3 material focuses on the senses. Each unit spans a ten-to-twelve week period of time, with learning experiences broken down into five phases.

This curriculum employs the problem-solving approach. Investigation, employment of creative learning styles, value clarification, and decision making are the principal means of teaching and learning. The curriculum emphasizes the use of a variety of methods and equipment. Microscopes, books, dramas, experiments, and multiple teaching

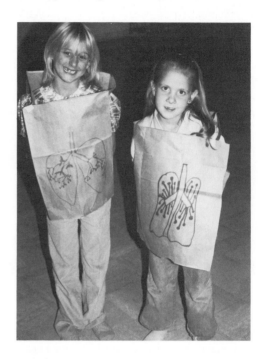

Recently developed curriculum models use a variety of creative activities. Children can learn how their respiratory systems work and what happens during an asthma episode.

and learning resources are employed. Multimedia, including films, slides, movies, records, radio, and television, are also incorporated into the program.

Children are encouraged to learn by doing. Learning centers provide a variety of teaching and learning strategies. Classroom teachers must be trained to use this curriculum. The Growing Healthy Curriculum Project is designed for use by regular classroom teachers, not just specialists trained in health education. However, before the curriculum can be used, all teachers must enroll in a sixty-hour training session. Usually spanning two weeks, the training sessions familiarize the teachers with the subject matter and the various methods and materials of the curriculum. They also participate in the same educational processes that the children will experience.

To ensure the success of the project, it is important to identify a team from the school or school district who will work well together. Funds must be appropriated to pay for the training and materials.

Surgeon General Calls for Teaching of Sex Education in Schools Starting at Grade 3

In a speech given in late 1986 Surgeon General C. Everett Koop stated that " . . . we need sex education in schools and that it must include information on heterosexual and homosexual relationships." The motivation for this strong statement of support for sex education in the school curriculum was the increasing concern about Acquired Immune Deficiency Syndrome (AIDS). It had become increasingly imperative to the medical and political leaders of the United States that the public needs to become more informed about AIDS—its cause, prevention, and treatment.

The surgeon general suggested that this instruction should begin as early as third grade (about eight years of age). It was his contention that school-age children, as well as the adult population, must learn how AIDS is contracted and how it can be prevented.

Such a statement calling for comprehensive school sex education raises problems, questions, and opposition. Is it appropriate to include instruction on AIDS in curriculum material on sexuality? At what age is it appropriate to teach children about human sexuality? Won't such instruction only increase the desire on the part of children to experiment with sex? Is it appropriate for the federal government to provide funding for such a program that includes strong value overtones?

These are just a few of the questions that must be answered if the schools are to respond effectively to the challenge of the surgeon general.

The cost of this training and of the materials, however, has reduced the number of curriculum adoptions. Today, school districts are economically hard-pressed and can ill-afford to implement such a costly program.

Thus, school districts must be willing to provide funds for implementation of the curriculum. The Growing Healthy Curriculum Project has received support from numerous agencies, foundations, and governmental units to develop materials, train teachers, evaluate, and disseminate the curricula.

Controversial Issues

The school health curriculum involves instruction in a number of controversial topics. Possibly the most controversial has been sex education. Many believe that young people, particularly teenagers, must be taught about human sexuality, reproduction, male and female growth and development, family life, and related topics. Attempts to develop a health curriculum that incorporates these topics have met with a great deal of opposition and occasional hostility. This opposition is largely a vocal minority of individuals in the community.

Sex Education

Family life education, human reproduction, venereal disease education, and even health education are all names for sex education. Unfortunately, many important learning experiences that could be of benefit to children are lost in the emotional response to the single word "sex." It is doubtful that an instructor would discuss sex techniques or emphasize coitus in the curriculum of elementary and secondary school children. Yet, these interpretations are argued by opponents of school sex education programs.

Human reproduction and sexuality are most often taught as an integrated part of some basic subject in the school curriculum. Usually these learning experiences are a part of health education, biology, or home economics courses. Though some school districts have developed separate school sex education programs, this isolated approach is the most susceptible to opposition.

In the past, attempts have been made to prohibit the teaching of human sexuality either as a separate sex education course or as part of some other subject. These efforts have even extended to proposed legislative action to ban such courses. However, no state presently has legislation that would prohibit such teaching.[10] In fact, thirty-one states either require, encourage, or permit school districts to include sex education in the curriculum. The remaining states have no legislation or regulations prohibiting sex education.[11]

Sex education has been challenged in the courts on several occasions.[12] Those who introduce such litigation argue that religious freedom, right of privacy, and constitutional rights are infringed upon by exposing children to the subject. The courts have ruled in favor of the schools and found the teaching of sex education to be constitutional and legal.

Opponents also argue that such instruction causes immorality; it has a detrimental effect upon the morals of young people. That such instruction actually leads to sexual activity and experimentation is another view often expressed by those seeking to have sex education removed from the schools. Others simply feel that such instruction will create an unwholesome environment.

A great deal of opposition is based upon religious and political positions. Conservative religious groups are usually the most vocal in arguing against school sex education. They feel that such instruction will undermine morals and values.

The conservative political spectrum has also been vocal in opposition. In the opinion of many opponents, school sex education has been considered part of a communist conspiracy to subvert the young people of America. For example, the John Birch Society in its promotional material linked supporters of school sex education programs with the international communist movement.[13]

It is estimated that about 80 percent of the population supports sex education.[14] Though sex education is considered legal and its opponents are in the minority, many school administrators are hesitant to incorporate more than basic human anatomy and physiology into the curriculum. Topics such as birth control, abortion, alternative marital life-styles, and other sex-related issues are kept out of the curriculum for fear of controversy.

Considering the problems of teenage pregnancy, teenage sexual activity, and young people's need for information, it is reasonable to suggest that human reproduction and human sexuality should be part of the school curriculum. Sex education programs have been shown to reduce the level of sexual activity by teenagers. Also, sex education programs supplement rather than undermine the influence of parents on matters relating to sexual beliefs and practices.[15] Failure to provide such instruction in the schools may result in continued ignorance and greater problems in sexual adjustment in the future.

Drug Education

Another controversial topic often found in health programs is drug education. With the increase in drug use during the 1960s and early 1970s, the schools developed drug education programs to curb the drug abuse problem. Most states have now passed legislation mandating such instruction.[16] Thousands of school districts include classes, lectures, talks, assemblies, and other activities concerning the dangers of drug use. Law enforcement personnel, reformed drug users, and government-funded curriculum have been used to increase young people's awareness of the problems associated with drug use.

All too often though, these school drug education efforts have failed to have any effect upon the drug use of school-age children. Many times, such instruction has involved only the cognitive level of education. The specific pharmaceutical facts about drugs are taught, but the relevance to the drug-taking behavior of the students is ignored. Educational efforts certainly increase the students' information levels about drug use, but the effect of such programs on drug-taking behavior is uncertain.

School children need accurate, updated information on drugs. Numerous school drug programs have been developed to educate young people about drug use and abuse.

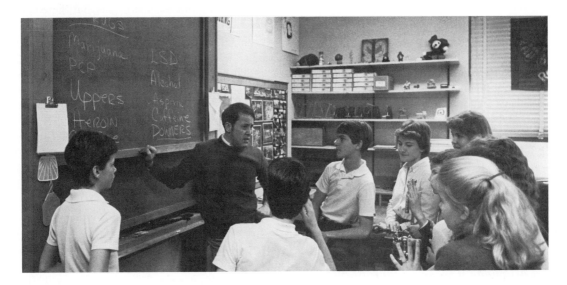

As with sex education, there are those individuals and organizations who are opposed to a drug education curriculum in the school. They argue that such information will result in additional drug experimentation and use. To some degree, they have a valid point. It has been shown that some drug education efforts have resulted in increased drug use.[17]

The approach of an effective drug education program is open to question. What should be the goal of such instruction? Should the drug education curriculum have as a goal the elimination of all drugs of abuse? Who should determine the purposes of the curriculum for a local school district? Whatever the objectives, the fact that current drug education has been less than effective must be taken into account. Greater emphasis needs to be placed on individual responsibility and decision making. The reasons why people use drugs must be focused upon, and procedures to meet these needs must be sought.

Another reason drug education programs have been less than successful is that many teachers are not knowledgeable enough to teach about drugs.[18] In fact, fallacies have often been taught in drug education classes. Many teenagers know more about the various drugs than do the teachers. For those students, the drug education class is a total waste of time.

The development of a useful drug education curriculum must involve a variety of community agencies and experts. It should draw upon a pool of resource people, including those involved in drug intervention and treatment services, the medical profession, law enforcement personnel, parents, and students, as well as teachers.

Other Programs

Drug and sex education are probably the most controversial topics included in a health education program. However, the teacher must be careful in the handling of other topics. For example, teaching that implies a negative opinion about chiropractic medicine can cause a serious conflict in many communities. Because of the differing views on nutrition, weight control, and diet, the health education teacher can easily be drawn into conflict and controversy. A simple question about health food stores can lead to the expression of conflicting positions.

Death education is often included as part of a health education curriculum. However, the variety of sensitive discussions and value-clarification strategies on the topics of death and dying are opposed by parents in many communities. Opposition to death education is also centered on a concern that such instruction will involve focusing upon religious beliefs and concepts about death.

This potential for controversy is one reason a comprehensive school health curriculum needs to be developed and supported by the school administration. Some agreement needs to be reached as to how to deal with these issues and how teacher support can be provided. Failure to address these controversial topics in the classroom denies the children exposure to basic human experiences. They need knowledge and skills to cope with these often very difficult and sensitive problems.

School Attendance by Children with AIDS

A recent issue of controversy has developed as to whether children with AIDS should be permitted to attend school. In several states, school officials have excluded children with AIDS from the schools. Where they have been permitted to attend school, some parents have boycotted the schools by withdrawing their children from the school. Also, lawsuits have been filed to restrain attendance of AIDS children on the grounds that they are a public health menace.

Parents who object to school attendance of children with the AIDS antibodies point out that states exclude pupils from schools due to other illnesses. It is their belief that such regulations should also apply to AIDS. Also, in 1986 the Centers for Disease Control announced that no one with AIDS would be permitted immigration into the United States from another country. As a result, parents have pointed out that if the government feels that AIDS is of sufficient danger to prohibit entrance as an immigrant, then the school population should be protected by exclusion of the AIDS patient.

The two principal causes of AIDS in school-age children are blood transfusion and birth to a mother having AIDS. Most school-related cases result from the former—blood transfusions, but there have been relatively few cases of AIDS among school-age children. Of concern to many parents is the child whose blood tests show the presence of the AIDS antibody, called "pre-AIDS." It must be understood that the presence of the antibody does not mean that the disease will eventually develop. Between 20 and 30 percent of those so affected develop the disease.

There is no evidence that AIDS can be communicated on a casual basis. It cannot be transmitted by person-to-person contact, such as drinking from a glass, using the same utensil, hugging or touching an AIDS patient, sneezing, or coughing. There is no evidence of sibling transfer of the HIV virus that causes AIDS.

State departments of education are rapidly developing policies for the local school districts regarding this matter. The states of Connecticut and Massachusetts were the first. In 1985, both states adopted guidelines that advised schools to handle AIDS cases on a case-by-case basis.[19] The National Education Association also recommends that the decision to permit children with AIDS to attend school should be on a case-by-case basis.[20]

In 1985, the Centers for Disease Control issued guidelines for schools that recommended that these children be allowed to remain in school. Each case should be judged separately. The Centers for Disease Control guidelines did recommend that preschool-age children not attend school because of their lack of control of body secretions.

Education of the public is vitally important to help overcome this very emotional and controversial issue.[21] Parents must receive accurate information about AIDS. Also, teenagers need information about the causal relationships of AIDS with sexual intercourse and IV transfusion among drug users, since the teen years are a time of experimentation by many with both drugs and sex. Teachers—as well as the child and family with the AIDS virus—need to be properly educated so as to be able to support the school policy.

School-Based Health Clinics

Should birth control information be provided for teenagers in school-based clinics?
Should contraceptives be made available in such clinics?

These questions have resulted in much controversy in several large cities in the United States in recent years. The first school-based health clinic designed to provide contraceptive information and contraceptives to teenagers was established in 1974 in St. Paul, Minnesota. This clinic provided immunizations, venereal disease treatment, contraceptive advice, and contraceptive prescriptions. Since then other communities have sought to develop such facilities. Usually, the services at these clinics are provided by a nurse practitioner.

The growth of school-based health clinics has risen from about a dozen in 1984 to over forty in 1986, with another sixty in the planning stages.[1]

Those who support the development of such school-based clinics point out that many pregnant teenagers did not have access to appropriate information regarding birth control and the provision of contraceptives. In one Chicago high school, one-third of the female students had babies during a calendar year.[2] Yet this school's clinic aroused much opposition by people in the community, most of whom did not have children in the specific school.

There has been extensive opposition to the development of these school-based clinics. Many opponents feel that the schools are not an appropriate place to provide contraceptives and birth control information. Among the specific points of opposition that are raised is the fear that such clinics will eventually become a place where abortions will be provided.

Do you feel that the school-based clinic is an appropriate health service to be provided in the schools of your community? What would be the reaction in your community if such clinics were to be established? Is there a need for such school-based clinics in your school district?

1. *Clinic News,* Support Centers/C.P.O., Washington, D.C.: 1, no. 4, (December, 1985): 3.
2. Ibid., 5.

Health Services

How comprehensive should health services provided by a school district within the school setting be? Should physicians, dentists, nurses, and other health care providers be employed by the schools? How much money should be spent in developing health facilities at the schools? These and similar questions have been raised when the scope of a school health service program is discussed.

Although health services have been part of the school program since the early years of this century, a broad range of medical care provided within public education facilities has met with only limited acceptance. Most Americans feel that the schools should educate young people, not provide medical care. They do not see a relationship between the provision of health services and the educational process. This has resulted in limited funding of health services in the schools, so rarely do school districts employ dentists, physicians, dental hygienists, or other health care providers (with the exception of nurses) on a full-time basis. It is also unusual for schools to provide a broad scope of health (medical) care in school clinics.

In comparison to other industrial countries in the world, the United States has a relatively underdeveloped system of school health services. In Sweden, 95 percent of the school-age children receive dental care through schools. In New Zealand, the rate of service is 98 percent. Dental nurses care for the school children, including such services as cavity preparation and fillings. The school dental services are not always provided in the school buildings, but in district dental health clinics. The program, however, is school-managed and school-based. The school-based dental health program provides this comprehensive dental care to all children, regardless of economic status, age, or other considerations. In addition, dental health education is integrated with the actual dental care.

By comparison, in the United States there are few school districts that provide dental health care. Instead, most children obtain dental care through private dental practice. Some children do receive dental care at local health departments; however, these visits are rarely coordinated with school programs. At best, dental hygiene is discussed in the school setting.

There are some isolated examples of medical services offered in the context of educational programs. One case involves a mini-clinic operated within a high school. Several health care disciplines are united to provide a variety of services. These services included dental care; nutrition counseling and education; and the services of an obstetrician/gynecologist, social worker, drug counselor, public health nurse, and nurse practitioner. The mini-clinic is operated as an outreach of a community health center and is funded by a government grant. A number of screening procedures, such as breast examination, pap smears, and hemoglobin and urinalysis tests, are provided. As a result of this mini-clinic, the services of the community health center have been made more accessible to school children.[22]

Other programs involve the use of nonmedical health care providers in school health service activities.[23] The schools involved with these projects have developed relationships with local medical schools and clinics. Usually, the focus of these projects is directed to people from low socioeconomic levels of the community. Of great importance to these medical service programs in schools is the financial support of the federal or state government. With the reduction of such funds in the 1980s and the inability of most school districts to support extensive health services with local school taxes, the future of medical services offered in the schools is doubtful.

The community agency that is most likely to become involved in the provision of school health services is the local health department, which provides nursing services to the schools and so plays a major role in the health appraisal of school children. The nurses become involved in the screening of vision, hearing, and other functions so that physical and emotional deviations can be identified and treated.

In addition, the local health department becomes involved with the school health program by monitoring local and state environmental health and safety regulations.

Immunizations and Physical Examinations

School health services were established at the turn of the century to combat childhood communicable diseases that were a major cause of death and debilitation in school children at that time. In an effort to protect the health of children, schools began to require the immunization of children for certain diseases. Also, children were required to have physical examinations prior to entering school.

Today, immunization is mandated in most states. Though some variance does occur from one state to another, the most commonly required immunizations are for diphtheria, pertussis, tetanus, polio, rubella, and rubeola. A child cannot attend school unless these immunizations have been received.

Immunization requirements are normally enforced by the school nurse and the local health department. It is the nurse's responsibility to obtain the immunization records of the school children, which requires communication with the home and family. When children have not been immunized, the school nurse must work in conjunction with the family, the family physician, or the local health department to see that the regulations are met.

Through the years, many individuals have challenged the legality of school immunization requirements. These people oppose such requirements because of religious beliefs, or because they view them as the government's attempt to control private lives. The courts have ruled that state statutes, health department regulations, and school district rules and regulations mandating immunization for school admittance are legal and constitutional, even though state law also requires school attendance.[24] Supporters feel such requirements ensure the protection of the health of the public.

Additionally, periodic physical examinations are also required by the schools. These, too, are monitored by the school nurse. Most school policies stipulate that, in addition to an examination before entering school, children are expected to have other examinations periodically throughout their school years. One national commission has recommended that all school children have a minimum of four fifteen-minute physical examinations at various times throughout their school years.[25]

One purpose of such examinations is to identify health problems in the growing child. It is also hoped that by encouraging young children to obtain periodic examinations, a life-long habit will develop. Today, some difference of opinion exists as to whether periodic physical examinations are necessary, and there is little evidence that such behavioral patterns do, in fact, develop in childhood.

For physical examinations obtained during the school years to be most useful, they should be conducted by a family physician. The chances of follow-up when health problems are found is greater than if mass examinations are conducted in a school or public health department. However, when it is not possible to obtain a physical examination from a family physician, for economic or other reasons, the child usually can use the services of a local health department.

Emergency Care

Injuries, accidents, and sickness are common occurrences within the school. It is imperative that school districts take appropriate measures to meet such emergency situations. Policies that specify procedures to be followed during injury or sickness should be developed by the school administration in consultation and cooperation with school health personnel, community medical personnel, legal counsel, and appropriate community agencies. The policies should be available in writing, and all school personnel should be aware of their provisions.

Regardless of the policies developed, it is obvious from legal precedent that school personnel have a responsibility to aid sick or injured children during school hours. Failure to do so has been considered negligent behavior.[26] Concern over the possible legal consequences should never keep a school teacher or other responsible person from caring for a sick or injured student.

The pattern of relying upon the school nurse, the physical education teacher, or the school secretary to administer emergency care is not acceptable policy. All too often, the nurse is not in the building or the physical education teacher is not available. The secretary, though usually available, may not be at the site of injury, or may not be properly trained to give the needed care.

Though not commonly required for teacher certification, it seems reasonable that all school personnel should be required to have training in first aid and cardiopulmonary resuscitation (CPR). In addition, appropriate first-aid equipment and supplies should be accessible throughout the school. They should not be kept locked in cabinets where they are difficult to secure in emergencies.

Health Assessment Screening

Several health appraisals are usually part of the school health program. No health appraisal should be conducted without an effective follow-up. The health assessment should also have an educational value for both the child and the parents, who should be informed of the results and the significance of the testing. Where a potential health problem is identified through the screening process, follow-up medical attention, treatment, and care must be obtained. The responsibility of the school is to assist parents in obtaining this care.

A common, early screening procedure is the weighing and measuring of children. This process, usually performed by the school nurse, the classroom teacher, or the physical education teacher, records the basic growth and development of the child.

Most children are screened for vision and hearing on several occasions during their school years. Both hearing and vision problems can develop gradually and sometimes are not noticed at all. The reduced ability to see or hear can affect learning and, ultimately, success in the classroom. Such conditions may also negatively affect school behavioral patterns. In addition to the formal vision and hearing tests, the classroom teacher can watch for behavioral changes that may indicate a developing problem.

Scoliosis, a lateral curvature of the spine, often becomes noticeable in the upper elementary grades. Early detection of students having scoliosis is important in controlling this health problem, and screening programs conducted by the school nurse, classroom teacher, or physical education instructor have been shown to be effective in identifying early cases.[27] It is important to conduct such screening, which involves little cost or time, before the adolescent growth spurt.

Though the school nurse conducts most health assessment activities, aides and other assistants, along with teachers, can also be trained to screen students. Regardless of who conducts the screening activity, the child's school health record should include the results of each procedure.

The School Nurse

The most visible person in a school health service program is the school nurse. Nursing services in the schools were introduced about the turn of this century as part of childhood disease control efforts.

Today, the services provided by school nurses have increased in number and scope. Most frequently, the school nurse provides direct care to children. The nurse is most often expected to care for a sick or injured child during the hours school is in session. Because such services obviously are not required full-time, the nurse spends much of her time keeping school health records of immunizations, screening results, and other pertinent data. These tasks are secondary, however, to the nurse's responsibilities for the care and supervision of student health.

The school nurse can and should be expected to perform a wider range of tasks than emergency care and record keeping. School nurses can play an important role in conducting immunization programs. Other measures designed to assess the health status of the children should be established and conducted by the nurse. All health assessment efforts should include components to interpret the findings to the parents and, in turn, help them find appropriate follow-up care in the community. The school nurse is in an important position to complete these health counseling tasks.

School nurses have become increasingly involved with special education students since the passage of PL 94–142, legislation that opened educational opportunities for handicapped children in the schools. The bill required schools to provide a normal education for all handicapped children within the structure of the regular school program. The nurse is part of the team that assesses the educational needs of the child and develops an individualized educational program (I.E.P.) for each handicapped child.

Many handicapped children need specialized physical care while at school. This may involve the administration of medication or using a special apparatus. Nurses can provide such services, help the child to become self-sufficient, and assist teachers in overcoming fears and concerns about having handicapped children in their classes.

The school nurse is not normally certified to teach health classes. Usually, a health instructor must have a state teacher's certificate and, unless the nurse has taken course work in teacher preparation, it is unlikely that she will have earned the necessary credentials.

Nurses do, however, serve as facilitators to the health teachers. In addition to this, they can be helpful resource persons for both the teachers and the students. Because of these functions, any time that a school district is developing a health education curriculum, the school nurse should be included in the planning process.

School nurses usually serve in the schools under one of two administrative patterns: (1) they may be employed by the school district and, as such, work full-time under the control and supervision of the school administration; or (2) public health nurses employed by the local health department may be placed in the schools as part of their work assignments. Usually, public health nurses work in several schools in the community, and so are unable to become closely acquainted with the children, faculty, and school administration. Although the district-employed nurse frequently works in several schools, she usually develops a close relationship to the school system, its personnel, children, and overall program.

The economic problems being faced by many school districts in the 1980s have introduced many problems in school nurse service. Many school districts and public health departments have been forced to cut back the number of nurses assigned to schools. As a result, in many communities the availability of school nurses ranges from minimal to non-existent, and so school health services suffer. Part-time nurses, mothers, school secretaries, and other under-trained personnel are forced to perform the most urgent nursing tasks, while other school nursing duties remain unattended.

The School Environment

The school environment can have a direct effect upon student health and well-being. The school is not a vacuum, protected from adverse elements. The environment, physical as well as emotional, must be considered when devising a comprehensive school health program. School buildings need to be clean, properly ventilated, well lighted, and adequately maintained. Conditions within the school building and on the school grounds must be free of hazards that could lead to accidents.

Safe School Setting

It is the responsibility of the board of education to provide a safe and healthful environment for students. Often local codes and regulations establish standards for school safety. Then it is the responsibility of the community health department sanitarian to inspect school facilities to make certain the standards are maintained. The food service facility is an example of one part of the school environment that must meet numerous health department regulations. The sanitarian inspects the food preparation facilities, as well as those for serving and eating, on a regular basis. Other state and local regulations assure proper sanitation and a safe water supply. In addition, heating, ventilation, and electrical system regulations, and various fire prevention codes must be met by school districts. These all require periodic inspections by the appropriate community agency.

A major problem in many communities, particularly in large urban settings, is the relatively poor physical condition of school facilities. Schools often are old, poorly maintained, and dirty, with litter covering the school grounds. Monies often are unavailable to repair damaged walls, ceilings, sidewalks, and other parts of the buildings. As school districts find themselves with increasing budget deficits, these adverse environmental school conditions will probably worsen.

A report from one school district told of a situation in which a tax referendum for building maintenance and repair was defeated by the taxpayers. This particular district needed funds to repair chipped paint, poor lighting, and a number of other problems. Several days after the referendum defeat, a portion of the ceiling plaster fell on one classroom, injuring several students.

Schools not only have responsibility for children while on school grounds, but also during transport to and from school. Every day, thousands of American school children ride a bus to school. Considering the great number of miles covered each year

The environment can affect the learning atmosphere of the classroom so most communities have established school standards. Periodic checks by the health department sanitarian assure compliance with these regulations. This sanitarian checks the classroom for proper lighting.

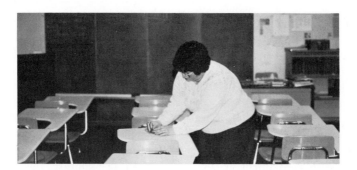

by school buses, school bus transportation is basically safe; however, over ten thousand injuries occur in school bus accidents annually.[28] In one recent year, approximately 125 people were fatally injured in school bus accidents.[29] Of these fatalities, twenty were passengers on the buses, sixty-five were pedestrians getting on or off the buses, and the other sixty-five were struck by school buses.

These statistics indicate that measures are needed to assure a safe school bus program. Thus, the selection, training, and supervision of competent school bus drivers is very important. These drivers must maintain control and discipline on the buses to avoid accidents. Children must be taught to follow directions for safety while on the bus and while waiting for the school bus.

It would seem appropriate to consider the lack of mandate that school buses be required to have seat belts. As of 1987, only two states had enacted seat belt laws for school buses, such legislation was pending in several other states, and seat belt laws had been defeated in sixteen states.[30] Although the majority of fatalities resulting from school bus accidents are not passengers, it would seem reasonable to suggest that seat belt use would reduce the likelihood of injury or death.

School responsibility for student safety also extends to field trips, extracurricular events, and other school-related activities. The teacher, coach, or activity sponsor is responsible for the safety and well-being of children while involved in such activities. Not only must school districts establish policy for transportation in these situations, but all school personnel should be covered by liability insurance to protect against possible litigation.

Asbestos in Schools

During the 1950s and 1960s, hundreds of new school buildings were constructed throughout the United States. In most of these buildings a hydrated mineral silicate, asbestos, was used as a soundproofing and fireproofing agent. Asbestos was applied to ceilings, floor tiles, roofing, shingles, cement, and insulation.[31] It was used in the construction of many different types of rooms.

As early as the 1960s, concern began to be expressed about the relationship of asbestos and cancer among workers exposed to high levels of the substance. Studies of individuals in the manufacturing and construction industries, who were exposed to asbestos for long periods of time, revealed that they were experiencing increased incidences of asbestiosis, lung cancer, and cancer of the esophogus,

The removal of asbestos from a school building is a rather complex and costly activity. Total removal is the most time consuming of the three procedures used in coping with the problem of asbestos in schools. The procedure necessitates isolating from the surrounding rooms the area where the asbestos is to be removed. Personnel involved in the removal process must wear protective clothing.

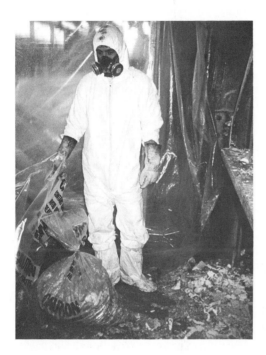

stomach, and colon.[32] These concerns led the Occupational Safety and Health Administration (OSHA) to establish exposure regulations in 1971. In 1973, the Environmental Protection Agency (EPA) banned asbestos for use in fireproofing and insulation.

Concern developed as to the effect of exposure of school children to asbestos fibers in school buildings. This concern centered particularly around the fact that children are exposed by being in the same buildings over a period of several years throughout their schooling days. Since asbestos fibers are neither chemically or biologically degradable, the cumulative effect on children might be dangerous.

As a result, school districts have been encouraged to take measures to eliminate this potentially hazardous school environmental factor. In 1982, the Environmental Protection Agency issued a regulation requiring that schools be inspected for asbestos. If asbestos is found, the schools must notify employees and parents. However, regulations differ from state to state as to what measures must follow notification.

School administrators must decide whether to totally remove the asbestos or to encapsulate it in some way. Encapsulation may involve spraying the area with a chemical sealant or constructing a permanent partition to enclose the area where the asbestos is present. The procedure of total removal requires much care so that asbestos fibers are not released into the air, contaminating other areas of the schools.

There is no agreement as to which is the best procedure for the school district to take. Total removal is the most expensive. One report indicated that the average cost per school district to remove asbestos was $128,230 compared to $22,703 for encapsulation.[33] Encapsulation, though less expensive, still does not remove the asbestos from the school environment.

Numerous questions have been raised concerning this problem. In addition to concerns about cost and the most effective risk-reduction measures to take is the basic issue as to whether it is necessary. The general public has little concern about asbestos in the schools. There is no evidence that any child has developed cancer or any other ailment as a result of asbestos exposure during school attendance. The evidence linking human health with asbestos is centered upon individuals who work directly with the substance over a period of years. Nevertheless, it is a community health concern that needs further research and attention.

Emotional Climate of the School

The physical climate within a school and classroom is not the only environmental factor that affects the health and well-being of students. The emotional climate established by the teacher can have direct effects upon children, too. This is particularly important in the elementary schools where the same teacher interacts with the same children throughout most of the school day.

The importance of positive mental health among teachers and other school personnel is essential to the classroom environment. The maladjusted teacher with mental and emotional problems can have a very detrimental effect on the students. The teacher experiencing stress and family or personal problems may contribute directly to the emotional problems of children in the classroom.

Stress is a major problem for many school employees. This tends to produce a number of negative behavior patterns among teachers.[34] Instances have been noted where emotionally disturbed teachers have behaved inappropriately or have exhibited bizarre actions. These actions often take the form of improper discipline and punishment or inappropriate academic demands on children. These inappropriate behaviors may surface in a teacher's conversations with the children, reactions to the students, or attitude toward the class.

One student told of a teacher who placed a telephone on her desk and warned the second-grade students that she could call God on this phone if they misbehaved. The teacher was under severe personal stress and receiving psychiatric care. The trauma, fear, and disruption this caused had a serious effect on the personal and academic growth of the children. It was reported that some children were afraid to attend school.

Schools seldom have developed plans to assist the emotionally disturbed teacher. School administrators fail to have teachers removed from the classroom when early signs of emotional stress are noted. It is not until a serious episode occurs that such action is taken. By this time, though, the children may be suffering emotionally, too.

In spite of the difficulty in coping with the problem of the emotionally disturbed teacher, school districts need to implement measures for better mental health. Teacher in-service programs on positive mental health and adapting mechanisms would be useful. Also, school districts should grant sick leave for emotional problems, as well as for physical illnesses. Schools must also consider leaves of absence for teachers with mental problems.[35] This would perhaps serve as an incentive for the teacher under stress to seek appropriate care. The teacher's job security and income would not be jeopardized, and so the individual may be more inclined to seek help.

School Lunch Program

Providing nutritious meals for children at school is one of the most widespread programs in American educational institutions. Each day, more than twenty-five million school children are served lunch at school. This makes the school lunch program one of the largest "restaurants" in the world. As can be expected, a program this large creates many difficult and controversial issues.

The first school lunch program was developed in New York City in 1853.[36] Children attending a vocational school for the poor were served free meals. Early in the twentieth century, nutrition programs were started in many local communities. This was especially important during the depression of the 1930s, a time when many children received a major portion of the necessary daily nutrients through community school lunch programs.

The National School Lunch Program was authorized in 1946. Data obtained during World War II suggested that many American men of draft age had nutritional deficiencies. This, plus an available surplus of farm products, resulted in the passage of the legislation. This program was a means of both using surplus farm products and of promoting good nutrition and health in school-age children.

In the years since 1946, changes in federal involvement in the school lunch programs have occurred. Federal subsidies have made milk available to school children, too. In the mid-1960s, the program was expanded to provide breakfast at school, particularly for needy children. It was believed that many children arrive at school in the morning without having been given anything to eat, which has a negative impact on learning. The federal government made provision to assist local school districts with food service equipment.

By the early 1970s, large food surpluses were no longer available to give to schools. Thus, the distribution of surplus foods to the schools was replaced by a system of government funding to assist local districts in the operation of the school lunch program. As a result, the amount of federal support of school lunch programs rose dramatically during the 1970s.

With the advent of federal budget reductions and reduced involvement in social service programs in the early 1980s, the federal government cut subsidies for school lunches. The reductions have had far-reaching effects. Cash assistance for meals was reduced, causing the price of school lunches to rise. The American School Food Service Association estimated that 10 percent of the school-age population dropped out of school lunch programs during 1981, the first year of program reductions. Many of these children were from low socioeconomic backgrounds, and their parents found it difficult to qualify for free or reduced-price meals as a result of tighter school lunch regulations.

In addition, federal aid to schools for breakfast programs was greatly reduced, even though many of these programs provided a basic food supply for low-income children. Funding for school lunch equipment was also cut. With the severe budget problems of many schools, funds will continue to be sparse for replacing and upgrading school lunch equipment. The loss of this federal support places a severe burden on local school districts. These districts now must either charge more for meals, reduce the amount of food served for the same price, or eliminate the school lunch program altogether. Many school administrators fear that increasing numbers of school districts will be forced to take this last alternative. Within the first year of federal cutbacks, over five hundred schools had dropped lunch programs completely.

The goal of the school lunch program has been to provide at least one-third of a child's daily nutritional requirements as established by the Food and Nutrition Board of the National Research Council. The federal guidelines have required that this lunch, called Type A, include some food from each of the following food groups: milk and milk products, meat and meat substitutes, vegetables and fruits, and bread.

In 1981, the federal government proposed lowering the requirement from one-third of the child's daily nutritional requirements to no more than one-fourth. Because of public and political opposition, this recommendation was not implemented.

Despite its good intentions, the school lunch program has generated controversy. There is a great deal of food waste in the program. The United States Department of Agriculture reported that 15 percent of all food served to children in the schools is thrown away, primarily in the fruits and vegetables groups. Such waste may occur because unpopular foods are served, because food is served in an unappetizing manner, or simply because of the throw-away mentality in the United States today. Government estimates place the dollar value of this waste at over $600 million a year.

In an attempt to reduce this food waste, a method of food service known as "offer versus serve" has been implemented.[37] This system offers five food items, and the child is able to select as few as three of the food items, but not all five. It is assumed that children will not select those foods that they would throw away.

Should schools sell "junk foods" as part of the school lunch program? These foods include soft drinks, candy, chewing gum, and other low-nutrition items. The federal government passed regulations in 1980 restricting the sale of such foods in schools. Many people feel this is inappropriate; they suggest that local school districts, not the federal government, should ascertain whether foods lacking nutritional value are sold at school.

One major reason the banning of such sales is opposed is that the funds earned from selling these foods are often used to support school activities, including athletics, clubs, bands, and other extracurricular activities. Many nutritionists and health professionals believe that it is inappropriate for the schools to make available foods that do not contribute to positive health and well-being.

The school lunch program should extend beyond the mere provision of nutrients for children. School efforts should be designed to educate the students about proper nutrition. Such efforts, it is hoped, will influence eating behavior of school children.

Summary

The schools play an important role in the health status of a community. The school health program has traditionally been divided into three components: (1) health instruction, (2) health services, and (3) promotion of a healthful environment. A comprehensive school health program integrates activities that are a part of all three components.

The school health instruction program introduces the students to health concepts, information, and knowledge. Health instruction is included as part of the total school curriculum at both the elementary and secondary school levels. The school health instruction curriculum should be developed to meet the needs and interests of the children. Even though health instruction is usually not considered a basic subject in the school curriculum, it is required by all state education regulations.

There have been efforts to establish a national curriculum in health education at various times in history. The School Health Education Study Curriculum in the 1960s was one such attempt. In recent years, a variety of health education models have been developed and disseminated throughout various parts of the country. The Growing Health Curriculum Project has received the most widespread attention and use. Most of the recently developed curriculum models make use of a broad range of materials and methods, including various audiovisual material. Teachers must usually attend special in-service training before the curriculum can be used in a school.

A variety of controversial topics are part of the health curriculum. The educational area that is most vehemently opposed is sex education. Opposition stems from morality, values, fear, and student readiness. This controversy makes it vital that the school curriculum include a carefully planned school health education program that considers the attitudes and feelings of the local community.

The issue of whether students with AIDS should be permitted to attend school has arisen in recent years. Even though there is strong feeling that each individual case must be evaluated independently, it must be understood that children with AIDS are not a danger to other children at school. There is no evidence that AIDS can be spread by casual contact.

A variety of health services are provided in many school settings. Some health services, such as the enforcement of immunization requirements, are developed to protect against childhood communicable diseases. A number of screening activities designed to assess the health status of children occur at school. Vision and hearing loss and postural deviations are commonly identified by these school screening programs. In addition, the school district must care for all children who become sick or injured while at school. Not only must teachers have the knowledge and skills for emergency care, but the school district should have a written policy that is followed when injury or sickness occurs.

The school nurse is important to the health service program. The nurse can provide a number of services at school, with the families of the children, and in the community. The school nurse is not just a bandage dispenser, provider of first aid, and record keeper. The nurse's skills and training prepare for a broader role as health counselor, facilitator, and educator within the school and community.

The environment within which children spend several hours of each day should be as safe and healthful as possible. The physical environment of the school building and grounds has a profound effect upon the students' well-being. Not only is the physical setting important to the education of the children, but the emotional climate established by the teacher has direct effects that must not be overlooked. Measures need to be taken to help teachers experiencing stress, emotional upset, and family problems.

Many schools have had to cope with the presence of asbestos in their buildings. This substance has been linked with several health problems, although none in school settings. Nevertheless, schools have been encouraged to either remove asbestos from the buildings or to encapsulate areas where it is present.

The schools have served lunches to school children for years. The school lunch program provides nutrients for many young people, particularly the economically disadvantaged. In spite of the value of the school lunch programs, many questions and issues have arisen relating to the program. These questions concern the quality of food served, the nature of the educational experience, the acceptability of government involvement, and the costs of these programs.

Discussion Questions

1. Explain the three phases of a school health program.
2. What does the concept of a comprehensive school health program mean to you?
3. Discuss some reasons why school health instructional programs have not affected the behavioral patterns of students.
4. What is the Growing Healthy Curriculum Project?
5. Identify the main features of several health education curriculum models developed in the past few years.
6. Describe some of the reasons why people have opposed the teaching of human sexuality in the schools.
7. What other controversial subjects and topics are often found in a school health instructional program?
8. Discuss the issues involved in the debate as to whether children with AIDS should be permitted to attend school.
9. What position has the Centers for Disease Control taken regarding school attendance for children with AIDS?
10. What immunizations are usually required by the states for admittance to school?
11. Who has the responsibility of caring for an injured child while at school?
12. What items would you include in a school policy for emergency care?
13. Define some screening procedures that are usually part of a school health service program.
14. Identify some of the skills that school nurses use in the school health program.
15. At what point does the school have responsibility for children coming to and going home from school?
16. What are some of the concerns regarding asbestos?
17. Identify the measures that school districts can take to eliminate the potential hazard relating to asbestos.
18. What are some measures that a school district could take to help teachers with emotional problems?
19. Describe some of the effects that government budget cutbacks have had on the school lunch program.

Suggested Readings

American Academy of Pediatrics. *School Health: A Guide For Health Professionals.* Evanston, Ill.: American Academy of Pediatrics, 1981.

Brophy, Helen. "School Nursing Services: A Century of Change." *Health Values: Achieving High Level Wellness* 6, no. 1, (January/February, 1982): 36–40.

Connell, David B.; Turner, Ralph R.; and Mason, Elaine F. "Summary of Findings of the School Health Education Evaluation: Health Promotion Effectiveness, Implementation, and Costs." *Journal of School Health* 55, no. 8, (October, 1985): 316–21.

Connell, David B., and Turner, Ralph R. "The Impact of Instructional Experience and the Effects of Cumulative Instruction." *Journal of School Health* 55, no. 8, (October, 1985): 324–31.

Cronin, Godfrey E., and Young, William M. *400 Navels: The Future of School Health in America.* Bloomington, Ind.: Phi Delta Kappa, 1979.

Education Improvement Center. *Recommendations for School Health Education: A Handbook for State Policymakers.* Report No. 130, Denver, Colo.: Education Commission of the States, 1981.

Fors, Stuart W., and Doster, Mildred E. "Implication of Results: Factors for Success." *Journal of School Health* 55, no. 8 (October, 1985): 332–34.

Fulton, Gere B.; Metress, Eileen; and Price, James H. "AIDS: Resource Materials for School Personnel." *Journal of School Health* 57, no. 1 (January, 1987): 14–18.

Gilbert, Glen G.; Davis, Roy L.; and Damberg, Cheryl L. "Current Federal Activities in School Health Education." *Public Health Reports* 100, no. 5, (September-October, 1985): 499–507.

Iverson, Donald C. "Promoting Health through the Schools: A Challenge for the 80s." *Health Education Quarterly* 8, no. 1 (Spring, 1981): 6–10.

Kane, William M. "Advocacy: Political Action for School Health Education." *Health Values: Achieving High Level Wellness* 6, no. 1 (January/February, 1982): 48–53.

Kenney, Asta M., and Orr, Margaret Terry. "Sex Education: An Overview of Current Programs, Policies, and Research." *Phi Delta Kappan* 65, no. 7 (March, 1984): 491–96.

Miller, Dean F., and Wiltse, Jan. "Mental Health and the Teacher." *Journal of School Health* 49 (September, 1979): 374–77.

Miller, Dean F. *School Health Programs: Their Basis in Law.* New York: A. S. Barnes, 1971.

Owen, Sandra L., and others. "Selecting and Recruiting Health Programs for the School Health Education Evaluation." *Journal of School Health* 55, no. 8 (October, 1985): 305–08.

Pine, Patricia. *Critical Issues Report: Promoting Health Education in Schools—Problems and Solutions.* Arlington, Va.: American Association of School Administrators, (1985).

Porter, Philip J. "Realistic Outcomes of School Health Service Programs." *Health Education Quarterly* 8, no. 1 (Spring, 1981): 81–87.

Price, James H. "AIDS, the Schools, and Policy Issues." *Journal of School Health* 56, no. 4 (April, 1986): 137–40.

Reed, Sally. "AIDS in the Schools: A Special Report." *Phi Delta Kappan* 67, no. 7, (March, 1986): 494–98.

Zimmerli, William H. "Organizing for School Health Education Programs at the Local Level." *Health Education Quarterly* 8, no. 1 (Spring, 1981): 39–42.

Endnotes

1. Cronin, Godfrey E., and Young, William M. *400 Navels: The Future of School Health in America.* Bloomington, Ind.: Phi Delta Kappa, 1979.

2. Castile, Anne S., and Jerrick, Stephen J. *School Health in America,* 3rd Ed. Kent, Ohio: American School Health Association (1982) 9.

3. *School Health Education Study: A Summary Report, 1964.* Washington, D.C.: School Health Education Study, 74 pp.

4. Pine, Patricia. *Critical Issues Report: Promoting Health Education in Schools—Problems and Solutions.* Arlington, Va.: American Association of School Administrators, (1985): 33.

5. Listing of over 120 models is available from the Centers for Disease Control, Atlanta, Georgia.

6. School Health Evaluation Study

7. Connell, David B., and others. "Summary of Findings of the School Health Education Evaluation: Health Promotion Effectiveness, Implementation, and Costs." *Journal of School Health* 55, no. 8, (October, 1985): 316–21.

8. Pine, Patricia. *Critical Issues Report,* p. 32.

9. Department of Health and Human Services, Bureau of Health Education. *The School Health Curriculum Project.* Washington, D.C.: U.S. Government Printing Office, 1980, 4.

10. "School Sex Ed Required in Three States and D.C., But Most States Allow Local Districts to Decide." *Family Planning Perspectives* 12, no. 6 (November/December, 1980): 307.

11. Ibid., 307–10.

12. Miller, Dean F. *School Health Programs: Their Basis in Law.* New York: A. S. Barnes and Co., 1971.

13. The John Birch Society. *Innocents Defiled,* filmstrip. San Marino, Calif.: John Birch Society, Public Relations Department.

14. Cassell, Carol. "The Opposition." *Impact* 1, no. 1 (October, 1978): 19.

15. Forstenberg, Frank F., and others. "Sex Education and Sexual Experience Among Adolescents." *American Journal of Public Health* 75, no. 11 (November, 1985): 1331–32.

16. Castile and Jerrick. *School Health in America,* 10–11.

17. Bard, Bernard, "The Failure of Our School Drug Abuse Programs." *Phi Delta Kappan* 57, no. 4 (December, 1975): 251–55.

18. Ibid.

19. Reed, Sally. "AIDS in the Schools: A Special Report." *Phi Delta Kappan* 67, no. 7 (March, 1986): 494.

20. Ibid.

21. Price, James H. "AIDS, the Schools, and Policy Issues." *Journal of School Health* 56, no. 4 (April, 1986): 137–40.

22. Bluford, John W. "Clinic Expands Adolescents' Access to Care." *Hospitals* 53, no. 19 (October 1, 1979): 125.

23. Cronin and Young. *400 Navels.*

24. Miller. *School Health Programs,* 104.

25. National Committee on School Health Policies. *Suggested School Health Policies.* Chicago, Ill.: American Medical Association.

26. Miller. *School Health Programs,* 67–68.

27. Miller, Dean F., and Lever, Carol Sue. "Scoliosis Screening: An Approach Used in the School." *Journal of School Health* 52, no. 2 (February, 1982): 98–101.

28. National Safety Council. *Accident Facts, 1986.* Chicago: National Safety Council, 1979, 90.

29. Ibid., 90.

30. Information provided by the Automotive Safety Foundation, 1986.

31. Stavisky, Leonard P. "State Responsibility for the Control of Asbestos in the Schools." *Journal of School Health* 24 (August, 1982): 358–64.

32. Ibid., 359.

33. *Asbestos in Schools: Inspection and Abatement.* American Association of School Administrators, Arlington, Va. 22209 (1985).

34. Brodbelt, S. "Teachers' Mental Health: Whose Responsibility?" *Phi Delta Kappan* 53 (1973) 268–69.

35. Miller, Dean F., and Wiltse, Jan. "Mental Health and The Teacher." *Journal of School Health* 49 (September, 1979): 374–77.

36. Means, Richard K. *Historical Perspectives on School Health.* Thorofare, N.J.: Slack, Inc., 1975.

37. National Dairy Council. *Dairy Council Digest* 53, no. 6 (November / December, 1982): 33.

14

Health Education/Health Promotion: The Forefront of Preventive Health and Wellness

Figure 14.1

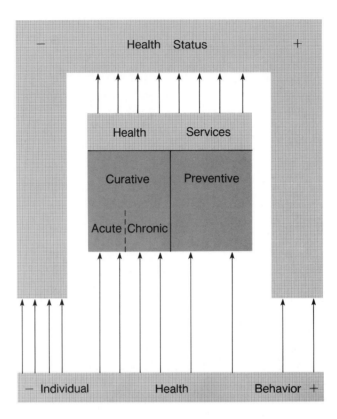

The health behavior patterns of many individuals do not contribute to optimum, positive health and well-being. For example, poor eating habits lead to weight problems for many Americans. Throughout the world, people smoke despite the evidence linking smoking to respiratory disease and cancer. Stress is also common in the lives of many individuals in our society. These and numerous other behaviors are part of the life-style of the majority of Americans, although they have detrimental effects on health.

Health Education and Behavioral Change

Traditionally, health services have focused upon curative health care. Most people consult the available health service (the doctor, the hospital, or the clinic) when they are sick with either an acute or chronic problem. Some leave the available health care service with improved (more positive) health and well-being; others do not experience significant improvement. Usually, few people enter health care systems for preventive purposes.

This relationship of individual health behavior to health services use and eventual health and well-being is depicted in figure 14.1. The health of an individual ranges on a continuum from very good (positive) to very poor (negative). As seen here, health status is related to individual health behaviors.

Some education about health is part of all phases of a community health program. However, most aspects of a community health program are focused elsewhere, so inadequate attention is given to effecting behavioral changes through education.

Figure 14.2

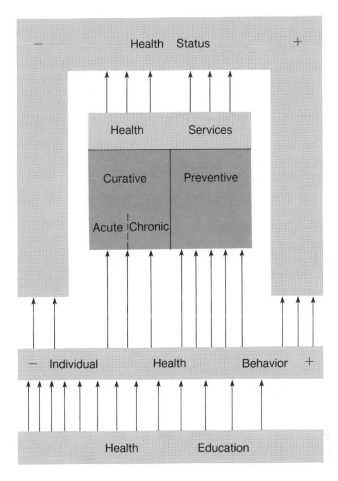

Community health education must develop planned experiences to positively influence health behavioral patterns, since a structured, effective program of health education is not currently a priority. Health education strategies can be designed to meet people's needs, regardless of where they might lie on the health continuum: from good (positive health and well-being) to bad (negative health, sickness, and debilitation). It is most likely, however, that health education activities will focus on the negative health behaviors.

This model, emphasizing health education, is depicted in figure 14.2. Education should make people more aware of and involved with preventive health. This will reduce the need for curative medical services and lead to a more positive health status.

The ultimate goal of any health education activity is to change behavioral patterns or to reinforce already positive activity. Influence of health behavior, not just acquisition of additional knowledge, should be the focal point of health education programs. Traditionally, the purpose of education has been to impart specific knowledge about a matter, which would result in the desired behaviors. Many health education instructors still adhere to this practice and impart factual knowledge about a topic to their audience using films, pamphlets, handouts, flip charts, or brochures. There has been little effort to learn if a specific strategy is effective for the population group or the topic under consideration, since behavior often is not influenced by cognitive learning experiences.

Possibly the best example of the ineffectiveness of this approach is the smoking habit. Thousands of people in the United States are very knowledgeable about the potential health hazards associated with smoking cigarettes, yet they continue to smoke. Until *attitudes* can be influenced, certain psychological needs fulfilled, and social influences overcome, the desired behavioral changes may never take place.

Research into human behavior has added to the health educator's available information. Sociological theories of learning behavior and behavioral change can help us to understand how changes in health behavior take place. It is important that those conducting a health education program understand how each audience can be persuaded to make certain changes in health behavior. The instructor must be flexible, too; a certain communication strategy that works with a given population is no guarantee that it will be successful with another group. Increasingly, community health educators are creating programs based on behavior dynamics research, not solely upon the techniques of teaching materials and methods used in the past.

Attitudes, cultural beliefs and value systems, teaching and learning strategies, and communication skills all affect the learning process. As a result, each is important to the development of health education programs.

Attitude Formation

An instructor must be aware of the attitudes of the population before planning and conducting a health education program. Any cultural group has established attitudes and values about the topic under consideration, as well as the educational process. Thus, the instructor should ask "What is the general attitude toward the issue under consideration?" and "How will the audience accept me or what I have to say?" Education involving attitude formation and influence can be effective in health modification, but only when the instructor has asked and answered these and other similar questions about the audience and the teacher-student relationship.

Cultural Dimensions

Documented studies have concluded that the cultural mores and background of a group of people must be considered in establishing any successful health education program. However, all too often those who plan and conduct the health education program are unfamiliar with the values, beliefs, language, or life-style of the population. Until the particular cultural group identifies a need and programming becomes part of their values, it is doubtful that a program will be accepted.

Educational Strategies

An educational strategy or communication skill that has been used to teach health concepts for years is not necessarily the best. Research and experience can tell us much about the most effective ways to present information that will likely result in the desired behavior.

In order for the community health educator to communicate effectively, it is important that the most effective methods and procedures for working with or educating particular groups are used. This necessitates a thorough knowledge of the consumers and their concerns, interests, background, value systems, and language. Many health education programs are ineffective because they are poorly planned or fail to take into consideration the background and the value systems of the prospective population.

Health Promotion

With greater interest in health maintenance and disease prevention, public interest in health education has increased. There are many who feel that through the process of education, health and well-being can be enhanced. But such a development requires a variety of approaches with the same focus: behavioral change. Strategies should consider not only education, but also societal structure and environmental considerations.

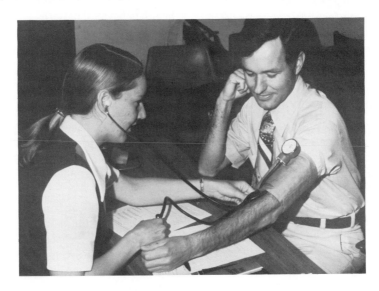

As a result, a broadened concept of health education known as *health promotion* has been developed and accepted. Health education and health promotion are not synonymous. Health promotion includes education plus related political and economic considerations. Health promotion has been defined as

. . . Any combination of health education and related organizational, economic or political interventions designed to facilitate behavioral and environmental changes conducive to health.[1]

The American Hospital Association has defined health promotion as:

. . . the process of fostering awareness, influencing attitudes, and identifying alternatives so that individuals can make informed choices and change their behavior in order to achieve an optimum level of physical and mental health and improve their physical and social environment.[2]

Health promotion implies that health education has multiple goals. Health education is increasingly turning to the behavioral sciences for a basis for operation. There is increasing focus on behavioral outcomes, with emphasis on how knowledge, attitude, and beliefs contribute to health behavior.

The health educator, more than a dispenser of knowledge, becomes a health advocate to different groups of people, often in the political realm. The health educator might work with community authorities to influence legislation or to establish environmental standards for health protection. Many important health improvements have been thus engineered and have resulted in better sanitation, proper sewage disposal, and a safe water supply. The health advocate also works with disadvantaged people, such as the elderly, the poor, the homeless, or a foreign-language-speaking group. Representing the concerns and needs of these people at important decision-making levels in the community is part of health promotion.

The health educator's role has expanded to include program development. This requires skill in setting goals, organizing a project, managing its operation, and then evaluating the effectiveness of the project. Since the funding for such programs often is obtained only through the grant process, the community health educator must also be skilled in grant development and writing.

Federal Government Involvement

President's Committee on Health Education

In the early 1970s, an extensive study on health education in the nation was conducted. The study committee, commissioned by President Richard M. Nixon and known as the President's Committee on Health Education, submitted its final report in 1972.[3]

The report noted that federal involvement in health education had been minimal. Only one-half of 1 percent of the total health care expenditures in the United States was for health education.[4] Even worse, about one-fifth of 1 percent of the federal allocation for health was expended on health education.

The study also reported that health education throughout the country was fragmented among many agencies. Even though it is an accepted fact that many major illnesses can be prevented by individual behavioral patterns, health education was a neglected phase of health care.

The committee identified many health needs that could be addressed through health education. Five specific population groups were noted as having unique health education needs: low-income families, mothers, school children and teenagers, middle-aged middle class, and the elderly.

The relationship between low income and poor health, as discussed earlier, is a recognized condition. The poor suffer from malnutrition, have higher rates of infant mortality, and experience a higher incidence of respiratory, emotional, and other disorders than the average population.[5] The ramifications of these health problems are social and political, as well as medical.

Mothers were singled out by the President's Committee as an important audience for health education. The mother has significant influence on the health and well-being of her young children.[6] Many health behavioral patterns such as nutrition of family members are influenced most by the mother.

Although most young children and teenagers attend school, the commission found health education in the schools extremely poor and ineffective. In the schools, health is often taught as part of another subject, such as biology, home economics, or physical education. There was little evidence that school health education was effective in improving eating habits, reducing teenage smoking, reducing incidence of venereal disease, or stopping the spread of drug usage.[7]

The middle-aged middle class was singled out by the commission because of its low fitness level. Poor nutrition was specifically identified as a negative factor. Obesity, lack of exercise, smoking, and high cholesterol food intake are common parts of this population's life-style. These conditions lead to a variety of chronic conditions.

Senior citizens have a number of different health needs.[8] The necessity for concern and health education for this population sector was amplified by this report. Living conditions, as well as health counseling, were noted as being important areas to address in improving the life-style of the aged.

The Presidential Commission made several important recommendations, one of which was for the establishment of a national office for health education. As the result of that recommendation, in 1974 the Bureau of Health Education in the Center for Disease Control was established. A year later the National Center for Health Education became a reality. This center was incorporated so as to operate in the private sector to improve health education.

Congress later passed the National Consumer Health Information and Health Promotion Act in 1976, which established an office of health promotion and health information within the Department of Health, Education, and Welfare (HEW). This office is now a part of the Department of Health and Human Services (HHS) and is known as the Office of Disease Prevention and Health Promotion.

Center for Health Promotion and Education

A major recommendation of the Presidential Commission was a national center for health education having five operational departments:[9]

1. Department for research in health education
2. Department for demonstration programs in health education
3. Clearinghouse for health information and education
4. Department for communications in health education
5. Department for community health education centers

As a result of this study, the Bureau of Health Education, composed of these five departments, was established. The mission of this governmental agency, located within the Center for Disease Control, was to strengthen health programs at the local, state, and national levels.

With the reorganization in 1981 of the Centers for Disease Control, the Bureau of Health Education combined with two other federal agencies and is now known as the Center for Health Promotion and Education (CHPE). The Center has maintained the same mission and program objectives as the original Bureau. The Center, in conjunction with other agencies, enters into contract arrangements for funding of a variety of health education and health promotion projects.

Office of Disease Prevention and Health Promotion

A federal law passed in 1976 mandated the establishment of a federal office of health information and health promotion. This office, known today as the Office of Disease Prevention and Health Promotion, has been reorganized several times since 1976. It is now part of the Department of Health and Human Services directly responsible to the Assistant Secretary for Health.

The major focus of the Office of Disease Prevention and Health Promotion is centered on promoting health and preventing diseases through various preventive program activities. Specific program initiatives are directed toward nutrition, school health, worksite health promotion, preventive services, and community/media health promotion.[10] This office has the principal responsibility to review and maintain progress reports of the 1990 health objectives for the nation. The various activities of this office focus on implementation of the national objectives. Among the many activities relating to these national health objectives has been the midcourse review of the objectives to ascertain the extent of movement toward achieving the objectives by 1990.[11]

The Office's goal of coordinating health promotion efforts throughout the nation is achieved through a series of activities that involve conducting regional forums on various community health promotion issues. The Office has provided technical assistance, as well as federal funds, for various community health promotion efforts.

An important project supported by this office is the development of the National Health Information Clearinghouse, a referral system that identifies health information resources. The information provided by these resources is made available upon request to the public, as well as to health professionals. A variety of information on health-related topics is produced and disseminated. The Clearinghouse operates a library for the public and maintains a data base of health-related groups, agencies, and support groups. Questions concerning rare diseases are answered through the Clearinghouse.

Another national program supported by this office has been a national health promotion media campaign. The goal of this project has been to inform the public, with special emphasis on minority groups, of action that would maintain or improve health by reducing health risks. Several mass media approaches have been used—television, radio, newspaper, magazines, as well as public posters and advertising. Each health message encourages people to write to the National Health Information Clearinghouse for more information on good health. These media health promotion messages have been directed toward the general public, toward mothers and children, and toward senior citizens.

National Center for Health Education

Established as a national agency in the private sector to improve health education, the National Center for Health Education has sponsored conferences, workshops, and seminars on a number of topics for many different audiences. It has been prominent in piloting, revising, and updating the Growing Healthy Curriculum Project. The Center also was a leading force in the role delineation project, an attempt to identify health educator competencies. The Center's plans for the 1980s have included activities in two areas of primary program emphasis: (1) involvement in school health and (2) an expanded focus on health in the workplace.

In addition to the federal funding that has been made available through the Centers for Disease Control, operational monies for the National Center for Health Education are made available from a number of sources in the private sector. The Kellogg Foundation and the Ittleson Foundation of New York are the primary backers, although funds have also been received from Aetna Life and Casualty, Bristol Meyers, United States Steel, and the Prudential Life Insurance Foundation. Voluntary agencies, such as the American Cancer Society and the American Heart Association, also contribute to the National Center. Donations from the American Dental Association and the American Hospital Association demonstrate the support of professional health organizations.

All of the organizations have become victims of political change and budgetary reductions in the 1980s. Funding for the National Center has been reduced, thus affecting programming, staffing, and overall effectiveness.

Of the three offices discussed, it is likely that the National Center for Health Education is the most viable because it operates in the private sector and receives a good deal of funding from nongovernmental sources. The Center corresponds with the federal government's current concept of encouraging the private sector to assume responsibility for health and social welfare programs.

In 1982, the Secretary of the Department of Health and Human Services established a health promotion awards program. The purpose of this program has been to recognize exemplary local and state community health promotion programs. Nearly two hundred programs throughout the nation have been recognized since the inception of the program. Awards have gone to programs in all categories of the 1990 national health objectives.

Health Education/Health Promotion in Operation

Health education and health promotion occur in many community settings. They may involve teaching classes in a school, in an industrial setting, or to some neighborhood group. Speaking to different clubs, agencies, or classes may be the means of imparting health concepts. Health promotion activities occur in such locations as hospitals, occupational settings, schools, the mass media, and health fairs.

The Hospital

Hospitals throughout the United States have become increasingly involved in health promotion programming. Hospitals are providing not only patient educational services, but wellness and health promotion activities for residents of the entire community. Nearly 90 percent of hospitals in the United States today offer patient education or community health promotion programs to at least one target population.[12] Most hospital-based health promotion programs are targeted for inpatients, hospital employees, patients on an outpatient basis, the general community population, and employees of corporations and industries.

Hospital-based community health promotion programs are a recent development. Prior to 1978, few hospitals had such programs.[13] Most hospital-based community education activities that did exist provided first-aid instruction and conducted health fairs and occasional seminars. Increasingly, these programs are providing instruction relating to wellness and improved individual life-style. Even though hospital-based community education programs are conducted for all age groups, most are directed at adults.

Hospital-Based Health Promotion Programs

Target Population	Most Common Programs
Inpatients	Diabetes, preoperation education
Hospital employees	CPR, orientation to hospital
Outpatients	Diabetes, nutrition
Community residents	CPR, prenatal
Corporations	CPR, stress management

Source: American Hospital Association. *Hospital-Based Health Promotion Programs: Report and Analysis of the 1984 Survey*. Chicago, Illinois: American Hospital Association, 1984.

Selected Titles of Hospital-Based Health Promotion Programs

Aim Well
Be Well
Health Awareness
Healthwise
Health Check
Life Check
Lifewise
Project Life
School of Good Health
Well Aware
Wellness Place
Wellness Institute

Source: Personal Communication with Center for Health Promotion. American Hospital Association, 840 North Lake Shore Drive, Chicago, Illinois 60611.

The primary purpose of these activities is to promote positive health habits. By conducting health promotion programs, the hospital creates a more positive image in the community. As a result, there is increased community support for the hospital and its activities. Individuals come to accept the hospital as a positive contributor to health and wellness—not just a place to go when injured, sick, or dying. The American Hospital Association has encouraged hospitals to become involved in such community health education efforts:

Hospitals have a responsibility to take a leadership role in helping ensure the good health of their communities.[14]

Focus on Wellness

These developments expand the hospital's focus from curative treatment for sick and disabled people to health promotion, disease prevention, and improved life-style.

Hospital-based community wellness programs employ a variety of approaches. One such program screened members of the local unions for hypertension and presented information about positive health behavior. People were encouraged to make life-style adaptations to reduce high blood pressure. Another hospital created health promotion messages for use on cable television. In one city, a wellness center, complete with exercise facilities and classrooms, was established in a shopping center. In yet another location, a school, closed because of reduced enrollment, has been rented by a hospital to house community health, nutrition, fitness, and related programs. These approaches are variations of an attempt to convince all sectors of a community to analyze and change their life-styles to promote health.

Patient Education

Hospitals, along with other health care institutions, continue to expand their patient education programs. These programs, available for both the patient and the family, are designed to inform all concerned about specific health problems. Most patients need more information about their condition than has been traditionally given. Patient education programs provide information about the condition of the patient, the treatment being rendered, the purposes of medication, and clarification of specific directions given the patient. These educational efforts help the patient to cope with a situation and to make any life-style adaptations that might be needed. Patient education sessions may be conducted on a one-to-one basis or in group settings.

Though any disability or health problem can be the focus of a patient education program, two of the more common programs are for diabetic and cardiac patients. Diabetic education programs help the patient understand how to control insulin levels and diet. Cardiac rehabilitation programs assist the heart attack victim in learning how to adjust to a new life-style. The patient is taught to live with heart disease.

One creative diabetic program was a summer camp sponsored by a local hospital for young diabetics. During the one-week session, the children learned about diabetes, how to cope with this condition, and developed skills to enhance their life-styles. Appropriate physical activities and skills were also taught.

An important tool in patient education programs is the learning resource center in hospitals or other health care institutions. This center might include a library with a variety of health education materials, as well as audiovisual equipment available for patient use on an individual basis. Learning carrels for independent study and areas for small-group teaching are often available, too. Hospitals have also found the use of closed-circuit television and in-house telephone circuits to be effective procedures for conducting patient education programs.

Patient education is likely to continue to expand in the future. The cost of some patient education programs is currently covered by insurance benefits, and further expansion will occur as other companies extend their benefits to include reimbursement of the cost of patient education services.

Occupational Health

With the rising cost of health insurance coverage for employees, more and more companies are investigating health promotion programs. Realizing the cost benefit of preventive health programs, several companies have employed health promotion and health education specialists, constructed facilities for conducting these programs, and taken measures to encourage life-style changes that are conducive to health and wellness.

From the employer's point of view, there are several advantages to health promotion programs: employees involved in such programs perform better on the job, individuals are more productive, and fewer days of work time are lost due to illness and accident. This, in turn, lowers the cost of health care coverage.

Health promotion programs also help employees to cope with stress, a major problem for both labor and management. Not only is stress management helpful, but employee morale increases and positively affects the company's output. Where health promotion programs have been established, employees feel that the company is interested in them as persons and not just as "cogs" in the machinery of industry.

The programs that have been developed vary from one locality to another and from one company to the next. Physical fitness programs are one very common component of industrial health programs. Opportunities for the workers to exercise regularly in such facilities as tennis courts, basketball courts, fields for team games, running tracks, and indoor racquetball courts are made available. This availability is an incentive for learning the skills necessary to participate in these fitness activities.

Wellness and health promotion programs include small- and large-group activities. Aerobic fitness classes often involve a number of individuals.

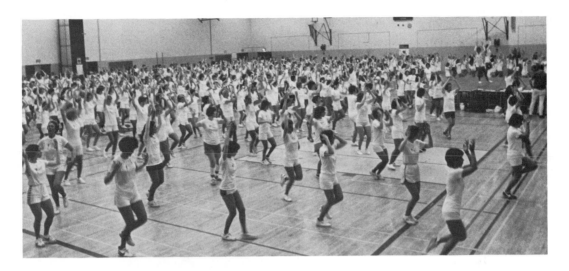

With W. K. Kellogg Foundation support, a pilot health awareness program has been launched in New York's lower Manhattan to prevent young people from adopting negative health behaviors. It is conducted by The Door—A Center of Alternatives, a project of the International Center for Integrative Studies. The program targets inner-city youth who are at high risk for substance abuse, nutritional deficiencies, and other health problems.

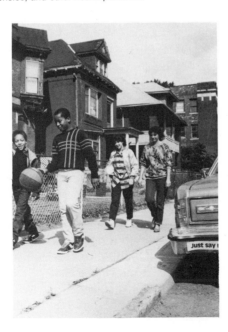

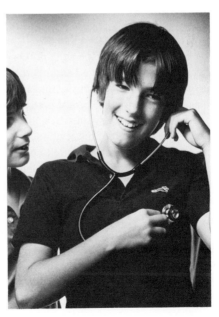

Some occupational health programs focus on reducing the risk of cardiovascular disease. Hypertension screening has revealed numerous individuals who are at risk for heart attacks. Education and risk-reduction planning following a screening program can reduce the possibility of a heart attack and help the employee to feel better and so live a more productive life.

Weight reduction programs have been instituted by many companies. Such programs include not only instruction about proper nutrition and nutrition intake surveys, but, in some cases, a revamping of the food service facility at the industrial site. In one instance, employees recommended, after several nutrition classes, that the company cafeteria change its menu to include more salads and nonfattening foods.

Safety instruction required by OSHA rules and regulations is an important component of an occupational health promotion program. Instruction in first aid, cardiopulmonary resuscitation (CPR), and accident prevention is often provided.

Regardless of the type of program, the most important component must be health promotion. Industry may create such programs because of economic incentives, but the employees actually benefit by improved health.

The School

Health education has been part of the school curriculum since the 1860s, when Horace Mann,[15] the noted education commissioner in Massachusetts, emphasized in his annual reports the need for effective physiology and hygiene (health) instruction in the schools. Principally as a result of his reviews and urging, Massachusetts became the first state to pass legislation requiring that physiology and hygiene courses be part of the school curriculum. School health programs now include health services in addition to health instruction. The presentation and study of health concepts are a part of the education process from preschool through college. However, coordinated, comprehensive school health education programs are few, and those that do exist lack uniformity.[16]

Before one can begin an effective health improvement program it is necessary that some assessment measures be conducted. A number of different health assessment tools are available to help the individual get started in a health promotion program. It is important to understand exactly what kinds of information the particular assessment instrument can provide.

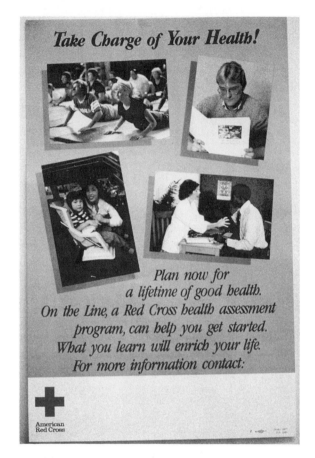

The curriculum for health education in schools is usually developed at the local level by educators within the school district and is designed to meet the particular needs and interests of students in the community. Though some states require that health education be part of the educational program, the development of comprehensive, statewide school health programs rarely occurs.

Though health education has not been a priority in schools in the United States, it still has the potential, when well organized and well taught, to have lasting positive effects upon the health and well-being of school-age children. In order for this to happen, support must be gained at the community level from various important decision makers for the school health program. The importance of school board members, superintendents of schools, principals, curriculum coordinators, and community medical and health leaders must be emphasized in designing school health programs that are effective in the lives of children.

To encourage district-wide school health program development, team efforts involving a broad range of personnel working together seem to be the most effective. An approach that has been found to be useful in motivating school districts and getting multidisciplinary teams to begin to work together to set goals has been to bring a team together for a concentrated conference. Here goals are implemented and plans initiated. This approach has been found to be successful in such states as Oregon, with the Seaside Conference, and in Ohio, with the Lake Hope Conference.

Mass Media

The mass media have a tremendous influence on the life-style of the United States citizen. Television, radio, and the printed page reach into every home in the United States.

The media can have both positive and negative effects on health behavior. From a negative standpoint, mass media, particularly television, often portray unhealthy life-styles. Such portrayal may amplify drunkenness, obesity, drug use, or habitual smoking.

Another media-related contributor to negative health behavior is advertising of products that have detrimental health effects. Though cigarette smoking advertising is banned on television, such advertisements do still appear in print. Advertising is also misleading in its presentation of many health-related products. Health education strategies need to be developed that assist the average citizen in discerning truth in advertising from that which is misleading.

In spite of the negative impact on health behavior made by mass media, a number of possibilities exist for using television, radio, and periodicals to teach positive health concepts. Simple, one-minute

health messages on such topics as accident prevention, immunizations, nutrition, and family planning have been developed and presented. These public-service announcements are often presented by local health departments or voluntary health organizations.

Popular television programming sometimes offers exercise and fitness programs. The viewer is expected to follow the leader in doing a series of exercises in the home. Though interesting to watch and usually well produced, the value of such a program in weight reduction, fitness, and the development of ongoing positive health behavior is doubtful.

With increased public interest in health issues, both television and radio have produced special prime-time health programs on topics such as abortion, health care costs, teen suicide, teen pregnancy, and world hunger. Such programs add to the awareness and health knowledge of citizens about such important issues. However, little behavioral effect on individuals is evident from such presentations.

The use of mass media in isolation usually will not bring about positive behavioral change. Such efforts must be reinforced by follow-up activities. One approach to the problem is to relate the message to an appropriate local health agency. The viewers, listeners, or readers are made aware that they can contact the agency for additional information on the topic or for personal counseling and/or services. The mass media message should also encourage listeners and readers to be screened for a health problem when appropriate, particularly concerning diabetes, hypertension, and physical fitness.

Not every media message is effective with all groups. However, it is important that a health message be as widely effective as possible. For instance, the health message should be comprehended by speakers of different languages where appropriate. Although mass media campaigns have been effective with varying age groups, the adult population is most often targeted.

The Health Fair

An interesting approach to community health education is the health fair. This exhibition or carnival may be held at an educational institution, a shopping center, as part of a larger county or regional

The National Health Screening for Volunteer Organization's Health Fair model incorporates four important services into every health fair event: screening, education, review, and follow-up. Pictured here are six of the basic screenings offered at every health fair site: (a) height and weight, (b) blood pressure, (c) anemia, (d) visual acuity, (e) blood chemistry, and (f) counseling and referral. These screenings, coupled with educational learning centers and follow-up, complete a health promotion project designed to increase the public's awareness of health topics, to encourage personal responsibility for health practices, and to detect potential disease in early stages.

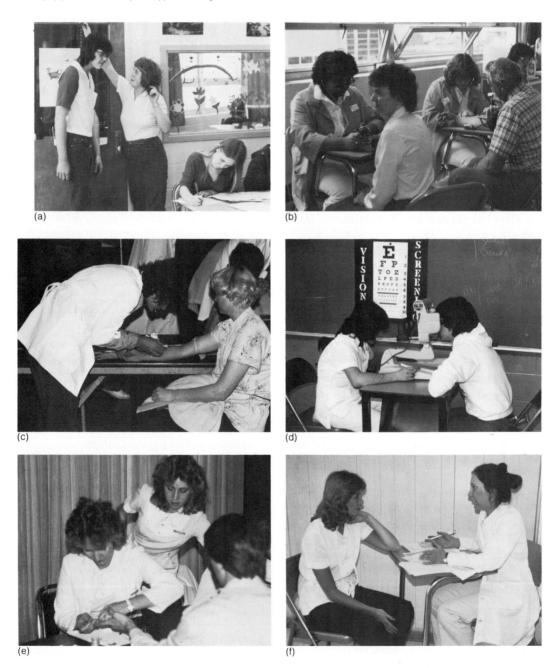

(a)

(b)

(c)

(d)

(e)

(f)

fair, or in any number of other community settings. Many people are exposed to health ideas and concepts in these settings. In this country, nearly two million people visit at least one health fair annually.[17]

Health fairs provide an opportunity to integrate health education activities with multiphasic health screening activities. Representatives from the community health agencies, health care providers, and consumers are brought together in these informal settings. This often leads to improved communication within the community.

An important benefit of the health fair is that it often commands media attention. Local newspapers will often present a story or picture from the fair. Also, television finds the health fair an interesting item to show on the local segment of the newscast.

Since learning is best facilitated by doing, health fairs usually provide experiential types of activities. A person may perform a simple exercise to see the effect of the exercise on the pulse rate. A health fair for school-age children may have the participants move through a maze of activities, each designed for some learning objective. Audiovisual aids accompany many of these activities.

The health fair stimulates interest in health by providing information and reinforcing already existing positive health behaviors.[18] It is an effective tool that challenges individuals to be informed about community resources.

Though the health fair stimulates a lot of interest and exposes individuals to a great deal of health information, its effect on long-range health behavior has not been documented. In fact, there is some evidence that many people who participate in these activities are already aware of their health status. For example, blood pressure screening is common at health fairs. But those volunteering to be screened are often already aware of their hypertension.[19]

Screening tests are very popular among those attending a health fair. They are most effective when targeted at a specific health risk population. Many kinds of screening procedures can be found. Those tests that have been shown to be reasonably justifiable have included weight measurement, skin fold thickness measurement, blood pressure, serum cholesterol and glucose tests, and stools for occult blood in people over fifty.[20]

Regardless of problems associated with health fairs, they offer an opportunity to expose people in the community to issues relating to wellness and an improved life-style. The interest and creative approach found in these settings may benefit some individuals who may not be reached in more structured educational settings.

Health Education/Health Promotion Financing

Health promotion activities have received much interest in the past few years. Though many reasons can be cited for this development, the increase in health care costs is primarily responsible. Health promotion is viewed by many as an effective means of reducing the incidence of long-term, expensive health problems.

If health promotion activities are to receive even wider acceptance, insurance coverage for these services must be expanded. Some health education and health promotion activities and services are covered today by health insurance programs. The services most likely to be covered include the following:[21]

1. Education services delivered to patients as part of the treatment plan for an existing condition
2. Preventive education services delivered to patients to avoid future illness
3. Education services delivered to nonpatients (the "well" community) to promote good health and prevent illness

Most coverage is part of the payment for hospital inpatient and outpatient care. Health education is not separately identified for reimbursement, but it is part of the overall hospital service coverage. In the future, if people are to be oriented to the importance of preventive health, third-party payment must be made more widely available for health education and health promotion services. This is particularly the case where these services are offered apart from the hospital or health care institution.

It is logical that tax incentives should be developed to encourage the purchase and construction of equipment and facilities used in health promotion programs. Maybe the cost of purchasing a stationary bicycle for use in the home could be a tax deduction. The cost of attending sessions on stress management or fitness might also be made tax deductible.

Regardless of the economic incentives, the future role of health education and health promotion in community health seems well established. Focusing upon positive life-style and wellness is much more personally rewarding than centering activities upon medical care and curative medicine.

Summary

Health education and health promotion activities are major factors in health prevention. Health education provides learning situations designed to positively affect people's health behavior. A broadened concept of health education now includes the role of political and economic interventions. This focus has been termed health promotion. Health promotion involves program planning, evaluation, and health advocacy in a variety of settings.

In the past, the United States federal government has shown some interest in health education and health promotion activities. The President's Committee on Health Education noted the relatively low state of health education programming as it existed in the early 1970s. As a result of the recommendations of the study, the Bureau of Health Education was established. Within the Department of Health and Human Services, the Office of Disease Prevention and Health Promotion has played an important role. In the private sector, the National Center for Health Education has played an important role in the expansion of health education and health promotion programs.

Health promotion activities take place in a number of settings, under the sponsorship of different kinds of organizations. Special emphasis should be given to such programming in the occupational setting, in schools and universities, and in the hospital or health care institution. Hospital programs focus upon patient education, as well as community health education activities. Mass media have been used to deliver health messages to the general public. These measures, along with the informal learning environment of the health fair or carnival, reach many people not usually contacted through more structured health programs.

Health care cost containment is the major impetus for the increased interest in health education and health promotion programs. To ensure that interest in this area expands in the future, economic incentives must be established.

Discussion Questions

1. What is the goal of any health education program?
2. Discuss the relationships between knowledge, attitude, and cultural determinants in establishing an effective program of health education.
3. What is implied by the various definitions being given to health promotion today?
4. In what ways do health promotion and health education complement each other?
5. How does health promotion relate to health prevention?
6. Discuss the findings of the President's Committee on Health Education.

7. Discuss some of the program activities of the Office of Disease Prevention and Health Promotion.
8. How does the National Center for Health Education differ from the Office of Disease Prevention and Health Promotion or the Center for Health Promotion and Education?
9. Why have hospitals become increasingly active in health promotion programming?
10. What is patient education?
11. Identify some of the kinds of activities being carried out by hospital-based health promotion programs.
12. Give an example of a health condition for which patient education strategies could be developed.
13. What are some benefits of health promotion programs to industry and business?
14. Identify ways in which the mass media could be used for health promotion.
15. What are the most effective activities carried out at health fairs in terms of individual health behavior?
16. Should health insurance coverage include the cost of health promotion interventions? If so, why? If not, why not?

Suggested Readings

American Hospital Association. *Hospital-Based Health Promotion Programs: Report and Analysis of the 1984 Survey.* Chicago, Illinois: American Hospital Association (1984) 110 pp.

Ardell, Donald B. "The History and Future of Wellness." *Health Values* 9, no. 6, (November/December, 1985): 37–57.

Cruz, Jon, and Wallack, Lawrence. "Trends in Tobacco Use on Television." *American Journal of Public Health* 76, no. 6 (June 1986): 698–99.

Freudenberg, Nicholas. "Shaping the Future of Health Education: From Behavior Change to Social Change." *Health Education Monographs* 6, no. 4 (Winter, 1978): 372–77.

Germer, Polly, and Price, James H. "Organization and Evaluation of Health Fairs." *Journal of School Health* 51, no. 2 (February, 1981): 86–90.

Green, Lawrence W. "How to Evaluate Health Promotion." *Hospitals* 53, no. 19 (October 1, 1979): 106–08.

Kelly, Kathryn E. "Building a Successful Health Promotion Program." *Business and Health* 3, no. 4 (March, 1986): 44–45.

Lange, Mary E., and Ardell, Donald B. "Wellness Programs Attract New Markets for Hospitals."*Hospitals* 55, no. 22 (November 16, 1981): 115–19.

Levy, Susan R. "Worksite Health Promotion." *Family and Community Health* 9, no. 3 (November, 1986): 51–62.

Office of Disease Prevention and Health Promotion. *Screening in Health Fairs: A Critical Review of Benefits, Risks, and Costs.* Washington, D.C.: U.S. Government Printing Office, 1985, 53 pp.

Pellegrino, Edmund D. "Health Promotion as Public Policy: The Need for Moral Groundings." *Preventive Medicine* 10 (1981): 371–78.

Riska, Elianne. "Health Education and Its Ideological Content." *Acta Sociologica* 25 (1982, Supplement): 41–46.

Sofalvi, Alan J., and Drolet, Judy C. "Health-Related Content of Selected Sunday Comic Strips." *Journal of School Health* 56, no. 5, (May, 1986): 184–86.

Stein, Jane. "Promoting Health by Video." *Business and Health* 2, no. 9 (September, 1985): 47–49.

Stewart, Gordon. "With a Little Innovation, Health Promotion Need Not Be Costly." *Occupational Health and Safety* 55, no. 4 (April, 1986): 84–87.

Watts, Albert C., and Breindel, Charles C. "Health Education: Structural vs. Behavioral Perspectives." *Health Policy and Education* 2 (1981): 47–57.

Wikler, Daniel I. "Persuasion and Coercion for Health." Milbank Memorial Fund Quarterly, *Health and Society* 56, no. 3 (1978): 303–38.

Endnotes

1. Green, Lawrence. *Promoting Health: A Source Book*. U.S. Office of Health Information and Health Promotion, Department of Health, Education, and Welfare, (1979): 5.

2. American Hospital Association. *Policy and Statement on the Hospital's Responsibilities for Health Promotion*. Chicago, Illinois: American Hospital Association, (1979).

3. *The Report of the President's Committee on Health Education*. New York: The Committee, 1971.

4. Ibid., 31.

5. Issues related to the health problems of the economically disadvantaged are discussed in chapter 15.

6. Issues related to maternal and child health are discussed in chapter 16.

7. Issues related to school health are discussed in chapter 13.

8. Issues related to health problems of the elderly are discussed in chapter 17.

9. *The Report*, 28–30.

10. Office of Disease Prevention and Health Promotion. *Fact Sheet*. Washington, D.C.: Office of Disease Prevention and Health Promotion, (July, 1985).

11. Office of Disease Prevention and Health Promotion. *The 1990 Health Objectives for the Nation: A Midcourse Review*. Washington, D.C.: Office of Disease Prevention and Health Promotion, (1986).

12. American Hospital Association. *Hospital-Based Health Promotion Programs: Report and Analysis of the 1984 Survey*. Chicago, Illinois: American Hospital Association (1984): 110 pp.

13. Lange, M. E., and Wolfe, A. *Promoting Community Health Through Innovative Hospital-Based Programs*. Chicago, Illinois: American Hospital Publishing Inc., (1984).

14. American Hospital Association. *Policy and Statement on the Hospital's Responsibilities for Health Promotion*. Chicago, Illinois: American Hospital Association, (1979).

15. Means, Richard K. *Historical Perspectives on School Health*. Thorofare, New Jersey: Charles B. Slack, Inc., 1975: 87.

16. Issues related to school health are discussed in chapter 13.

17. Office of Disease Prevention and Health Promotion. *Screening in Health Fairs: A Critical Review of Benefits, Risks, and Costs*. Washington, D.C.: U.S. Government Printing Office (November, 1985): 5.

18. Germer, P., and Price, J. H. "Organization and Evaluation of Health Fairs." *Journal of School Health* 51, no. 2 (February, 1981): 87.

19. Wassertheil-Smaller, S., et al. "An Evaluation of the Utility of High Blood Pressure Detection Fairs." *American Journal of Public Health* 68, no. 8 (August, 1978): 770.

20. Office of Disease Prevention and Health Promotion. *Screening in Health Fairs: A Critical Review of Benefits, Risks, and Costs*. Washington, D.C.: U.S. Government Printing Office, 1985, 53 pp.

21. Bureau of Health Education. *Focal Points*. Atlanta, Ga.: Center for Disease Control, June, 1980: 1.

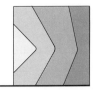

UNIT FOUR

Special Target Groups

15

Health of Minorities: Socioeconomic Factors Affect Health Status

> Blacks, Hispanics, Native Americans, and those of Asian/Pacific Islander heritage have not benefited fully or equitably from the fruits of science or from those systems responsible for translating and using health sciences technology.[1]

There are numerous socioeconomic aspects to community health programs. These must be considered if the programs are to be used by those for whom they are intended. All too often, cultural differences are not taken into account in establishing health care or community health service programs. It is vital, however, that cultural and sociological factors are considered if the program is to be a success. Ethnic differences and racial variations, in addition to language barriers, determine the particular medical service approach appropriate for a population. Value systems must also be understood before effective health care can be made available to all.

Emphasizing the importance of sociological considerations, the late Dr. John H. Knowles, former president of the Rockefeller Foundation, said in a speech to the American Public Health Association in 1972 that the next major advances in health in our nation would depend on the accomplishments of social science rather than medical research. He suggested that it is necessary for community health to deal with issues such as housing, pollution, overpopulation, civil injustices, and other social problems.

Within our society in the United States the provision of health care has been geared to middle- and upper-class values and standards. However, there are many racial, economic, and ethnic groups whose values, education, and health habits are quite different from the "mainstream." It is also important to understand the nature of poverty and its effects on our nation's health. Only as such understanding takes place will effective programming for these groups result.

Poverty

Much has been said and written about the relationship between poverty and the status of health and well-being in the United States. The poverty level, as established by the United States government, varies depending on such factors as family size, sex and age of family head, number of children under the age of eighteen, and location of residence. The poverty level is the measurement of income developed by the Social Security Administration in 1964 and revised in 1969. In the mid-1980s, for example, the poverty level for a family of four was $10,178.[2]

It is well known that the poor in this country usually do not experience the same level of health as do those individuals who have the financial means to receive proper health care. The problem is more than an inability to afford the cost of health care. The poor person tends to feel less at ease in medical care settings than does the more affluent individual. The poor, as a group, usually have less understanding of how the medical system operates and are less likely to seek treatment or preventive care.

As a result of this discomfort, the poor tend to make less use of health facilities. They seek the services of a physician less often than do those in the middle and upper classes. In many areas where the economically disadvantaged reside, particularly in metropolitan areas, the primary source of health care is the emergency outpatient department of the city hospital or at the public health department clinic. Poor citizens usually do not have physicians who can be contacted when there are health needs. They often are thrust into the health care system at a time of urgent need, with little or no familiarity with the health care provider.

Vital statistics amplify the disparity in well-being between the economically disadvantaged and the middle and upper class in our society. Mortality rates for the poor are more than a third greater than those for the nonpoor. Birth rates are greater among the poor and minority populations. Among the economically disadvantaged (particularly the black population) infant mortality is twice that of the middle- and upper-class white population, and maternal mortality is three times greater.[3]

The rural poor in the United States experience a number of health problems. A retired clinical psychologist administers tests to the unemployed and underemployed in West Virginia.

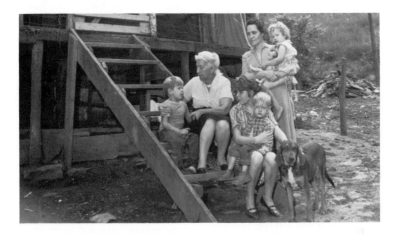

Poor people are not usually oriented to preventive health. Instead, these individuals tend to be crisis-oriented. Too often the poor are reluctant to seek health care because of a feeling of not needing or not being able to afford the care. The person may deny that he or she is susceptible to a specific condition, or may not even perceive the seriousness of the situation. When poor people become ill and need proper medical care, they are likely to try some home remedy or to ask the advice of friends and relatives, rather than go to a doctor or a health clinic.

Health usually does not rank as a high priority item among the poor. Instead, finding acceptable living conditions and the opportunity for employment have top priority. Only when health limits activities through debilitation or pain does health become a priority consideration.

The child born in poverty is often handicapped from birth because the mother suffered from malnutrition or did not have proper prenatal care. Mothers who have inadequate prenatal care are much more likely to give birth to a premature baby or a child with below-average birth weight. Premature births are those in which the child at birth weighs less than twenty-five-hundred grams or five-and-one-half pounds.[4] These infants are more likely to experience serious health problems needing extensive medical care and treatment.

Malnutrition is fairly common among the poor. Two population groups are particularly affected by malnutrition: children and the aged. Studies have shown that the normal growth of children from low socioeconomic environments is often impaired by as much as six months to a year because of poor nutrition. This is of particular concern during the early years when normal brain development is affected. It is now believed that retardation occurs as the result of malnutrition during early childhood.

Closely related to problems of malnutrition is dental health. Tooth decay and periodontal disease are very common problems among children living in poverty. Some statistics suggest that two out of every three children living in poverty in the United States never see a dentist for preventive purposes.

A number of other health problems afflict the poor. Some of these will be examined specifically as we look at selected sectors of our society. An examination of these poverty-stricken minority groups will also provide a better view of the importance of sociological and health factors in establishing community health programs.

Minorities

The United States is a nation of ethnic groups. As such, many citizens can trace their heritages to several foreign countries. However, there are population groups that can be identified by singular traits and so are known as minorities. Interest in the health status of several minorities has increased in recent years, principally because these groups are more likely to be poor. They also tend to have specific value systems and beliefs that affect their use of the health care system. Thus, in providing health care for the poor, it is often necessary to have an understanding of minority cultures.

The largest minority group in the United States is the black population, representing about 11 percent of the national population. The second largest minority is Hispanic and constitutes the most rapidly growing population in the United States, now about 6 percent. Many of these Spanish-speaking people trace their roots to Mexico, although Puerto Ricans, Cubans, and other Spanish-speaking Latin Americans are also classed as Hispanic. A third population group considered an important minority includes the Native Americans and Alaskan natives, descendants of the first people to inhabit the North American continent. Many unique health problems are found among this minority population.

The living conditions of many minorities often are not conducive to good health and well-being. These people are more likely to live in overcrowded conditions. Frequently, they are not home owners and, as a result, encounter many problems caused by renting property owned by absentee landlords. Minorities tend to spend a larger proportion of their income on rent than do other individuals.

Unemployment is much higher among minorities than among the general population. Unemployment breeds discontent, frustration, and lack of self-esteem, and often results in lawless actions. Even more crucial, because unemployment results in less available money, items such as food and health care often are not available.

Additionally, the educational level of minorities is not as high as that of the general population. Literacy is an important tool in adapting to American life, but most minorities cannot read as effectively as non-minorities.

Health and Human Services Task Force

In 1984, the Secretary of the Department of Health and Human Services established a task force on black and minority health concerns. The report, released in 1985, reported a disparity in key health indicators among blacks and other minorities.[5] The Task Force identified six causes of death that account for 80 percent of excess mortality over that in the white population. These six health problems that were identified as needing special priority for programming among minorities were: (1) cancer, (2) cardiovascular disease and stroke, (3) chemical dependency with special emphasis on deaths due to cirrhosis, (4) diabetes, (5) homicide and accidents, and (6) infant mortality.

The report indicated a 16 percent excess mortality among black males and 10 percent among black females from cancer over what is found among the white population. Significant differences were noted in mortality from cancer of the esophagus, larynx, lung (males), cervix, and prostate gland.

Cardiovascular heart disease mortality rates are similar in black and nonblack males. The incidence of cardiovascular disease is greater among black females than whites. The death rates for cardiovascular disease among blacks is more than twice to three times greater than for whites under forty-five years of age.

Both hypertension and stroke were found to occur more often among the black population than the white. Though cardiovascular disease is a major cause of death among Hispanics and Native Americans, it is a proportionately smaller contributor to deaths.

Chemical dependency is a serious factor among minority populations. The task force particularly addressed the problem of deaths related to cirrhosis

Cancer Mortality (per 100,000 Population)

Site	White	Black
Esophagus	2.6	9.2
Larynx	1.3	2.5
Lung (Male)	69.3	91.4
Cervix	3.2	8.8
Prostate	21.0	43.9

Source: *Report of the Secretary's Task Force on Black and Minority Health*. U.S. Department of Health and Human Services. August, 1985. p. 93.

Heart disease death rates: per 100,000 population under 45 years of age

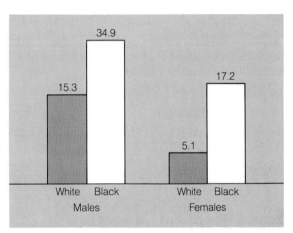

Source: Report of the Secretary's Task Force on Black and Minority Health, *U.S. Department of Health and Human Services, U.S. Government Printing Office, 1985.*

Cirrhosis of the liver death rates: per 100,000 population

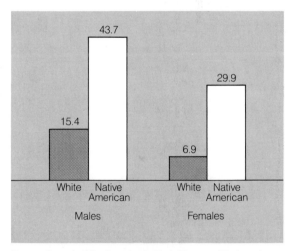

Source: Report of the Secretary's Task Force on Black and Minority Health, *U.S. Department of Health and Human Services, U.S. Government Printing Office, 1985.*

of the liver. This condition is associated with excessive alcohol consumption and is a major problem among the Native American population.

Diabetes is the seventh leading cause of death in the United States. Its prevalence is higher in the black population than among whites. The task force addressed the problem of diabetes particularly among Hispanic females, expressing concern regarding the relationship of diet, obesity, and diabetes in this group.

The problems of homicide, accidents, and infant mortality were also discussed and analyzed by the task force. As a result of the work of this task force, several recommendations were made. It was recommended that health information and educational strategies for minority populations should be implemented, and that those who develop patient education activities must be aware of the various cultural and language needs of minority populations.

Another recommendation was that access, delivery, and financing of health services to minority populations should be improved. Related to this is the importance of improving the availability and accessibility to health professions for minorities.

The report stated that local and community agencies should be encouraged to develop programming to meet the health needs of minorities. At the federal level, there should be better coordination among governmental agencies in administering existing programs for minorities. A special office in the Department of Health and Human Services has been established to manage implementation of the report's recommendations.

Finally, the report indicated that improved data collection and research regarding minority health are needed. Research related to risk factor identification, effective educational interventions, and development of preventive and treatment services was recommended.

Blacks

Generally speaking, the health of blacks in the United States is not as good as that of whites. The principal reason for this is the lower socioeconomic level of many black citizens; many of the problems associated with poverty apply to blacks.

The death rates of blacks are higher for heart disease, cerebrovascular disease, malignancies, diabetes mellitus, and accidents than those of other ethnic groups.[6] Hypertension is greater among black adults than among whites. National statistics indicate that black women tend to be obese more often than white women. Black males smoke more cigarettes than white males. Tobacco is the greatest risk factor for cancer for the black population.[7] Many black children have not been immunized for the childhood diseases. There are many other similar comparisons, but the end result is always that many black individuals do not experience acceptable levels of good health and wellness.

Though many reasons can be given for these conditions, two are especially relevant to community health: (1) cost of the health care, and (2) lack of adequate transportation to obtain the needed health care.

The majority of blacks live either in the inner core of urban cities or in rural, isolated communities. Both of these geographical locations have few resources in terms of readily available health personnel and facilities. As a result, it becomes difficult for people to obtain needed medical attention, and individuals do not seek preventive medical care. Not until a major health need arises will a physician be consulted.

If such a need exists, transportation must be arranged and this can be costly. The cities offer public transportation, but this is not a viable solution when one is ill and in need of medical care.

A lower proportion of the black population than the white population has insurance coverage. Without this insurance, the poor are unable to pay for needed health care. Medicaid, the federal medical insurance program for the needy, does provide some financial support for certain of the economically disadvantaged, however.

Sickle-Cell Anemia

One affliction that is not confined to poverty-stricken blacks is sickle-cell trait and sickle-cell anemia. Sickle-cell victims are predominantly black; however, other people whose ancestry is Mediterranean, Caribbean, or South American can also be affected. About 8.5 percent of the black population in the United States have sickle-cell trait. Sickle-cell anemia, the disease itself, is found in approximately 1 percent of the United States black population.[8]

Sickle-cell anemia is an inherited disorder of the red blood cells. These cells become sickle-shaped and, as a result, can block normal blood flow in the blood vessels. Any part of the body can be affected by this blockage. Sickle-cell disease initially causes pain in the bones, the joints, or other body organs. This pain, called *sickle-cell crisis,* is often precipitated by infection. Death may occur, depending upon the extent of the blockage and the organs of the body that are affected.

A necessary part of sickle-cell screening is counseling. Couples need to discuss the screening results with a knowledgeable health professional or counselor in order to make life-determining decisions.

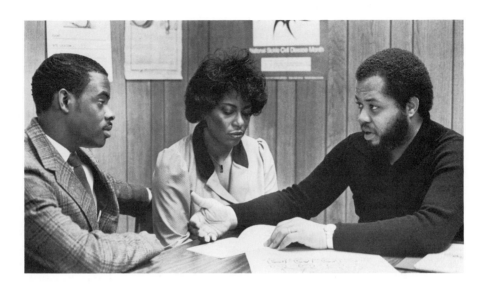

The importance of screening for sickle-cell trait and counseling individuals with the trait have led to many sickle-cell community health programs. Programs have been designed to educate people, particularly blacks, regarding sickle-cell anemia and sickle-cell trait. These programs also see that as many people as possible are screened. Counseling individuals with sickle-cell trait is important. They must be made aware of the potential threat to their offspring created by this genetic condition.

Sickle-cell programs also instruct individuals and their families on appropriate action in times of sickle-cell crisis. Because of the importance of maintaining a good level of overall health and well-being, many sickle-cell programs include assistance in good nutrition, dental care, disease prevention, and other general health measures.

Federal funds for sickle-cell conditions have been made available on two fronts. First, research efforts have provided greater understanding of the biological and physiological origins of this problem. Second, programs designed to screen, educate, and assist the black population concerning sickle-cell trait or sickle-cell anemia have been put into operation throughout the nation. Both of these activities have resulted in screening and educational programs.

Hispanics

Several million Spanish-speaking persons, a majority of them of Mexican-descent, live throughout the United States. The greatest number of Hispanics reside in the southwestern part of the country and in Florida. In several major cities, such as Miami, San Antonio, and Los Angeles, the Spanish-speaking population has major influence.

Many of these individuals, particularly those from Cuba and El Salvador, enter the United States as refugees. Others, particularly those from Mexico, enter the United States as illegal aliens. They cross into the United States in hopes of finding employment and a better way of life. When caught, these illegal aliens are returned to the Mexican-United States border, but many attempt to return another day.

So that health programming for the Hispanic population in the United States is effective, the health worker should be fluent in Spanish. An understanding and acceptance of cultural mores, beliefs, and behavioral patterns are also vital to this programming.

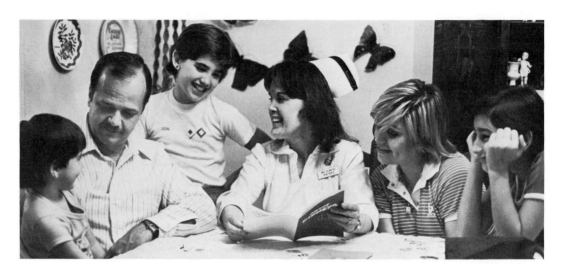

The refugees, as well as the illegal aliens, are usually unemployed and lack access to the social services that offer health care. Many of the Hispanics who are legal residents are laborers, moving from area to area as the seasons change. Because of poverty, high mobility, and cultural differences, the health of this population is not good. Their nutritional and overall health status is worse than that of the general population.

Hispanics in the United States tend to be a youthful population. Their median age is twenty-three, and nearly 20 percent are children less than ten years of age.[9] Hispanics in the United States have a relatively high fertility rate.

The likelihood of having diabetes was found to be two to five times greater in the Hispanic population than in the general population.[10] There also tend to be elevated rates of obesity in this population group.[11] Grain products are dietary staples, while leafy vegetables are not typically a part of their diet. Hispanics in the United States tend to have a relatively low consumption of dairy products.[12]

Many Hispanics have a different concept of disease than that of scientific medicine. The germ theory of disease transmission is often misunderstood or unaccepted. Instead, many believe that the body must maintain a balance of the "hot" and "cold" qualities associated with the four humors: blood, phlegm, the yellow bile of anger, and the black bile of depression.[13] A "hot" ailment is treated with "cold" medications, and a "cold" disease is treated with a "hot" medication so that the all-important humoral balance is maintained.

Many migrants rely on traditional folk medicine. These traditional healing measures reflect the influence of custom and religious belief. Folk medicine employs herbs, liniments, diet regulation, massage, and a number of other practices. The dispensers of folk medicine, the *curanderos,* are the most important traditional healers in the Spanish-speaking culture. Thus, integrating these traditional folk medicine practices with modern medical practices is a most difficult problem.

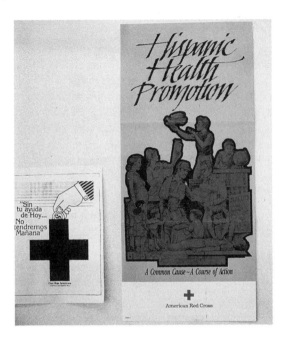

If health promotion programs are going to be effective for minority populations, it is often necessary to provide information and announcements in the principal language of that group. In many parts of the United States the use of Spanish is very important.

Other cultural problems make programming health services for the Spanish-speaking population extremely difficult. Often they are reluctant to approach a health agency for assistance because of apprehension about governmental agencies and authority in general. Another very important barrier is language. It is difficult to communicate health problems through an interpreter. Many community health agencies currently do not have Spanish-speaking personnel to communicate with these people. Increasingly, however, health organizations are seeking to employ community health personnel who are bilingual.

Another difficult problem is helping the Hispanic people solve their health problems without changing their culture. The family structure of the Spanish-speaking population is complex, with family ties being particularly important. When an individual becomes ill, the health worker must deal not with a single person, but with an extended family.

This family structure includes the nuclear family, the extended family, plus others, selected by the parents, who serve as a type of godparent. The elderly members of the family are highly respected, and an illness quite often cannot be treated unless the head of the family is convinced that there is a need and gives approval for medical care.

The need for hospitalization presents the Hispanic with some very difficult decisions. The individual may resist hospitalization because it means leaving the family. For many people, not just the Hispanic, having to go to the hospital is a traumatic experience. Some believe a hospital is the place where a person goes to die. As a result, hospitalization often must include the entire family. Accommodations must be made for other members of the hospitalized individual's family.

The Hispanic culture views childbearing as both a privilege and an obligation. As a result, Hispanic women often resist family planning. During pregnancy, they are very careful to avoid emotional upsets and unpleasant sights, believing this will affect the unborn child. This concern, however, does not extend to procurement of adequate prenatal care. As a result, many complications occur in childbirth, and there is a high rate of miscarriage.

As for all economically disadvantaged people, the cost of health care is a particularly heavy burden for the Spanish-speaking population. Unemployment is high among this group of people, which is one reason why they have the lowest level of health insurance coverage. Because of the inability to pay for health care and because of a lack of trust and understanding of the health care system, it is not unusual for these people to rely on the traditional medicine and healing procedures of their cultural heritage.

The Migrant Worker

Many Hispanics, particularly Mexicans, are migrant workers. The migrant worker is likely to experience most of the health problems found in society in general. It has also been found that respiratory diseases, especially tuberculosis, are major health problems of migrant workers. Because of poor sanitary conditions and inadequate water supplies, diarrhea and dysentery plague the migrant. The migrant accident rate is nearly three times the average national rate. Also, the rates of heart disease, diabetes, hepatitis, and cirrhosis of the liver are higher among this population group than for the nation as a whole.

Migrants receive less preventive care than that which other groups in the United States obtain.[14] Preventive health measures are not practiced by many migrants. They fail to obtain adequate vision care, dental care, and physical examinations.

Many states have established programs to help meet some of the health needs of the migrant. Since 1962, the federal government has provided funds designed to help local communities meet migrant health needs. Some of the projects that have been effective include: (1) family clinics where health services can be obtained, (2) services of the public health nurse, (3) health education stressing basic personal health, and (4) sanitation services directed at a more healthful living environment.

As with all federally funded programs, rather extensive reductions in these migrant programs have been made during the 1980s. The federal government expects the individual states to pick up the support of these programs.

The great mobility of migrant families creates a difficult problem in administering the various health and social services. All too frequently, the moves from one location to another make it impossible for the migrant to qualify for local resident status. As a result, health care may not be available when and where the individual needs it. Medicaid eligibility is also often unobtainable because of the migrant's lack of stability.

In order for a health care facility to be used by Spanish-speaking persons, it is important that their individual health needs be well defined. Members from the Hispanic community should be involved in the planning process. This will provide the opportunity for the people to have a voice in the type, organization, and quality of health care that will be provided. It will also provide a sense of community involvement for this minority population group.

Female migrants are more likely to visit the health care facility than are the males. Regardless, appropriate treatment is often delayed due to a variety of factors. These include costs, times, fear, working hours, and disbelief in the medical profession.[15]

The necessity for providing bilingual health professionals in those localities with Spanish-speaking residents should not be overlooked. Such a measure is important in communicating not only symptoms of illness, but also feelings, which are often lost when communicating through a translator. Also, use of a translator distances an individual from the health professional. The lack of adequate health care providers who speak Spanish often serves as a barrier for getting needed health care.

Native Americans

Health care for the Native American and Alaskan native population has been far from adequate. Their health status lags some fifteen to twenty years behind that of the general American population.[16]

Federal health care programs for the nearly 960,000 Native Americans living on reservations are made available through the Indian Health Service. It is the only federal program that provides direct health services to Native Americans. The Indian Health Service operates hospitals and health centers throughout the nation; most are in Alaska and the western part of the United States where the majority of the Native American population lives.

Native Americans experience a number of major health problems. The leading cause of death on many Indian reservations is accidents. This is partially the result of the extensive distances over which many must travel. Towns and villages on the reservations are separated by many miles, and connecting roads are often dangerous.

No doubt accidents are also related to the problem of alcohol consumption. Alcohol-related deaths are five times that of the general United States population. Alcoholism is a very serious problem among all age groups of Native Americans. For many, the consumption of alcohol is a means of escape from unemployment, poverty, and frustration. Excessive drinking also leads to malnutrition,

Comparisons Between Native Americans and the United States Population as a Whole

Alcohol-related deaths	459% higher among Native Americans
Accidents	155% higher among Native Americans
Diabetes	107% higher among Native Americans
Homicide	51% higher among Native Americans

Source: "The Runner is the Message," *Public Health Reports* 101, no. 4 (July/August, 1986): 437.

Many personal problems confront the Native American teenager living on a rural reservation. Stressors that are common to teenagers, as well as conflicting cultural values, changing cultural patterns, and poverty, often result in alcoholism, suicide, or other mental health problems.

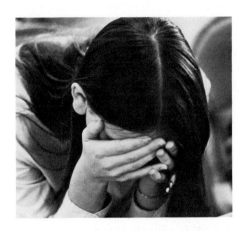

infection, mental health problems, and cirrhosis of the liver. Extensive programming at the community level has been established in an attempt to help reduce this heavy alcohol consumption.

The Native American tends to have the various health problems associated with poverty—respiratory illnesses, dental concerns, lack of health education, and malnutrition. Tuberculosis, although a major problem in the past, is not so threatening to the health of Native Americans today. In 1955, there were 55 deaths per 100,000 population from tuberculosis. At the end of the 1970s, that statistic had been reduced to 6.1 per 100,000 population.[17]

Adequate maternal and child health care services among Native Americans have not been available traditionally. Statistics indicate that the birthrate among Native Americans is nearly twice that of the national average.[18] Both maternal and infant mortality are also higher than the national average. However, there has been an improvement in these mortality rates in the past decade. Increased efforts at providing maternal and child health care services in the home and in the community have contributed to this reduction. Programs designed to improve water supply, sewage disposal, and other related environmental factors have also directly contributed to improvement of child health among Native Americans, although the problem continues to exist.[19]

Infant diarrhea is a major problem on many reservations. This is often due to the fact that the water supplies are not always sanitary. Many residents of reservations must obtain their water from some distance since they do not have tap water in their homes, and the purity of this imported water is often unacceptable.

Otitis media, an inflammation of the middle ear, is another major health problem among many Native Americans. In comparison, otitis media is not even considered to be a minor problem for the general United States population. Seventy-five percent of the cases found among Native Americans occur in preschool children.[20] This condition is a specific concern because it can result in permanent hearing impairment. The cause of this problem is uncertain. There is some evidence that poor sanitation in the home environment may be a predisposing factor. Without proper screening for hearing deficiencies and with little knowledge of the problem, many Native Americans develop serious and permanent loss of hearing. Therefore, training in the proper care of the ears is a priority for Native Americans.

Mental health problems are also much greater among Native Americans than the national average. Although hospital days in mental health facilities have increased in recent years, this is not an indication of increased incidence of mental illness. Rather, it probably signifies the fact that Native Americans are less resistant to seeking help for mental disorders today than was the case in the past. The most common mental health disorders found among Native Americans are alcoholism, drug abuse, schizophrenia, neurosis, personality disorders, and organic brain syndrome.[21]

Homicide and suicide occur with alarming frequency on many reservations. Suicide is a special problem among teenagers. Conflicting values, expectations, and changing cultural patterns produce stress that results in a variety of maladaptive behavioral patterns.

The only available health service for many Native Americans is provided by the Indian Health Service. The difficulty in providing health care to many clients, however, is compounded by the distances that separate homes from medical facilities. It is not unusual to find people living fifty to a hundred miles or more from the nearest health clinic. Many communities, isolated by miles from a clinic or a hospital, may be visited by a physician or a nurse. Such visits occur sporadically, resulting in a critical problem if medical help is needed in an emergency.

There have been some efforts made to improve the health status of Native Americans. In 1976, the federal government passed the Indian Health Care Improvement Act. The purpose of this legislation was to authorize funds for the improvement of the health status of Native Americans. As a result, health services on the reservations have expanded, safe drinking water and sanitary disposal facilities have been constructed, and the number of Native Americans trained to serve as health providers has increased. But the future health status of Native Americans is dependent upon even more extensive measures.

Refugees

The United States has always been a nation to which people migrated for a life free of oppression. The founding fathers of this nation came to the new world seeking freedom and independence. These opportunities have encouraged a renewed influx of refugees, particularly since the latter part of the 1970s.

The greatest number of refugees have come from Southeast Asia. Laotians were the first Asian group to arrive in rather large numbers in the 1970s. Then thousands of Vietnamese people immigrated, after the war, seeking freedom and protection from the new totalitarian government in Vietnam. Most of these people endured extreme physical hardships, many coming on overcrowded boats, experiencing hunger and thirst, piracy, and the loss of relatives and friends. A number of these people also experienced total economic loss. During the previous regime, many of these immigrants were merchants, businessmen, government employees, soldiers, and educated professionals. Because of their role in the former society and their affiliations with the United States government in some instances, the new Vietnamese government sought to kill or "retrain" these people. Many lost their positions, their possessions, and even their families.

Following the victory of the Khmer Communist government in Kampuchea (Cambodia) in 1975, thousands of people sought refuge in Thailand. Here these people experienced extreme malnutrition, among other traumas. Some of these Kampucheans have left the Thai refugee camps and have been admitted into the United States. Thousands still remain at the camps, with little hope for an early resolution to their refugee status.

Refugees have come to the United States from other parts of the world. The most recent influx has come from Central America, where civil war has uprooted many people. Many refugees have also come from Cuba and Haiti. In 1980, approximately 125,000 refugees came to Florida from Cuba in what was called the "freedom Flotilla."[22] However, resettlement of these individuals throughout the country met with numerous problems. Refugees from Haiti have immigrated, hoping to find a better life, particularly food to eat, land on which to live, and an opportunity for employment. The entrance of these illegal aliens has had a serious impact on many health and social services in a number of communities, especially in the state of Florida.

As refugees come to the United States, they are faced with a variety of adaptation problems. Language presents a significant barrier that must be overcome. Health is another major concern. As refugees become a part of our communities, their health has a significant effect on the health of the community.

Malnutrition is a common problem faced by refugees. Those who are sponsored for admittance into the United States, however, usually are not malnourished by the time they immigrate. Many do experience food ingestion and diet problems though. Some refugees, particularly Asians, dislike milk and dairy products and often experience diarrhea and stomach cramps if they consume even small amounts of these products.

Refugees often come to the United States with a number of diseases. Tuberculosis, intestinal parasites, skin infections, and malaria are common. Very few refugee children have obtained the required immunizations for polio, DPT, and measles before their arrival in the local community.[23]

Many refugees are not familiar with the concepts of modern medicine. They find a visit to a physician or to a clinic to be very foreign. Therefore, it is important that someone on the medical staff of the health care facility be present to calm their apprehensions or that a translator be present to interpret the conversation with the patients. It is helpful if the medical staff is sympathetic and familiar with the various cultural beliefs that affect the health practices of the newcomers.

In many instances, reliance upon folk and traditional healing practices is a part of these cultural beliefs. This is particularly the case of the individuals who have come from rural localities. For example, Haitians who believe in voodoo have been difficult to treat in some medical settings.

Some refugee health problems and diseases are difficult to cope with in the United States because most medical providers have had little experience with them. One disease has been a most mysterious problem. Over a period of about two years in the early 1980s, some twenty-five Laotians died of a mysterious condition. These seemingly healthy young males suddenly became ill and died for no recognized reason. The exact cause still remains unresolved.

The influx of refugees from Southeast Asia has been supported by the federal Indo-Chinese Migration and Refugee Act. Under provisions of this program, the government provides support for a family to establish itself in a community. This support is discontinued after the English language and marketable skills are learned. After this, the family is expected to become self-supporting. Often this takes a period of months or even years. As a result, many refugees become the recipients of welfare. Medicaid and food stamps are included in the welfare payments. Unfortunately, since refugees are usually better off on welfare than they were in their home countries, some tend to remain on welfare even after they are able to function independently. The unemployment problems of the 1980s have contributed to the difficulty of many refugees in finding work and becoming self-sufficient.

Community Health Centers

A major public health program to improve the access to medical care by the poor is the establishment of community health centers. Primary health care for low-income families in both rural and urban settings is provided at community health centers (CHC).

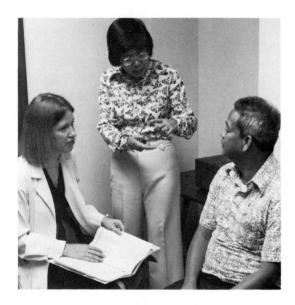

At the Neighborhood Health Center in the Kalihi-Palama area of Honolulu, Hawaii, this Vietnamese man is informed through a translator of the treatment the Center's physician has prescribed for him. This center was established in 1977 with the help of the Kellogg Foundation.

In many urban communities, the major health care facility for low-income residents has been the local hospital. The hospital, however, is an inappropriate source of primary health care. The services available at the hospital clinic are treatment oriented and not preventive in nature. The development of community health centers has helped to reduce this reliance on hospital care.

The community health center delivers accessible, comprehensive, integrated, and family-oriented health care. The kinds of services available vary from one locality to another, but medical, pediatric, surgical, nutritional, and dental services are usually available.

The central location of community health centers helps to overcome an important barrier to obtaining health care—travel. The proximity of the needed facilities encourages these residents to obtain health care when needed.

It is important that community residents understand what services are available and the procedures for obtaining them so that minor hospitalizations can be avoided. Many citizens often are not aware of the services available so they continue to use the more expensive outpatient department of the local hospital. They do not know that quality care can be provided at another location. It has been difficult to encourage people to turn from the traditional health care facility—the hospital—to a new facility, even though it can be shown that effective service is provided at the community health center.

Federal support of community health centers has changed in the 1980s. Congress has shifted administration and support to the primary care block-grant program. States are increasingly operating and funding these centers. They must match federal funds with their own monies. This reduction in federal support and the resultant financial problems faced by many state governments leave the future operation level of community health centers in question.

Summary

The economically disadvantaged portion of the United States population usually does not experience as high a level of well-being as does the general population. This lower level of health is evidenced by malnutrition, increased respiratory disease, and an overall lack of physical and emotional wellness. Health promotion and disease prevention measures are not particularly important to the poor, so illness and other medical problems are usually in the advanced stages by the time treatment is sought. Their limited financial resources are not spent on health unless it is absolutely necessary.

The poor often do not have access to needed health care facilities and services. For many, the emergency outpatient department of the hospital or the health clinic of the public health department is the entry point to the health care system.

In the United States, several minority populations are economically disadvantaged. Blacks, Hispanics, Native Americans, and refugees constitute specific groups most in need of community health programming. Each of these groups tends to have many of the health problems associated with poverty. In addition, each group has unique health concerns.

The health status of a majority of blacks in the United States is not what it should be. This is usually because of the lack of health care services in communities where many blacks live—the inner-city and rural localities. For many blacks, the health provider is not a person with whom they can easily identify.

A specific health problem of major proportion among blacks is sickle-cell disease. Screening of blood cells for sickle-cell trait is very important in coping with this problem. Education and counseling measures are needed so that people understand the results of this screening activity.

The United States is home to a growing Spanish-speaking population. Their health problems are compounded by language and cultural barriers. The mobility of Spanish-speaking migrants also makes ongoing comprehensive health care very difficult.

Several health problems can be noted among Native Americans. One of the most serious is alcoholism. Various efforts have been initiated to help the Native American population with this problem. Other health problems that afflict these people include diarrhea and otitis media.

In recent years there has been a large influx of refugees into the United States. They have brought various health problems with them, including respiratory diseases and digestive problems. Treatment of these problems and instruction in preventive measures are hampered by the refugees' unfamiliarity with western medicine.

An important community health measure designed to meet the health needs of the economically disadvantaged is the community health center. These centers, located in medically underserved areas, often provide the only health care available to many minority people. The reception these health care centers receive from the minorities is often dependent upon good planning. This takes into consideration the medical needs and interests of the citizens. Citizen involvement in this planning process is more likely to make the cultural background of the specific community a factor in planning.

Discussion Questions

1. Discuss some of the relationships observed between poverty and the status of health and well-being of a population group.

2. What is the level of poverty as identified in the United States?

3. Why do the poor tend to make less use of health care facilities than do the middle and upper class?

4. Explain why health is not a high priority among the poor.

5. In what ways does transportation play a role in the health care of the economically disadvantaged?

6. What were some of the reported findings of the Secretary's Task Force on Black and Minority Health as it relates to health of the black population?

7. Discuss the future impact of the recommendations made by the Secretary's Task Force on Black and Minority Health.

8. What are the differences between sickle-cell trait and sickle-cell disease?

9. What unique dimensions are presented in working in health facilities that serve Hispanics?

10. Discuss some of the specific cultural considerations that influence the concept of medicine among Hispanics.

11. What are specific problems that present themselves in providing health care to migrants?

12. What kinds of services are provided by the Indian Health Service?

13. Discuss the problem of alcoholism among Native Americans.

14. What is otitis media and to what degree is it a problem among Native Americans?

15. What are some considerations that must be taken into account when providing health care to refugees in the United States?

16. What health problems do refugees from Southeast Asia experience?

17. Discuss the importance of folk medicine to refugees.

18. How do community health centers meet the health needs of low-income families?

Suggested Readings

Anderson, Ronald M., and others. "Access of Hispanics to Health Care and Cuts in Services: A State-of-the-Art Overview." *Public Health Reports* 101, no. 3 (May/June, 1986): 238–52.

Chi, Peter S. K. "Medical Utilization Patterns of Migrant Farm Workers in Wayne County, New York." *Public Health Reports* 100, no. 5 (September/October, 1985): 480–90.

Coulehan, John L. "Acute Myocardial Infarction Among Navajo Indians, 1976–83." *American Journal of Public Health* 76, no. 4 (April, 1986): 412–14.

Dahlberg, Keith. "Medical Care of Cambodian Refugees." *Journal of the American Medical Association* 243, no. 10 (March 14, 1980): 1062–65.

Erickson, Roy V., and Hoang, Giao Hgoc. "Health Problems Among IndoChinese Refugees." *American Journal of Public Health* 70, no. 9 (September, 1980): 1003–05.

Goodwin, Melvin H.; Shaw, James R.; and Feldman, Clyde M. "Distribution of Otitis Media Among Four Indian Populations in Arizona." *Public Health Reports* 95, no. 6 (November/December, 1980): 589–94.

Heckler, Margaret H., Secretary. *Report of the Secretary's Task Force on Black and Minority Health.* United States Department of Health and Human Services, Washington, D.C.: U.S. Government Printing Office, 1985: 239 pp.

Marcus, Alfred C., and Crane, Lori A. "Smoking Behavior among U.S. Latinos: An Emerging Challenge for Public Health." *American Journal of Public Health* 75, no. 2 (February, 1985): 169–72.

Markides, Kyriakos S., and Careil, Jeanne. "The Health of Hispanics in the Southwestern United States: an Epidemiologic Paradox." *Public Health Reports* 101, no. 3 (May/June, 1986): 253–65.

Owens, Mitchell V.; Cameron, Charles M.; and Hickman, Patti. "Job Achievements of Indian and Non-Indian Graduates in Public Health: How Do They Compare?" *Public Health Reports* 102, no. 4 (July/August, 1987): 372–76.

Rhoades, Everett R., et al. "Mental Health Problems of American Indians Seen in Outpatient Facilities of the Indian Health Service, 1975." *Public Health Reports* 95, no. 4 (July/August, 1980): 329–35.

Rhoades, Everett R.; D'Angelo, Anthony J.; and Hurlburt, Ward B. "The Indian Health Service Record of Achievement." *Public Health Reports* 102, no.4 (July/August, 1987): 356–60.

Rhoades, Everett R.; Reyes, Luana L.; and Buzzard, George D. "The Organization of Health Services for Indian People." *Public Health Reports* 102, no. 4 (July/August, 1987): 352–56.

Rudov, Melvin H., and Santangelo, Nancy. *Health Status of Minorities and Low-Income Groups.* Washington, D.C.: U.S. Government Printing Office, 1979.

Endnotes

1. *Report of the Secretary's Task Force on Black and Minority Health.* U.S. Department of Health and Human Services: U.S. Government Printing Office, 1985: 1.

2. *Statistical Abstracts of the United States, 1985:* 429.

3. Rudov, M. H., and Santangelo, N. *Health Status of Minorities and Low-Income Groups.* Washington, D.C.: U.S. Government Printing Office, 1979, 6.

4. Topics are discussed in chapter 16 and 20.

5. *Report of Secretary's Task Force.*

6. Comparative data presented in this section is from the Division of Vital Statistics, National Center for Health Statistics, Washington, D.C.

7. *Report of Secretary's Task Force,* 88.

8. Lin-Fu, Jane S. *Sickle-Cell Anemia: A Medical Review.* Rockville, Md.: Department of HEW, Bureau of Community Health Services, 1978, 2.

9. *Report of Secretary's Task Force,* 53.

10. Markides, Kyriakos S., and Careil, Jeanne. "The Health of Hispanics in the Southwestern United States: An Epidemiologic Paradox." *Public Health Reports* 101, no. 3 (May/June, 1986), 258.

11. *Report of Secretary's Task Force,* 54.

12. Ibid., 54.

13. Madsen, William. *The Mexican American of South Texas.* New York: Holt, Rinehart, and Winston, 1964, 71.

14. Slesinger, D. P., and Cautley, E. "Medical Utilization Patterns of Hispanic Migrant Farmworkers in Wisconsin." *Public Health Reports* 96, no. 3 (1981): 261.

15. Chi, Peter S. K. "Medical Utilization Patterns of Migrant Farm Workers in Wayne County, New York." *Public Health Reports* 100, no. 5 (September/October, 1985): 480–90.

16. Department of Health, Education, and Welfare. *Health, United States, 1979.* Washington, D.C.: U.S. Government Printing Office, 1979, 16.

17. Ibid., 16.

18. *Report of Secretary's Task Force,* 57.

19. Department of Health, Education, and Welfare. *Health, United States, 1979,* 16.

20. Goodwin, M. H.; Shaw, J. R.; and Feldman, C. M. "Distribution of Otitis Media Among Four Indian Populations in Arizona." *Public Health Reports* 96, no. 6 (1980): 589–94.

21. Rhoades, E. R., et al. "Mental Health Problems of American Indians Seen in Outpatient Facilities of the Indian Health Service, 1975." *Public Health Reports* 95, no. 4 (1980): 329–35.

22. Department of Health and Human Services, Office of Refugee Settlement. *Statistical Abstracts of the United States,* 1981, 90.

23. Erickson, R. V., and Hoang, G. H. "Health Problems Among Indo-Chinese Refugees." *American Journal of Public Health* 70, no. 9 (1980): 1004.

16

Child and Maternal Health: A Measure of a Community's Well-Being

> "Health problems related to infants and mothers are controllable and great strides have been made. However, the levels of control already attained can be reduced if vigilance is lowered or resources and efforts are cut back."[1]

The period of time from conception through pregnancy, childbirth, and until a child enters school is one of extreme importance to an individual's health and well-being. These years are a time of great growth and development that plays a large role in the future physical and emotional status of a person. Not only do congenital and environmental conditions influence the infant and young child, but the health status of the mother also has a profound effect on the health and well-being of her child.

A variety of maternal factors affects the health of a fetus. For instance, because the fetus is dependent upon the mother for food, water, oxygen, and the disposal of waste products, the physical and emotional state of the mother during this period of time has a direct influence on the fetus. The mother's nutritional status, her age, and the presence of infectious diseases all affect the condition of the fetus. Use of drugs, alcohol, or tobacco by the mother can result in low infant birthweight, a leading cause of infant mortality.

Child health has improved tremendously in the past fifty years. Infant mortality has been reduced significantly, as has maternal mortality. Many of the childhood diseases that caused much suffering and death in the early part of this century have been virtually eliminated by immunization programs. To a great extent, nutrition-deficiency diseases have been reduced. Yet in spite of these positive strides in infant and child health, many improvements still require the attention of community health programming and health policy planners.

Infant Mortality

Measures of the quality of infants' and mothers' health are an indication of the overall health of a society, a community, or cultural group. In a nation where the infant and maternal mortality rates are high, it is very likely that the inhabitants experience a wide range of health problems. If nutrition and health care are inadequate, communicable diseases cause even more sickness and debilitation. Infant mortality is thus closely allied to poverty.

History has shown that as infant and maternal health improve in a cultural group, so does the overall health of the people. This is evident in the history of the United States. At the turn of this century, the infant mortality rate within the first year of life exceeded one hundred deaths per one thousand live births. Communicable diseases were the leading cause of these deaths, although many resulted from poor prenatal care.

By 1950 the infant mortality rate had been reduced to about twenty-nine per one thousand live births, and by 1965 it had fallen to below twenty-five per one thousand live births. In the past two decades this statistic has been further reduced by more than one half; today the infant mortality rate is slightly below eleven (10.5) per one thousand live births.

It is not known whether this rate can be further reduced or, if possible, to what degree. The Surgeon General's Report on Disease Prevention and Health Promotion set as a national goal the rate of nine per one thousand live births by the year 1990.[2] This goal would seem to be attainable. However, the United States still ranks fourteenth among all nations in its infant mortality rate despite its great wealth and resources. A wide discrepancy in infant mortality rates exists among states, with three states having infant mortality rates less than eight (Wyoming, Montana, and Wisconsin) and three states having rates of more than fourteen (South Carolina, Mississippi, and Alabama).[3]

Infant Mortality, Worldwide

Nation	Rate
1. Finland	6.0
2. Japan	6.2
3. Sweden	7.0
4. Switzerland	7.7
5. Norway	7.8
6. Denmark	8.2
7. Netherlands	8.4
8. France	9.0
9. Canada	9.1
10. Belgium	9.2
11. Spain	9.6
12. West Germany	10.1
12. United Kingdom	10.1
13. Australia	10.3
14. United States	10.5

Source: World Population Data Sheet, Population Reference Bureau, 1985.

Even though there has been a measure of success in improving infant mortality rates and the health status of infants and children, not every economic and racial group in the United States has benefited. The infant mortality rate of black newborn babies is nearly double the national figure. The same is true among infants born to economically disadvantaged families of all races.

A significant public health problem in our society is teenage pregnancies. Nearly a half-million infants are born annually to unwed teenage girls, most of whom are economically poor and culturally disadvantaged. Unmarried black teenagers are five times more likely to become pregnant than white teens.[4]

Economically disadvantaged women often receive inadequate prenatal care. Prenatal care should begin as early in the first trimester of pregnancy as is possible so that potential risk factors can be minimized. The health status of the pregnant woman can be noted and appropriate obstetrical and gynecologic care can be planned. As many as 25 percent of all pregnant women in the United States do not receive adequate prenatal care in spite of its extreme importance.[5] The majority of these women are black, poor, and less educated.

Infants born to economically disadvantaged women are often not given adequate health care. This is the result of the uneven geographic distribution of health care facilities and providers, particularly in rural areas and in urban localities. Not only are health services often unavailable, but when available they are usually not utilized. Mothers may not use the health services for prenatal, postnatal, and early infant primary health care for such reasons as disinterest, a lack of money, or a poor understanding of the importance of such care. Often there are also racial or language barriers hindering the mothers.

Low Birthweight

Of all infant deaths, two out of three involve babies weighing less than twenty-five hundred grams (5.5 pounds) at birth. Low birthweight has been associated with a number of health problems. Not only is such an infant more likely to die within the first year, but future health can be adversely affected. There is an increased incidence of mental retardation, growth and development problems, birth defects, blindness, cerebral palsy, and various other neurological diseases.

A number of maternal factors contribute to low birthweight. The chances are three times greater for a pregnant woman to have a low birthweight infant when she has had inadequate prenatal care. This is quite often the case among teenage pregnancies and the poor.

Poor maternal nutrition has also been identified as a factor among those who deliver infants of low birthweight. Not only are nutritional habits during pregnancy important, but nutritional status before pregnancy is also relevant.

The premature infant begins life with several "strikes" against it including an increased risk of mental deficiencies, neurological diseases, and possible growth and developmental problems. Fortunately, medical technology has greatly enhanced the future of such infants in recent years.

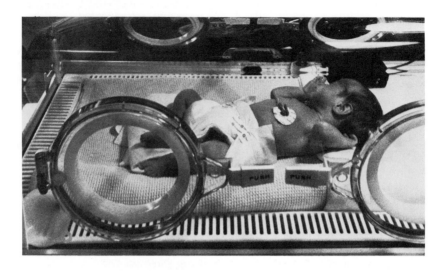

Other factors associated with low birthweight include maternal smoking and use of drugs and alcohol. Pregnant women who smoke have been found to be at higher risk for having a low birthweight baby.

Another concern is Fetal Alcohol Syndrome. This affects infants born to women who drink heavily during pregnancy. Such infants are often shorter and have low birthweight. Many are mentally retarded, have various body abnormalities, and have such problems as heart defects or eye and ear anomalies. At the present time there is no medical agreement as to what level of alcohol consumption can be considered safe. There is no absolutely safe level of alcohol consumption for the pregnant woman.[6]

The incidences of Fetal Alcohol Syndrome could be reduced by informing women through public education programs of the dangers of ingesting alcoholic beverages during pregnancy. Not only do pregnant women need such information, but men need to become better aware of the dangers to the fetus associated with drinking. They may be able to encourage their wives and/or other female acquaintances to refrain from the use of alcoholic beverages while pregnant.

Birth Defects

Second to low birthweight as a cause of infant mortality are birth defects. One out of ten births in the United States results in an infant with a birth defect. Information is continually being documented to add to the store of knowledge already completed on causes of birth defects. Environmental factors, especially, have received considerable attention in these studies.

The fetus is at special risk during the first trimester of pregnancy. During this period of time there are several recognized dangers associated with exposure to hazardous chemicals and radiation. Women who are exposed to such chemicals as lead, carbon monoxide, polyvinyl chloride, and anesthetic gas during early pregnancy may endanger their fetus's well-being.

Drugs taken during pregnancy have been linked to birth defects. One of the best documented cases is the effect of the sedative drug thalidomide on thousands of newborn babies during the 1960s. Thousands of women, principally in Europe, who used this drug while pregnant, gave birth to seriously malformed infants. Most babies were born without arms and/or legs.

Several drugs are known to cause birth defects. For example, use of the tranquilizer, chlormazanone, by pregnant women has been shown to increase the risk of infant malformation.[7] A hormone, diethylstilbestrol (DES), has been shown to have a relationship to birth defects when pregnant women are exposed to it. The fetus may also be affected by marijuana, and there is much evidence linking heroin use by pregnant women with the occurrence of heroin dependency in newborn infants.

Another high-risk factor related to congenital birth defects is maternal age. Teenage women and women thirty-five years of age and older are more likely to have infants born with birth defects. For example, the risk of having a Down's syndrome (a form of mental retardation) child increases when the mother is thirty-five years of age or older.

Several medical advances have helped to reduce the number of birth-related injuries and birth defects. One such medical development is electronic monitoring of the fetal heart rate, which can detect fetal distress during early labor. Such indications provide the physician with information that is helpful in delivering the baby. Potentially injurious complications can often be avoided.

Electronic fetal monitoring is not without its detractors. Some feel it leads to unnecessary cesarean operations. Others suggest that maternal infections are more prevalent when such procedures are used.

Amniocentesis has helped to reduce the incidence of birth defects in infants. By removing a small amount of amniotic fluid from the amniotic sac, certain birth defects can be identified early in pregnancy. Through genetic and medical counseling, decisions can be made about whether to continue a pregnancy or to terminate it.

Sudden Infant Death Syndrome

Nearly ten thousand infant deaths occur annually from Sudden Infant Death Syndrome (SIDS), usually during a child's first six months. The infant is put to bed in apparently good health and is later found dead in the crib, having stopped breathing for apparently no reason. This syndrome, then, has also been referred to as "crib death."

There are presently no known causes of Sudden Infant Death Syndrome, though several theories and relational observations have been noted.[8] Some feel that SIDS might be the result of a minor viral infection in the airway. Others have noted that SIDS occurs quite often among premature infants and in infants with central nervous system abnormalities. Abnormalities of autonomic regulation of respiratory and cardiovascular functions have been noted. Whether this is due to genetic or environmental factors is unknown.[9] There also seems to be a relationship with low socioeconomic status. Blacks and Native Americans have a two to three times greater risk of having SIDS than whites.[10]

Some reports suggest that SIDS may be associated with certain other risk factors. One associated risk factor is maternal age—being less than twenty at the first pregnancy. Other risk factors that have been identified are sex (more males die of SIDS than females), and certain prenatal problems. Many SIDS victims have had hypoxia (a condition where there is a reduced supply of oxygen) during this period. There are also increased incidences of Sudden Infant Death Syndrome during the winter months.

In addition to the trauma of losing an infant, most SIDS parents carry heavy guilt over the loss. They often wonder if in some way their seemingly normal child may have died as the result of their negligence. There is little that parents can be taught of a preventive nature due to the lack of information regarding the etiology of Sudden Infant Death Syndrome.

Parents and Birth Crisis

Parents experiencing a birth-related crisis, such as the death of an infant, a stillbirth, or the birth of a baby with a defect, need support and comfort. Such an experience is emotionally difficult. Parents of a retarded child or of an infant needing long-term hospital care are usually not prepared to cope with the situation. Therefore, it is important for communities to establish support programs for parents. Some hospitals have provided meaningful assistance activities. Volunteer groups in many localities come to the aid of grieving and distressed couples. Such aid must be extended over a period of weeks, months, or even years, until the mother and father have learned to cope with the crisis.

Immunization

For many years communicable diseases were the leading cause of death among children. But increased public health efforts at immunizing children of preschool age have resulted in a significant reduction in fatalities due to communicable diseases. There has also been a reduction in incidences of such diseases as diphtheria, pertussis, tetanus, measles, mumps, rubella, and polio.

Today all states require children to have certain immunizations prior to enrolling in school for the first time. However, there are various degrees of enforcement. In spite of school attempts, health department informational programs, and public media announcements, it has been estimated that as many as 40 percent of American children have not been immunized against one or more of the childhood diseases.[11]

The state health department in each state is responsible for establishing the standards of immunization. To assist the states the Centers for Disease Control has published a recommended immunization schedule for the states to follow. In 1986 the Centers for Disease Control made a major change in its recommended immunization schedule. Whereas previously CDC recommended that the DPT-4 (diphtheria, pertussis, and tetanus) and the OPV-3 (oral polio vaccine) be given at eighteen months, it now recommends that these be given with the MMR (measles, mumps, and rubella) vaccine at fifteen months. It is felt that this will reduce the number of necessary visits to the physician or health clinic and in turn will help to reduce costs.

Through the 1970s immunization levels for mumps, rubella, and measles increased. Mumps, though usually the least serious of these three diseases, has been known to cause serious complications. Central nervous system problems and deafness have occasionally resulted from mumps. In adults, mumps may cause sterility if the reproductive organs are affected.

Rubella is of great concern to pregnant women. The fetus may be affected if the woman has rubella early in her pregnancy. Immunization of young women should only occur when there is no chance of pregnancy.

Measles is considered the most serious of the childhood communicable diseases. The most dangerous measles complication is encephalitis, an inflammation of the brain that can cause permanent brain damage and retardation. In the mid-1980s an increase in the number of cases of measles was observed.[12] The actual number of cases increased over 100 percent from the previous year. The incidence

Recommended Immunization Schedule

Age	Immunization
2 months	DPT-1 (diphtheria, pertussis, and tetanus)
	OPV-1 (oral polio vaccine)
4 months	DPT-2
	OPV-2
6 months	DPT-3
15 months	DPT-4
	OPV-3
	MMR (measles, mumps, and rubella)
4–6 years	DPT-5
	OPV-4
14–16 years	Tetanus and Diphtheria Toxoid (for adult dose)

Source: Centers for Disease Control. "New Recommended Schedule for Active Immunization of Normal Infants and Children." *Morbidity and Mortality Weekly Report* 35, no. 37 (September 19, 1986): 577–79.

rate rose from .8 per 100,000 to 1.7 per 100,000 population in one year. The incidence rate was observed in all age groups with the highest incidence rate being among children of preschool age, 0 to 4 years. The greatest increase in incidence rate occurred among children of the 10-to-14-year age group. Over half (55.6 percent) of the cases were acquired at school. Nearly 60 percent were unvaccinated or had been vaccinated prior to their first birthdays. There are still many children of school age who are not adequately immunized for measles. A serious need exists to focus measles preventive measures on preschool-age children over fifteen months of age.[13]

Some public health concern has arisen over the decrease in immunizations for diphtheria, pertussis, tetanus, and polio over the last several years. The incidences of all four of these diseases have been reduced to very low levels.[14] But possibly because of these low incidence levels, parental concern for having children properly immunized has decreased. Greater public health and school health service efforts are needed to keep immunization levels at a safe and effective level.

As with many health problems, the preschool-age children who are not immunized are most likely the poor and those residing in the inner city. Immunization of these children is often made available through the programs of local health departments and community health centers. The parents need to be informed and educated as to when each procedure should be given. The combined efforts, then, of the public health agency and school officials can effectively increase immunization levels and decrease the number of communicable disease cases.

Teenage Pregnancy

One of the major public health problems in the United States today is teenage pregnancy. Over a million girls under the age of nineteen become pregnant each year. This averages to at least one in ten teenage girls becoming pregnant.[15] Four out of five teens who become pregnant are unmarried. Twenty-five percent of all teenage females in the United States have had at least one pregnancy and many of these have had multiple pregnancies before reaching the age of twenty. Among teenage mothers, more than 25 percent become pregnant again within the first year after their first delivery.[16] Teenage pregnancy is a problem of increasing intensity with little indication of abatement in the future.

The large number of teenage pregnancies can be attributed to several factors, but increased sexual experience by young adolescents is a major reason. At least twelve million adolescents between the ages of thirteen and nineteen are sexually active. Fifty percent of teenage girls in the United States have had premarital sexual intercourse. The average age at which teenagers begin to experience intercourse is about 16.4 for whites and 15.5 for blacks.[17]

Another reason for the increase in teenage pregnancies is that the most effective medical methods of contraception—the pill and the intra-uterine device—are not commonly used by teenagers. Instead, less effective contraceptive measures—the diaphragm, withdrawal, and rhythm—are being employed.[18] The reduction in the use of the pill and the IUD can be attributed to several factors, but primarily to the publicity given to the health risks of each. Nearly two-thirds of unwed teenagers do not practice contraception at all, or they are inconsistent in their use of a particular method. This ineffective use of contraceptives is highlighted by the fact that nearly one-half of all teenage pregnancies occur in the first six months after beginning sexual intercourse.

Most teenage pregnancies are not wanted. In fact, four out of every five (82 percent) are unwanted.[19] Such a dramatic figure points out the severe social problems caused by teenage pregnancy. Because of these consequences and because adolescents are not using effective contraceptives it seems important to educate them on birth control measures.

However, providing contraceptive information to young adolescents is a controversial issue. Most teenagers have little accurate information about birth control measures. What they do know has usually been obtained from friends, the movies, or other nonstructured sources. Thus any public health activity directed at preventing adolescent pregnancy should include sex education and information about contraceptives and their effective use.

The school would seem the likely place for the sex education classes that include instruction about contraception. However, many school districts fail to provide such instruction. In many school districts where sex education is part of the school curriculum, birth control information is expressly prohibited.

In 1985 the state legislature in Wisconsin passed legislation that provides funding for sex education instruction in public schools. In addition funds are provided for counseling of pregnant adolescents. The Wisconsin legislature also passed rather controversial legislation making grandparents of babies born to teenagers legally responsible for the babies' financial support.

Since the schools have been ineffective in providing appropriate contraceptive information to teenagers and because parents fail to inform their children about this matter, it becomes evident that community health agencies must fill this void. This has been one of the important services provided by various family planning agencies. Other agencies with programming for young adolescents help the sexually active teenager to make responsible decisions about birth control. Not only should educational and counseling services be available for females, but the adolescent male also needs information regarding contraception, pregnancy, and sexuality in order to make decisions on responsible sexual behavior.

Health Effects

There are many health problems associated with teenage pregnancy. Childbearing during the teen years is a high-risk experience. Infant and maternal mortality rates are much greater in teenage births than other maternal age groups. Infant mortality is twice as high in teenage births than in other age groups, while maternal mortality is nearly two and a half times as great.

Low birthweight infants are a serious problem. A teen mother is twice as likely to have a low birthweight baby as is a mother between the ages of twenty and thirty-five. Infants born weighing below twenty-five hundred grams (5.5 pounds) are more than twenty times as likely to die before the age of one year.[20] The number of premature infants born to teenagers has increased since 1980 with the majority being born to economically poor minorities.[21]

There are a number of factors that result in low birthweight babies born to teenage mothers. Lack of prenatal care and the expectant mother's poor nutrition are often the source of the problem. Also, the use of tobacco, alcohol, and drugs have been associated with premature deliveries.

In order to protect against low birthweight, the expectant mother needs improved prenatal health care and improved nutrition. Early prenatal medical care is very important. Such care should include pregnancy testing and then appropriate checkups during the pregnancy. Once the infant is born, both baby and mother should receive postnatal medical attention. Although for many young mothers the only medical services that are available are those of the local health department or of a community family planning agency, even these would improve the well-being of both mother and child.

Social Services

Many social problems are asssociated with teenage pregnancy and motherhood. Today it is very uncommon for an unmarried teenage mother to give up her baby for adoption or for care by friends or relatives. Ninety-six percent of unmarried teenage mothers keep their infants.[22] Various health and social services for both mother and infant and day-care services for the infant are needed in many communities as a result.

In all likelihood the child will be raised in a single-parent family. Because of a lack of education and job skills, the teenage mother is usually unable to financially support her family. As a result, many teenage mothers and their infants live in economic poverty and encounter related social problems.

Social services must include counseling, financial support, day-care services, and legal services. It is also important for the mother to have the opportunity to further her education, which has more often than not been interrupted because of the pregnancy. However, vocational training for the teenage mother is often not a reality in many communities.

Family Planning Services

Another important community service that assists not only pregnant teenagers but also individuals of all ages and social groups is family planning. Family planning services have come a long way since the early twentieth century when Margaret Sanger opened the first birth control clinic in 1916 in Brooklyn, New York. Operation of this clinic was illegal according to the laws of that time. On several occasions it was raided by the New York vice squad, and Sanger was frequently arrested and put into jail. In time, however, Margaret Sanger organized a group called the Birth Control League. This organization was the forerunner of the present Planned Parenthood Association which provides family planning services to the nation's communities.

Many women become pregnant and bear children who are neither planned nor wanted. Although the exact number of such pregnancies is unknown, accumulated data leaves little doubt that most of the nearly one million teenage pregnancies are not planned. Many other couples wish to plan their families and have some time space between children. For these parents contraceptive information and family planning services are very important. But others have not conceived for a variety of reasons. Information on conception is as important to those individuals as contraception is to others. All of these circumstances show why comprehensive family planning has become an important community health activity.

Ideally, all pregnancies should be wanted pregnancies. Therefore, family planning services must include information about how to space a family and

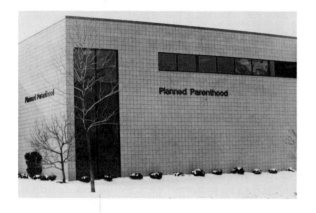

The services of Planned Parenthood include a broad range of family planning services. An individual can receive prenatal care, birth control information and contraceptives, educational services, and counseling, as well as preventive emphasis relating to family planning, at Planned Parenthood Centers throughout the nation.

how to care for infants, as well as providing information about contraception. The services provided for family planning should be viewed as a part of primary and preventive health care.

Family planning services are provided in many different settings. For many couples a personal physician, general practitioner, or an obstetrician may be the source of information, counseling, and service concerning these matters. The physician can help the couple to better understand contraception, family planning, child spacing, and infant care, and can provide needed services to the couple.

For other individuals and couples there may not be a physician to whom they can turn. As a result family planning services have been established in different community health agencies and programs. Local health departments and community neighborhood health centers usually provide these services. Hospitals or specific agencies such as Planned Parenthood affiliates offer family planning services. There are more than five thousand family planning clinics in the United States.[23] Most family planning clinics tend to serve primarily low-income individuals.

Family planning agencies provide a number of services, but education is the most important component of their family planning program. Educational activities include information about reproductive anatomy and physiology as well as about various contraceptive methods. Studies have shown that many young people, particularly teenagers, have little accurate information about human reproduction. This is due in part to the failure of parents and the schools to provide this information to young people.

Counseling is another important aspect of family planning. Counseling must be designed to help an individual or couple to make intelligent decisions concerning contraception, medical procedures needed during pregnancy, and other pertinent matters.

Many family planning centers perform pregnancy screening, a relatively simple procedure. This screening, however, should be accompanied by counseling. If a woman is pregnant, it is important that prenatal care is discussed. Appointments for periodic follow-up should be established. If the woman is not pregnant, counseling, particularly about contraception, is still useful.

Many teenagers will not consult with a family planning service out of fear of parental reactions. Either they do not want their parents to know of their sexual activity or the relationship of the two sexual partners is unstable.

The question of teenagers being given counseling and the services of a family planning center has created several complex issues. Most family planning clinics do not require parental consent or notification prior to providing such service to a teenager. The United States Supreme Court has ruled it unconstitutional to legally require parental consent before contraceptives can be given to teenagers. However, the federal government attempted to impose a regulation that would have required any federally subsidized health clinic to notify the parents of any teenager under eighteen years of age who applies for contraception. This regulation, referred to by many as the "squeal rule," has been opposed by many family planning specialists, educators, social workers, and young people. The assumption is that

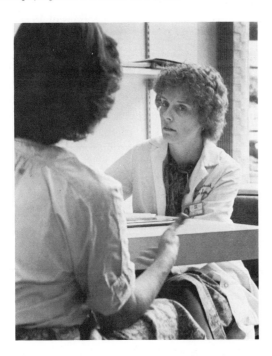

Family planning agencies have provided birth control information and contraceptives to young people. Without the opportunity to obtain this reliable birth control counseling, the number of teenage pregnancies would be even greater.

many teenagers needing contraceptives would not seek them because they do not wish their parents to be aware of their sexual activity. These people contend that such a regulation would lead to more unwanted pregnancies and have no impact on the level of sexual activity among teenagers. The position of the federal government in requesting such a regulation was that it would help to restore parental authority in the lives of teenagers and would thereby reduce sexual activity. This hotly contested governmental regulation has been overrruled by the courts.

Several medical services can be found in family planning centers. A pregnant woman may undergo a comprehensive physical examination that includes a complete health history, along with blood and urine laboratory analysis so that as much as possible is learned about the health status of the woman. Other tests available through family planning centers include Pap smears, gonorrheal cultures, serologic tests for syphilis, and tests for other sexually transmitted diseases.

Both male and female sterilization have become increasingly common in the past decade. This procedure is now the most commonly used form of contraception in the United States. These procedures are often performed in family planning centers. As with any major medical procedure, it is important that the individual is properly informed about the permanent nature of this action.

All too often the perceived role of family planning services is directed only toward the female. A need exists to also provide services to the male. The issue of male responsibility in adolescent pregnancy is often not dealt with by many family planning counselors and program planners. When one realizes that most sexual activity is initiated by the male, it becomes obvious that no major resolutions to problems of teenage pregnancy will occur without focusing on the male, as well as the female. Increasingly, the need to focus contraceptive and family planning educational programs on the key role the male plays is being considered by many family planning organizations and agencies.[24]

Not all family planning services involve pregnancy or contraception. Many couples are unable to have children. Because of this, it is often necessary for both the male and female to undergo infertility testing and to receive appropriate instruction and counseling. Though not as common, these services are available in some community family planning centers.

Abortion

Possibly the most controversial and emotional issue in public health today is abortion. Prior to the 1960s, it was illegal to obtain an abortion in the United States unless certain medical reasons made the procedure necessary. When an illegal abortion was performed, it usually resulted in complications, diseases, and sometimes death.

Throughout the 1960s there were several unsuccessful attempts to legalize abortion. But not until 1967, when the state of Colorado passed a liberalized abortion law, did states begin to change their laws to permit abortion. By January 1973, when the

United States Supreme Court declared existing state laws prohibiting abortion unconstitutional, sixteen other states had passed liberalized abortion laws. The Supreme Court announced its decision in the cases of *Roe v. Wade* and *Doe v. Bolton.*

In these landmark legal decisions it was concluded that the unborn is not a person and therefore has no rights under the law. The woman's right to have an abortion was supported by the Supreme Court; the state could not interfere with this right. This legal decision left the decision to have an abortion to the pregnant woman and her physician, but only during the first twelve weeks of pregnancy. After the first trimester, the state could permit abortion only in cases that would preserve and protect the health of the mother. Abortion during the third trimester was prohibited unless the measure was necessary to preserve the life of the pregnant woman.

Since the Supreme Court decisions, the number of abortions performed each year has increased dramatically. One-fourth of all pregnancies end in abortion. There are about 1.5 million abortions in the United States each year.[25] One in three was obtained by a teenager—supporting the statistics that women who had abortions were mainly young, white (69 percent), unmarried, and childless.[26] Three out of every four abortions take place in a nonhospital abortion facility.[27]

The availability of abortion services and facilities has met with increasing opposition, which has taken on political and religious dimensions. It has resulted in a clash between two groups with different value systems and viewpoints. Each is asking government to impose their viewpoint on the other.

The major opposition, or "pro-life" groups, voice theological or religious arguments. These opponents contend that abortion is an act of murder or the direct taking of life, since they believe that life begins at conception. An embryo has human characteristics and therefore is a person. Any action that destroys this fertilized egg is tantamount to murder and should be ruled unconstitutional.

In 1976 the United States Congress approved the Hyde Amendment. This legislation forbade the use of federal monies for funding abortions except when the woman's life was threatened. This action halted Medicaid reimbursement for abortions. As a result, many women, particularly indigent women, could not obtain legal abortions.

During the congressional elections of 1978 and the national presidential campaign of 1980 the question of abortion attracted much attention. In most political conflict there is a common ground between poles where a compromise can be worked out. However, it appears there is no such area of compromise when the conflict concerns abortion. For the antiabortion, or pro-life group, there simply is no room for compromise. Abortion is wrong and must not be permitted.

The pro-abortionists, or "pro-choice" group, argue the scientific and medical feasibility of the procedure and the issue of "the right of the mother." This group does not believe that a fertilized egg is a person, particularly during the first three months of pregnancy. Their concern is more toward an emphasis on individual rights than on reproduction. They believe that a woman's freedom rests in having control over her reproductive process. The woman has a right to make decisions regarding her bodily functioning.

In 1980 the Supreme Court upheld the constitutionality of the Hyde Amendment. Since 1980, with the election of an administration committed to the antiabortion position, major political activity concerning abortion has again surfaced. There has even been a constitutional amendment proposed in Congress that would ban abortion.

New advances in medical technology have compounded this issue. Physicians are able to save the lives of premature babies at earlier stages of the pregnancy. Today 24-to-26-week-old fetuses can survive with major life sustaining efforts. With the use of sonograms the medical profession can now view in much detail the developing fetus. Such technology has led many health care providers to have reservations about conducting abortions late in the first trimester and during the second trimester of pregnancy. In spite of the fact that most abortions occur during the first trimester, at times, due to improper timing, the abortion is done to a mid-trimester fetus. One is left with the question as to whether these fetuses are "viable."

An unfortunate development in this conflict has expanded recently with the opponents of abortion using violent tactics against abortion clinics. Demonstrations of harassment against those coming to abortion clinics have occurred. Picketing of abortion clinics, threats to doctors and nurses working in the clinics, and bombings of these facilities have taken place. Some clinics have difficulty getting physicians to perform abortions due to fear for personal safety. There have been a number of instances in which abortion clinics have been damaged or destroyed by fire bombs.

When the positions are so extreme and tenaciously held consensus is obviously unattainable and will not be reached in the near future. In many respects, it is unfortunate that a medical and health issue has turned into a political one. It can only be hoped that other measures of contraception will become so widely accepted that the need for abortion will be reduced. In theory this sounds good; in practice it is not likely to happen. The result? Continued bitter anamosity.

Cesarean Delivery

An operative procedure whereby the fetus is removed directly through the abdomen is known as cesarean section. This procedure is a relatively safe operation. It is necessary under certain circumstances, such as when there is a small pelvic opening in relation to the baby's head size, when there is malpresentation of the fetus for delivery, or when other obstacles are present, interfering with a normal delivery.

A dramatic increase in the number of cesarean deliveries has taken place in the 1980s. The number has increased fourfold between 1965 and the mid-1980s. One in five (20.3 percent) of all births is through cesarean delivery.

There are several concerns resulting from this development. Cesarean delivery is a more expensive procedure than a normal delivery. It requires a longer hospital stay—twice the time experienced by women having a normal vaginal delivery. Women without health insurance are less likely to have cesarean deliveries.

There is greater risk of injury or death to the mother from a cesarean delivery. Delivery complications are more common. There is increased risk of respiratory distress in infants born by cesarean section. The cesarean delivery must be considered a major operative procedure and as such the various potential problems associated with surgery accompany the birth process.

The important question being raised by this increase in cesarean deliveries is whether there is legitimate reason for such deliveries. Since for many women the operative procedure is covered by insurance, the reason for cesarean delivery may be economic. Hospitals with intensive care units for newborns and more sophisticated technology are more likely to perform cesarean deliveries. The possession of such equipment by many hospitals, some say makes it necessary to encourage its use from an economical point of view.[28]

Maternal and Child Health and the Government

The overall health of infants, children, and mothers has improved steadily throughout the twentieth century. Numerous reasons can be given for such improvement: increased medical technology, development of immunizations, improved nutritional status, and overall advanced knowledge relating to health. Some would suggest that improvement has been due in part to the increased involvement of government spending and programming in activities designed specifically to improve health.

The federal government has supported child health programs for many years. Several programs have made some positive contributions to the improved health of mothers and children. Though it would not be possible to review all public health accomplishments through the years, highlights should be noted.

Healthy Mothers, Healthy Babies Coalition

In 1982 a coalition of six organizations came together to improve maternal and infant health. The primary source of focus was to be accomplished through education. This coalition has expanded to include over eighty religious, health professional, and governmental organizations. The activities of this coalition are directed toward:

1. Providing information that encourages positive health habits for pregnant women
2. Motivating pregnant women to seek regular prenatal care and good nutrition
3. Informing women of health risks relating to childbearing

4. Developing understanding among men of the supportive role they play in pregnancy and infant care

State coalitions have been developed in over forty states. A broad range of programs bringing together private and public governmental agencies has been involved. Activities have been as widespread as conducting statewide television and radio media campaigns, providing crisis phone service and pregnancy hotlines for expectant women, working as lobbyists for increased funding for maternal-child health programs at the state legislative level, and establishing similar coalition programs in various cities.

Source: Arkin, Elaine Bratic. "The Healthy Mothers, Healthy Babies Coalition: Four Years of Progress." *Public Health Reports* 101, no. 2 (March/April, 1986): 147–56.

As early as 1935, under provisions of the Social Security Act, maternal and child health programs were funded. In the years since, several federal assistance programs have included child health.

During the 1960s a number of public programs not specifically designed for health included maternal and child health components. The Vaccination Assistance Act of 1962 made funds available to help local health departments immunize all preschool children. The Model Cities Programs established neighborhood health centers where preschool children could be given health services. Often these centers were the only source of health care for the poor and disadvantaged children.

The Head Start Program provided services to preschool children of low income families. The program included educational activities, medical provisions, social services, and nutritional services. Over 80 percent of the children enrolled in the Head Start Program also received medical screening. Most children who have had problems identified through these screenings have also received appropriate follow-up measures. Dental care and immunizations have also been provided.

Early and Periodic Screening, Diagnosis, and Treatment (EPSDT) for all young people under age twenty-one who are eligible for Medicaid was legislated in 1967. This program is a multiphase program of preventive health for children of low income families. The purpose of EPSDT is to detect health problems and take corrective action to improve the health status of children. EPSDT provides the following services: a health history, physical assessment, check on immunization status, various screening tests such as blood tests for lead poisoning and sickle cell, urine tests for albumin and sugar, tuberculosis tests, and hearing and vision screening. The purpose is to identify problems, not to diagnose disease.

Every child deserves as healthy a home environment as is possible. This sometimes necessitates the support and assistance of various community health and social services agencies.

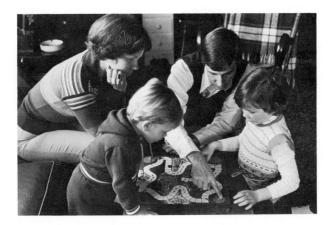

The effectiveness of EPSDT as an intervention in providing good health has been noted in a number of studies. It has been concluded that this program is a cost effective and beneficial program of child health.[29] Its value is evidenced by the periodic screening, which shows a decrease in the incidences of health problems requiring extended care.[30]

Several other federal programs have also had as a major goal the improvement of maternal and child health. The Supplemental Feeding Program for Women, Infants, and Children (WIC) has been administered by the United States Department of Agriculture. Realizing that maternal nutrition is a vital factor in infant health, the WIC program has provided supplemental foods and nutrition education to women who are at risk nutritionally. Similar federal programs include the Family Planning Program and the Maternal and Child Health Program.

The major source of public funding for prenatal and postnatal care and for delivery for low socioeconomic women is Medicaid. Over a half million deliveries are paid for each year by this federal health insurance program for the poor; nearly $1.2 billion were spent on Medicaid maternity care in a recent year.[31] The major component of these payments is for hospitalization.

As with most health and social service programs, federal budget reductions during the 1980s have led to significant reductions in maternal and child health program support. In the first half of the 1980s federal support of maternal-child health programs was reduced by 23 percent.[32] The Omnibus Budget Reconciliation Act of 1981 created the health block grants.[33] One of these was the maternal and child health care block. This block-grant program brought together several former categorical programs: maternal and child health care programming, genetic disease research, adolescent pregnancy services, Sudden Infant Death Syndrome research, hemophilia research, crippled children research, and lead-based paint poisoning research. Under provision of the maternal-child health block-grant program, individual states must match spending ($3 state share for every $4 of federal money received). The states now have greater control over maternal-child health programming. This places a great responsibility for programs relating to child health and maternal health on state and local health departments.

These developments shifted the emphasis from federal mandate, support, and control to specific state programming. Since the local health department is the prime provider of health care for many poor mothers and children, greater emphasis has been placed on providing comprehensive primary services and family planning services.

Many infant and child health services are most useful when available in the home. For this reason, local health departments must provide adequate personnel, particularly public health nurses, to enter the homes and provide these important maternal and child health needs and services.

Issue—Case Study

IUDs—No Longer Available Due to Corporate Economics

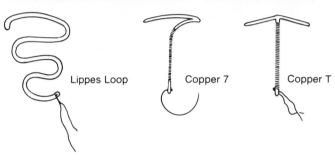

Lippes Loop   Copper 7   Copper T

In the early 1980s over two million American women were using the intrauterine device (IUD) as their primary means of contraception. The IUD has been a very effective contraceptive with a 95 to 99 percent effectiveness rating. Two-thirds of the IUDs in use were copper-bearing devices manufactured by the G. D. Searle Company. The Lippes Loop, manufactured by Ortho Pharmaceutical Corporation, accounted for 31 percent of the IUDs in use. Less than 3 percent of the remainder that were in use were manufactured by other companies.

In 1985 the Ortho Pharmaceutical Corporation announced they were stopping the production and marketing of the Lippes Loop. Several months later the G. D. Searle Company stopped United States distribution of their copper-bearing IUDs. The reasons given for these actions were basic economics. It was no longer economically profitable to continue production of these items.

Specifically this was due to financial risks brought on by lawsuits charging liability for injuries allegedly related to IUD use. The number of lawsuits had increased in recent years. Seven hundred and seventy-five lawsuits had been filed against the Searle Company. Four hundred and seventy had been solved out of court. Ten cases went to court with eight finding the company not liable for the charges leveled against them. Nevertheless, court costs and other related costs were continuing to escalate. It was reported that just four of the cases cost the company $1.5 million.

The cost of liability insurance had risen for these companies. This, accompanying the already increasing costs for court settlements, forced the action the companies took in stopping production of the IUD.

This action raised a number of serious questions and concerns:

1. What will this reduced choice of contraceptives on the marketplace do in the future to individuals seeking contraceptives?
2. For women who have relied on the IUD as a primary contraceptive measure, what can she do?
3. What does such an action as this portend for the future for other pharmaceutical products and medical devices?

Summary

The health and well-being of infants, preschool children, and mothers is an important factor in any culture. In the United States, maternal and child health has improved significantly in this century.

However, there are still many health problems related to maternal and child health. Infant mortality has been reduced to below eleven per one thousand live births. Yet this ratio is nearly double for the economically disadvantaged. The principal causes of infant mortality are low infant birthweight and congenital disorders.

Babies born with a low birthweight not only are more likely to die in infancy, but their future health status is often adversely affected. A number of maternal factors have been identified as contributing to low birthweight.

Birth defects are second only to low birthweight as a cause of infant mortality. Maternal health and environmental factors have been shown to result in certain birth defects.

Once a major cause of death among children, communicable diseases have been greatly reduced throughout the past several decades. This is due in large measure to the development of effective vaccines for several different communicable diseases. Today seven once fatal childhood diseases are of minor consequence due to immunization: (1) diphtheria, (2) pertussis, (3) tetanus, (4) polio, (5) measles, (6) rubella, and (7) mumps. In spite of these major improvements, parents must still be aware of the need to update all immunizations for their children.

One of the more rapidly expanding health problems in the United States today is teenage pregnancy. The increase in teenage pregnancy is due to many factors: increased sexual experience among adolescents, poor information regarding contraceptives, and a permissive society. Most teenage pregnancies are not wanted and as a result many social problems occur. Teenage pregnancies often involve low infant birthweight, poor maternal nutrition, and inadequate prenatal care.

Family planning services are available in communities throughout the nation. Educational services are important to improve family planning. Educational efforts include family planning counseling and other medical services.

One of the most controversial issues in public health is abortion. Since 1973, when the United States Supreme Court ruled abortion legal, thousands of abortions have been performed. However, many people are opposed to abortion. They view abortion as murder, suggesting that the fetus is a viable life. This has lead to extensive political and religious debate concerning the procedure. This issue will not be easily resolved in the near future.

Within the past decade a significant increase in cesarean deliveries has taken place. This major operative procedure produces greater risks to both the mother and the infant and is much more costly in terms of economics and use of medical resources.

The federal government has for many years supported and provided maternal and child health programs to various populations. Many public health observers suggest that this federal involvement has resulted in the improved status of maternal and child health care in the nation. But a change in government philosophy in the early 1980s has placed increased responsibility for maternal and child health programming on the local and state governments. Regardless of the source of the services, the vigilance, resources, and efforts in coping with health problems of infants, children, and of mothers should not be reduced.

Discussion Questions

1. Discuss what can be learned about the health status of a society by reviewing its infant and maternal mortality rates.

2. What are some of the dynamics that have resulted in a reduction in the infant mortality rate in the United States in the past fifty years?

3. What is meant by the term "low birthweight"?

4. Identify some of the maternal factors that have been identified as contributing to low infant birthweights.

5. Explain the relationship between Fetal Alcohol Syndrome and infant mortality and debilitation.

6. What is electronic fetal monitoring?

7. What are some of the possible causes of Sudden Infant Death Syndrome?

8. Discuss the effect immunization of preschool children has had on childhood communicable diseases.

9. Discuss some of the causes of increased teenage pregnancy.

10. Do you feel that sex education in the school curriculum could reduce the teenage pregnancy rate? Why or why not?

11. Why should family planning services be made available to males as well as females?

12. What are some social services available to pregnant teenagers in your community?

13. What are some of the services provided by family planning agencies?

14. Should nonmarried teenagers be given contraceptives without their parents' consent? Why or why not?

15. Explain the position rendered by the Supreme Court regarding abortion in 1973.

16. Discuss the arguments heard during a debate concerning abortion.

17. In what ways have new advances in medical technology compounded the issues relating to abortion?

18. What is the significance of the terms "pro-choice" and "pro-life"?

19. Discuss reasons why there has been an increase in the number of cesarean deliveries during the past several years.

20. Discuss the need for government involvement in maternal and child health programming.

21. Identify ways in which federal support for maternal and child health programming has changed since 1980.

22. What are the maternal and child health block grants?

Suggested Readings

Apte, Dipali V. "A Plan to Prevent Adolescent Pregnancy and Reduce Infant Mortality." *Public Health Reports* 102, no. 1 (January/February, 1987): 80–86.

Arkin, Elaine Bratic. "The Healthy Mothers, Healthy Babies Coalition: Four Years of Progress." *Public Health Reports* 101, no. 2, (March/April, 1986): 147–56.

Ashley, Mary Jane. "Alcohol Use During Pregnancy: A Challenge for the '80s." *Canadian Medical Association Journal* 125 (July 15, 1981): 141–42.

Brown, Sarah S. "Can Low Birth Weight Be Prevented?" *Family Planning Perspectives* 17, no. 3 (May/June, 1985): 112–18.

Donovan, Patricia. "The Holy War." *Family Planning Perspectives* 17, no. 1 (January/February, 1985): 5–9.

Dryfoos, Jay. "School-Based Health Clinics: A New Approach to Preventing Adolescent Pregnancy?" *Family Planning Perspectives* 17, no. 2 (March/April, 1985): 70–75.

Flick, Louise H. "Paths to Adolescent Parenthood: Implications for Prevention." *Public Health Reports* 101, no. 7 (March/April, 1986): 132–47.

Forest, Jacqueline Darroch. "The End of IUD Marketing in the United States: What Does It Mean for American Women?" *Family Planning Perspectives* 18, no. 2 (March/April, 1986): 52–54.

Harris, Stanley. "Services and Educational Approaches to Adolescent Pregnancy." *Journal of Community Health* 11, no. 1 (Spring, 1986): 31–34.

Lesser, Arthur J. "The Origin and Development of Maternal and Child Health Programs in the United States." *American Journal of Public Health* 75, no. 6 (June, 1985): 590–98.

Little, Ruth E., and Streissguth, Ann Pytkowicz. "Effects of Alcohol on the Fetus: Impact and Prevention." *Canadian Medical Association Journal* 125 (July 15, 1981): 159–64.

Maddox, Mary, and Edgar, Eugene. "Implementing EPSDT Screening in the Public Schools: Resolving Some Issues." *Journal of School Health* 53, no. 9 (November, 1983): 536–40.

Makinson, Carolyn. "The Health Consequences of Teenage Fertility." *Family Planning Perspectives* 17, no. 3 (May/June, 1985): 132–39.

Marsiglio, William, and Mott, Frank L. "The Impact of Sex Education on Sexual Activity, Contraceptive Use, and Premarital Pregnancy Among American Teenagers." *Family Planning Perspectives* 18, no. 4 (July/August, 1986): 151–62.

Philliber, Susan Gustavus, and others. "Age Variation in Use of a Contraceptive Service by Adolescents." *Public Health Reports* 100, no. 1 (January/February, 1985): 34–40.

Pitt, Edward. "Targeting the Adolescent Male." *Journal of Community Health* 11, no. 1 (Spring, 1986): 31–34.

Polit, Denise F., and Kahn, Janet R. "Early Subsequent Pregnancy among Economically Disadvantaged Teenage Mothers." *American Journal of Public Health* 76, no. 2 (February, 1986): 167–71.

Randolph, Linda, and Gesche, Melita. "Black Adolescent Pregnancy: Prevention and Management." *Journal of Community Health* 11, no. 1 (Spring, 1986): 10–18.

Torres, Aida, and Forrest, Jacqueline Darroch. "Family Planning Clinic Services in the United States, 1983." *Family Planning Perspectives* 17, no. 1 (January/February, 1985): 30–35.

Zelnik, Melvin, and Kantner, John F. "Sexual Activity, Contraceptive Use and Pregnancy Among Metropolitan-Area Teenagers: 1971–1979." *Family Planning Perspectives* 12, no. 5 (September/October, 1980): 230–37.

Endnotes

1. United States Department of Health and Human Services. *Surgeon General's Workshop on Maternal and Infant Health—Report,* (1981): 3.

2. Department of Health and Human Services. *Promoting Health, Preventing Diseases: Objectives for the Nation.* Washington, D.C.: U.S. Government Printing Office, Fall, 1980, p. 17.

3. National Center for Health Statistics, Monthly Vital Statistics Report. *Annual Summary of Births, Deaths, Marriages, and Divorces: United States,* October 5, 1984.

4. Randolph, Linda, and Gesche, Melita. "Black Adolescent Pregnancy: Prevention and Management." *Journal of Community Health* 11, no. 1 (Spring, 1986): p. 11.

5. Ryan, George. "Review and Assessment of the Current Status of Knowledge, Services, and Deficiencies," in the *Surgeon General's Workshop on Maternal and Child Health—Report* (1981), p. 27.

6. Kruse, Jerry. "Alcohol Use During Pregnancy." *American Family Physician* 29, no. 4 (April, 1984): 199.

7. Heinonen, O. P.; Slone, D.; and Shapiro, S. *Birth Defects and Drugs in Pregnancy.* Littleton, Mass.: Publishing Sciences Group, 1977: 516.

8. Pope, A. J. "A Status Report: Sudden Infant Death Syndrome-Cause and Effect." *Health Education* 14, no. 5 (September/October, 1983): 6–9.

9. "Premature Mortality Due to Sudden Infant Death Syndrome." *Morbidity and Mortality Weekly Report* 35, no. 14 (March 21, 1986): 169–70.

10. Ibid.

11. *The Status of Children, Youth, and Families.* Washington, D.C.: U.S. Government Printing Office, 1979, p. 37.

12. "Measles—United States, First 26 Weeks, 1986." *Morbidity and Mortality Weekly Report* 35, no. 33 (August 27, 1986): 525–33.

13. Ibid., 533.

14. *The Status of Children, Youth, and Families,* 25.

15. Alan Guttmacher Institute Report, *Teenage Pregnancy: The Problem That Hasn't Gone Away* (1981).

16. Surgeon General's Report on Health Promotion and Disease Prevention. *Healthy People.* Washington, D.C.: U.S. Government Printing Office, 1979: 48.

17. Zelnik, Melvin, and Kantner, John F. "Sexual Activity, Contraceptive Use and Pregnancy Among Metropolitan-Area Teenagers: 1971–1979." *Family Planning Perspectives* 12, no. 5 (September/October, 1980): 230.

18. Ibid., p. 231.

19. Ibid., p. 235.

20. Surgeon General's Report on Health Promotion and Disease Prevention. *Healthy People,* p. 24.

21. Friedman, Emily. "The Health Lifeline: Out of the Reach of Women and Children?" *Hospitals* (October 20, 1986): 46–51.

22. Alan Guttmacher Institute Report, *Teenage Pregnancy,* p. 27.

23. Torres, Aida, and Forrest, Jacqueline Darroch. "Family Planning Clinic Services in the United States, 1983." *Family Planning Perspectives* 17, no. 1 (January/February, 1985): 30.

24. Harris, Stanley. "Services and Educational Approaches to Adolescent Pregnancy." *Journal of Community Health* 11, no. 1 (Spring, 1986): 31–34. Pitt, Edward. "Targeting the Adolescent Male." *Journal of Community Health* 11, no. 1 (Spring, 1986): 45–48.

25. Henshaw, Stanley, et al. "Abortion in the United States, 1978–1979." *Family Planning Perspectives* 13, no. 1 (January/February, 1981): p. 6.

26. Ibid., p. 15

27. Ibid., p. 13.

28. "Who Receives Cesareans: Patient and Hospital Characteristics." NCHSR Publications, Information Branch, National Institutes of Health, Rockville, Md. (1985).

29. Currier, Richard. "Is Early and Periodic Screening, Diagnosis, and Treatment (EPSDT) Worthwhile?" *Public Health Reports* 92, no. 6 (November/December, 1977): p. 536.

30. Irwin, P. H., and Conroy-Hughes, Rosemary. "EPSDT Impact on Health Status." *Health Care Financing Review* 2, no. 4 (Spring, 1981): p. 39.

31. Kenny, Asta M., and others. "Medicaid Expenditures for Maternity and Newborn Care in America." *Family Planning Perspectives* 18, no. 3 (May/June 1986): 103–10.

32. Friedman, Emily. "The Health Lifeline: Out of the Reach of Women and Children?" *Hospitals* 60 (October 20, 1986): 46.

33. Block-grant programs are discussed in detail in chapter 2.

17

Senior Citizens: Needs, Services, and Hope for Life's Later Years

Medical advances have enabled many people to live longer lives than past generations. Not only are people living longer but for many the quality of the extended life is greatly improved compared to that experienced by their forefathers. Throughout the nation, communities have established senior citizen centers for this ever-increasing population of elderly (usually those considered to be at least sixty-five years of age). People who frequent these centers can meet for social events, educational experiences, recreation opportunities, and a variety of other services. The later years of life should be a time of positive activity that encourages a feeling of contribution and meaning.

In spite of the great potential that the elderly possess, a variety of factors, including increased mobility and separation of families, has resulted in numerous problems. This is particularly true when these individuals are faced with illness and disability that require some type of care. The situation has created a number of social responsibilities for communities, hence involving the field of community health for direction and action.

Old Age

When does old age begin? At what point is an individual considered elderly—a senior citizen? There is no magical day or year at which the status is attained. As with other factors in human development and life-style, all individuals vary.

In the United States, age sixty-five has been designated by the 1935 Social Security legislation as the time in life when an employee can retire and receive Social Security benefits. Because of this, many people consider sixty-five as that point in life when elderly status is achieved. And once this status is reached, our society assumes that life-style changes will occur.

But nothing magical occurs physiologically, emotionally, or socially at sixty-five that is different from earlier ages. Many individuals in their late sixties, seventies, and beyond can still be productive. History was made by leaders who achieved greatness and world renown after reaching the age of

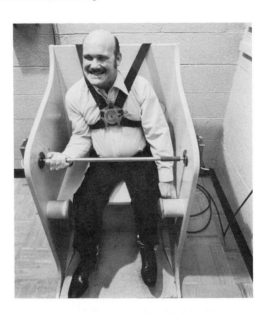

Researchers at the National Institutes of Health study the physiological changes that occur with age. More than six hundred volunteers visit the Gerontology Research Center of NIH to be involved in the research efforts. This particular test helps measure arm and shoulder strength.

sixty-five. For example, Winston Churchill was sixty-five before he became the Prime Minister of Great Britain and led his nation during World War II. Some of the great works of art were created by artists who were in their seventies. Michelangelo was over seventy when he completed his work in the Pauline Chapel in Rome. When Picasso died in 1973, at the age of ninety-one, he was still active in his artistic endeavors. The Chinese philosopher, Confucius, was teaching until his death at the age of seventy-two. In 1984, the people of the United States re-elected President Reagan, who was 73 at the time.

With today's increased life expectancy, it is important that people are not required to retire from productive, regular employment at the age of sixty-five. From an analysis of other cultures, it is obvious that the elderly can be very productive far beyond the traditional retirement age of sixty-five. In fact, in many nations, the elderly are highly respected and often consulted for the wisdom they have earned with age. They remain a very integral part of the family unit and lead very fulfilled lives.

This is usually not the state of affairs in the United States; the opposite is often true. Early retirement is a goal for many working people. However, upon retirement, retirees often find it difficult to find meaning and satisfaction in their lives. Their ideas are considered "old-fashioned" by the younger generation, and they are not sought out for their experiences and knowledge. Rather, they are encouraged to retire as soon as retirement age is reached.

The current status of the elderly in the United States indicates that they must be encouraged to lead a more productive life-style, and they must be provided with opportunities to do so. Such developments will necessitate a reorientation of our concept of aging and the redesigning of many social structures. This challenge requires creative thinking, but also offers great opportunity for the future of millions of Americans.

Demographics of the Elderly

Today one person in nine, approximately 11 percent of the American population, is over sixty-five years of age. There are over twenty-six million persons in this population group. The number of people reaching sixty-five years of age is increasing daily so that projections are that the percentage of senior citizens will double by the year 2020. The fastest growing segment of the American population is over eighty-five years of age.

Although the elderly account for a little more than 11 percent of the American population, they account for 29 percent of health care costs, they use 25 percent of all prescription drugs, make 15 percent of all visits to physicians, and account for 34 percent of all days in short-stay hospitals.[1]

There are many reasons for the projected increases in the over sixty-five population. Primarily, though, improved health status and health care have resulted in longer life expectancy.

With increased numbers of people expected to live beyond age sixty-five in the years ahead, many social issues need to be addressed. Will there be resources to meet the demands that this population group will create? Economic problems will plague many elderly citizens in the future. Inflation, which reduces the buying power of the dollar, will inhibit the elderly citizens' efforts to purchase food or obtain health care and other services.

Social Security, established in 1935, is a social insurance program for the elderly. It provides old-age insurance for retired workers and their dependents. Also eligible are the survivors of deceased or disabled workers and their dependents. For a number of people, Social Security has been a very helpful program. Even though many retired individuals have other retirement programs, some rely totally upon Social Security for financial support.

There are serious problems concerning the future of Social Security as it has existed for more than fifty years. Inflation, high interest rates, increasing Medicare costs, governmental spending, and, of course, the surge in the number of recipients have brought the Social Security System to the edge of bankruptcy. Some economic and political experts predict that the Social Security System will be broke in the very near future, possibly as soon as the early 1990s. Political discussions, debates, and legislative attempts have been undertaken to keep the program solvent, but no easy solution to the problem has surfaced.

Chaos would result if Social Security funds were not available for those who have paid into the system and planned to rely upon these retirement monies. In an effort to "save" Social Security, some have suggested reducing the benefits available to the recipient. Others suggest raising the costs to employers and employees and requiring groups not now paying into Social Security to do so. These two options would increase the amount of funds in the system. However, the American public is not supportive of increased taxation of personal income. Thus, these are not considered viable solutions. The demise of the Social Security System would have a dramatic effect on the ability of senior citizens to pay for their health care needs and services.

Three Major Problems Relating to Drug Use (Over-the-Counter and Prescription) Among the Elderly

1. Heightened drug effects because of aging
2. More frequent drug and alcohol-drug interactions
3. Toxic drug effects misdiagnosed as senility or mental illness

Source: Report of the Public Health Service Task Force on Women's Health Issues, Vol. I. "Issues Related to Alcohol and Drug Abuse and the Mental Health of Women: Executive Summary." *Public Health Reports* 100, no. 1 (January/February, 1985): 96.

Elderly Health Problems

The improvement in the general level of health in America has led to greater longevity. In spite of this overall improved health status, widespread provision of health care, and advanced health technology, certain health problems continue to plague the elderly.

Chronic Diseases

Chronic and degenerative diseases are the major health problems of the elderly. Arthritic conditions (particularly rheumatoid arthritis and osteoarthritis), hypertension, malignant neoplasms, and heart disease are the most prevalent chronic conditions experienced by senior citizens. Some of these chronic conditions are eventually fatal. The leading causes of death among the elderly are heart disease, neoplasms, cerebrovascular diseases, influenza, and pneumonia.

As people age, hearing and vision problems frequently develop. Since these problems often develop gradually, the individual is unaware of the loss until a serious problem occurs. An accident may result because the individual is unable to hear a warning sound. Limited vision and blindness can have emotional as well as physiological effects on the elderly. Cataracts, once a leading cause of vision loss in many senior citizens, are not as threatening anymore. Fortunately, surgical procedures to remove cataracts have improved and have helped many elderly to see and function productively in their later years.

Chronic diseases create adjustment problems for the elderly. Whereas most younger people are able to receive health care, medicine, and therapy to cure an illness or sickness, chronic diseases are longer lasting. Many are debilitating, with ongoing pain and discomfort. The long-term nature of chronic diseases is both costly and depressing to individuals.

Chronic illnesses result in an increase in the number of pharmaceutical drugs taken on a routine basis. The elderly consume 25 percent of all drugs used annually in the United States with an average of thirteen prescription drugs a year being consumed by each person over the age of sixty-five.[2] There is increasing evidence that as one grows older certain physiological changes affect the action of drugs on the individual. For example, there is often reduced efficiency of the kidneys, the primary mode of excretion of drugs.

There is no cure for most chronic conditions experienced by the elderly. Unfortunately, the exact cause of these conditions is often unknown (as in the case of cancer, arthritis, and heart disease). In spite of the fact that certain risk factors can be identified for these conditions, it is impossible to prescribe a pill, perform an operation, or provide therapy to cure the problem. The individual must adapt to the pain, debilitation, and other problems caused by the chronic conditions. Many elderly people resign themselves to the problem because they view it as "a sign of getting old" or "something with which I must learn to live."

Most chronic diseases are now known to originate in early life. The life-style of earlier years has a very definite effect upon the development of chronic conditions later in life. Diet, the use of alcohol and tobacco, and activity are just a few of the life patterns that relate to chronic diseases.

Nutrition

The nutritional status of the elderly is a major public health concern because many senior citizens are malnourished. The healthy senior citizen needs about the same amounts of essential nutrients as do younger people. However, they usually require fewer calories to maintain satisfactory weight levels. In an attempt to reduce calorie intake the elderly often will not eat nutritionally balanced meals.

Economics are a major factor in elderly malnutrition. The rising cost of food makes it necessary for many senior citizens on fixed incomes to purchase less nutritious foods. Thus, the high food costs have a definite negative effect on the health and well-being of the economically disadvantaged elderly.

Other factors, isolation and loneliness, also lead to poor eating patterns. The individual living alone is not likely to prepare nutritious, well-balanced meals. It seems unimportant or a waste of time to prepare a nutritious meal when there is no one with whom to share it. Because of this reasoning, the elderly are more likely to snack on less-nutritious, inexpensive food that does not contain needed vitamins and other nutrients.

For this reason, many communities have social centers where the elderly can meet and eat with others for a relatively low cost. These services are provided in schools, churches, union halls, and community centers. This opportunity to socialize leads to improved intake of nutritious food.

Reduced mobility is another major factor that affects shopping and cooking habits of the elderly. Many people with arthritic handicaps are fearful of cooking for fear of spilling hot food on themselves. Others do not have the energy or capacity to stand in the kitchen to prepare a full meal.

Chronic diseases also affect the nutritional status of the elderly. These conditions impede physiological processes such as digestion and absorption. Drugs, too, will sometimes undermine the nutritional status of an individual. For example, prolonged use of laxatives can alter the absorption of vitamins, or result in diarrhea, weight loss, and fatigue.[3]

As individuals grow older, certain taste buds do not function as efficiently. Foods often taste more sour and bitter than they did before. For this reason, foods are not as appealing and so many senior citizens lose their appetites. Though it is possible to adjust to this problem, many elderly refuse to eat certain nutritious foods that now do not taste as they did in earlier years.

Dental problems also prevent the elderly from having a well-balanced diet. Dental caries and periodontal disease, important health problems for the elderly, are major causes of tooth loss among senior citizens.[4] Dentures, the only alternative when teeth are lost, make it difficult to eat certain foods. Those elderly who cannot afford dentures are forced to eat only liquids and soft foods. Not only do they fail to eat well-balanced meals, but certain nutrients are not as readily available.

Osteoporosis

Another physiological development that affects the elderly, particularly older women, is a thinning of the bones. Beginning in the mid-thirties slight bone loss begins and continues throughout life. This gradual bone loss occurring over a period of years usually goes unrecognized until a bone is broken, resulting in pain and disability. Healing of the fracture often is very time consuming. This condition is known as *osteoporosis*.

Osteoporosis, a serious debilitation for many, requires prolonged medical and therapeutic care. Thin, small-framed females are more at risk for osteoporosis than larger females. Because of denser bone structure, males are less likely to get this condition. Early indication of having osteoporosis is loss of body height. The vertebrae become compressed with age due to a weakening of these spinal bones. A curvature of the spine is often noted in elderly females.

The cause of osteoporosis is not known. Several factors may play a role in its development.[5] These include decrease in hormone levels—it is principally found in post-menopausal females, inadequate calcium in the diet, inadequate exposure to sunlight, and inactivity.

Treatment of individuals with osteoporosis involves taking measures to prevent further bone loss. Diet is an important preventive factor. People should eat foods that are high in calcium. In addition Vitamin D will often be added to the diet as it helps in calcium absorption. Calcium and Vitamin D may slow the rate of bone loss but they will not cause new bone to form. Excess protein should be avoided as it can lead to bone loss.

Regular exercise can be helpful in prevention of osteoporosis and in the treatment of the patient. Exercise may stimulate formation of new bone and helps by maintaining strength of the skeletal system. Estrogen also slows the process of bone loss. For this reason some physicians prescribe this hormone to females with osteoporosis.

Accidents

Falls are a leading cause of fatal injury among the elderly. Most falls, both fatal and nonfatal, occur in the home.[6] Nonfatal accidents result in serious injury, hospitalization, and lengthy disability and rehabilitation.

The greatest incidence of falls among the elderly has been attributed to several different factors:[7]

1. Loss of muscle strength and endurance
2. Loss of vision and hearing acuity
3. Slowed adjustment to light-dark changes
4. Postural imbalance
5. Altered gait
6. Slowed reaction time

All of these factors usually develop as part of the aging process.

As a person grows older the ability to drive an automobile is often impaired. Slower reaction time, reduced adaptation to darkness, and a lessening of depth perception all contribute to poorer driving skills. Senior citizens must recognize these changes and be willing to adapt driving patterns. The elderly individual may need to drive more slowly, reduce night driving, drive fewer miles at one time, and adapt to winter driving conditions.

Health-Related Social Problems

Many problems faced by the elderly are not primarily health concerns. However, these problems do have an impact on the ability to obtain health care, on the emotional health of the individual, and on the quality of life experienced. Two such health-related social problems are transportation and housing.

Transportation

Mobility is a problem for many senior citizens. As long as a person is able to drive and can afford to operate an automobile, that person is usually able to care for personal needs. However, advanced age frequently forces an individual to rely on others for transportation to appointments, for obtaining the essentials of life, and for recreating outside the home. Independence is lost.

Inadequate transportation, in addition to the loss of independence, affects the health of the elderly. They need transportation in order to grocery shop and to travel to medical facilities. But in many communities, there is no comprehensive transportation system so it becomes extremely difficult to go to the physician's office when care is needed.

Reliance upon others for transportation has a negative effect upon the emotional health of the elderly. Psychologically, it tends to produce an attitude of dependence. Not only is the person dependent upon others for transportation, but this characteristic often carries over into other areas of living as well.

Some community social service agencies provide transportation for the elderly. However, this usually is limited to travel to and from a specific agency. Within some communities there are several agencies providing transportation, but unfortunately, this, too, is usually limited in destination and route. Measures need to be designed that would provide unrestricted mobility within the community for the elderly.

Mass transportation in urban communities is often the only means of travel for the senior citizen. In many communities, public transportation offers reduced fares to this age group. In spite of this, many people are hesitant to use public transportation because they fear crime, because of inappropriate time schedules, or because of unacceptable routes.

Housing

In spite of the belief that most elderly live in an institutional setting, the vast majority of senior citizens, in fact, live in a house, an apartment, a condominium, or some type of public housing within the community. Only 5 percent of those over sixty-five years of age are institutionalized.

Often the elderly reside in older houses that have structural deficiencies. The United States Senate Special Committee on Aging reported that at least 30 percent of the elderly population live in substandard, deteriorating housing.[8] This is particularly the case in urban communities among the economically disadvantaged. As a home becomes older, major repairs are often needed to maintain the structure. But the costs of construction, building repair, and maintenance make it very difficult for the poor to maintain a home. These rising construction and maintenance costs, along with the rising expenditures needed to heat a home and the potential for crime, pose serious problems for many elderly citizens.

Rent and property taxes have increased dramatically in recent years. For the elderly living on fixed incomes, this increase has forced them to sell their homes and move to less desirable locations. But rental property is often not maintained at an acceptable level, thus exposing the elderly to a number of the same health problems encountered in their own homes.

Housing quality has a direct relationship to the health and well-being of people. Not only is this related to physical well-being, but in the case of the elderly, also to emotional health. Emotional health often deteriorates when an individual is forced to move from an area where he or she has lived for many years.

In order to help provide good living conditions for all citizens, including the elderly, many local health departments have units that conduct housing inspections. These activities assure that housing meets local building codes. These health department employees also inspect facilities where the residents have complaints about conditions. Such inspections usually result when the landlord fails to make repairs requested by tenants.

Mental Health

The emotional health of the elderly is a concern of community mental health services. The Presidential Commission on Mental Health (1978) identified in its report the need for improved mental health services for the aged.[9] An estimated 15 percent of the elderly population in the United States have some mental disorders.[10] Many experiences in the later years of life have such a profound effect upon mental and emotional health that individuals need help in order to cope.

Mental illnesses among the elderly may be functional, organic, or a combination. Functional illnesses are caused by emotional stressors. Organic illnesses result from physical impairments such as cerebral arteriosclerosis.

Depression

A common cause of functional mental illness is depression. During the later years, the death of a spouse or close friend has an emotional effect with which the elderly find difficult to cope. The nature of chronic illnesses and the uncertainty of cure can also depress people. The trauma of retirement can lead to depression and psychological problems since many people no longer feel wanted or productive after retirement. Economic pressures during the senior citizen years have contributed to the emotional instability of many. Some individuals are uncertain about how they can pay for the necessities of life, such as food, housing, and medicine. Because of these problems, depression and schizophrenia are the most common causes of psychiatric admissions among the elderly.[11] Depression may affect as many as one in four persons over the age of sixty.[12]

In days gone by, the elderly were often placed in state mental health institutions if they had emotional and pyschological problems. This often occurred when the family physician was unable to provide the needed medical care for a patient. Once placed in such institutions, they were often forgotten, received poor or inadequate care, and seldom received the psychological rehabilitation that would permit them to return to their communities.

The development of community and mental health centers has been a positive step in upgrading the care for the elderly.[13] Much of the needed care is available on an outpatient basis so the individual is able to live at home with relatives or friends; it is unnecessary for the person to be institutionalized for long periods of time.

In spite of the potential for improved psychiatric care for the elderly, many community mental health centers have not been successful in meeting the inpatient needs of many elderly.[14] Psychiatric treatment is often long-term and can have detrimental effects on the patients. The treatment of depression often uses drugs that, in turn, may result in the loss of appetite, insomnia, or even personal withdrawal. As a result, clinical care for the elderly mental health patient sometimes compounds the individual's health problems.

Suicide

The loss of a spouse, separation from family or loved ones, and feelings of hopelessness and uselessness are common experiences among the elderly. These factors, along with many others, result in depression, and all too often, in suicide among many senior citizens. Twenty-five percent of reported suicides are committed by the elderly (more than ten thousand per year).[15]

Coping with this problem is no easy matter. Programs and activities designed to prevent suicides among the elderly are needed. These activities should include not only community counseling agencies, but also therapeutic services.

Senility

It is not uncommon for an elderly individual to experience memory loss to some degree. In some instances, this may be simply the inablity to remember a person's name. For others it may be a more complex and serious problem involving forgetfulness, confusion, and/or changes in personality and behavior. Although it is often assumed that senility affects all elderly, it actually does not affect the vast majority of senior citizens.

Numerous conditions have been referred to as senility problems. The two most common forms of mental impairment of the elderly are (1) senile dementia and (2) Alzheimer's disease.

Senile Dementia

It has been estimated that approximately 5 percent of all people over sixty-five are affected by senile dementia.[16] This condition is the result of a series of minor strokes that cause a narrowing of blood vessels that supply the brain with oxygen. This impediment to the oxygen supply disrupts brain functioning and results in death of brain tissue. Some problems referred to as senile dementia can be treated and cured, whereas others can only be treated. Lost brain function cannot be restored.

Alzheimer's Disease

A disorder common to many senior citizens that produces memory loss and disorientation is Alzheimer's disease. It has been estimated that this impairment is present in some 2.5 million adults in the United States.[17]

A German pathologist, Alois Alzheimer, first described this disease in 1906. No particular population is at risk; it affects all races, geographical groups, and cultural populations. The cause is not known, but those afflicted by Alzheimer's disease have neurofibrillary tangles (clumping and distortion of fibers in the nerve cells) of the cerebral cortex.

Recent research has also discovered that scattered throughout the cortex the Alzheimer's patient has groups of degenerated nerve endings. These areas of degeneration are called plaques. They disrupt the passage of electrochemical signals between the cells. The greater the number of tangles and plaques the more serious is the disturbance of intellectual function and memory in the individual.

An early indication of Alzheimer's disease is forgetfulness, particularly of more current events. As the disease progresses memory loss increases, often accompanied by confusion, restlessness, and various personality and behavioral changes. In the most severe stages the patient becomes incapable of self-care.

Research supported by the National Institute of Aging has been studying three potential factors in the development of Alzheimer's disease.[18] These are (1) traces of aluminum in the brain, (2) viral infections of the central nervous system, and (3) genetic defects. The brains of people with advanced cases of Alzheimer's disease have been found to contain high amounts of aluminum.

So far the most consistent finding is that the activity of certain chemicals in the brain changes. This is known as the *cholinergic system* and is involved in memory and learning. The change that is most commonly found in Alzheimer's disease occurs in the proteins of the nerve cells of the cerebral cortex.[19] Changes in these proteins lead to an accumulation of neurofibrillary tangles that are associated with memory loss and disorientation. Some studies suggest that drugs can be used to block the breakdown of the cholinergic activity in the brain and so improve the memory and learning in Alzheimer's patients.[20]

Long-Term Care Facilities

The very nature of illness experienced by the elderly frequently results in long-term care and treatment. This medical care often must continue even after leaving the hospital. As a result, long-term health care facilities are very important in meeting these needs.

The present long-term institutional concepts originated in the late 1800s and early part of the twentieth century. Before the depression of the 1930s, the major form of government-supported institutional care for the elderly was the county poorhouse. These facilities were known as "almshouses" or "county farms." They were financed by local government. The poorhouses were often known for their poor living conditions. Most disappeared following passage of the Social Security legislation of 1935. This legislation provided income maintenance for the elderly and the disabled and specifically denied payment to "inmates of public institutions" to prevent the program from supporting residents of county poorhouses.[21] Since the passage of the Medicare and Medicaid legislation in 1965 the number of beds in nursing homes and the number of elderly living in long-term institutional settings has increased. However, it is important to note that the vast majority of senior citizens will never live in a long-term care facility. Only about 5 percent of the United States population over sixty-five years of age reside in long-term care institutions.[22] It is estimated that by the year 2000 there will be a need for 1.2 million beds in long-term care facilities. The projected cost of this need will exceed $60 billion.

There are several types of these facilities, including nursing homes, extended care facilities, home care services, and community-based services. These facilities provide medical and rehabilitative care, and various social services for those individuals who either cannot obtain the needed care in the home or who are in situations where there are not adequate support systems for them.

Even though most senior citizens are able to receive the care they need while living in a noninstitutional setting, conditions may arise that require long-range, around-the-clock nursing and medical care. Also, many elderly do not have family or friends who can provide the necessary support.

Thus, placement in a long-term care facility is necessary and often creates a major life change for an individual. For this reason, placement in an institution must result from careful decision making.

Several factors are important in this process:[23]

1. The physical and emotional care needs of the individual
2. The person's degree of support from family, friends, and neighbors
3. The attitude of the patient regarding institutional placement

The needs of the elderly are a primary factor in determining the type of care and services required. Assessment of these needs must include a medical evaluation, a functional ability evaluation, a psychological evaluation, and a social evaluation.[24]

Placement in a long-term care facility should be a decision reached only after all alternatives have been discussed. It should not result simply as a matter of convenience for the health care providers or the person's family. This action must be taken only out of concern for the well-being of the patient involved.

Even though elderly persons are placed in long-term care facilities for a variety of reasons, two types of problems in particular result in the most admissions.[25] These are (1) the need for rehabilitative care following an acute illness and (2) chronic disabling disease. These conditions require the services of personnel who cannot work effectively in the home setting.

Nursing Homes

The principal health care facility providing long-term care is the nursing home. Nursing homes are licensed to care for individuals who must have nursing care on a daily basis. Although people of any age may be admitted to a nursing home, the majority of nursing home patients are senior citizens, and 75 percent are over the age of seventy-five.[26]

Though nursing homes have been in existence for decades, the Medicare and Medicaid legislation of 1965 stimulated a growth spurt in the nursing home industry. This legislation created two programs of federal health insurance for the elderly. Regulations were established governing the provision of nursing home care, guaranteeing a specified level of care for people in nursing homes paid for by Medicare and Medicaid.

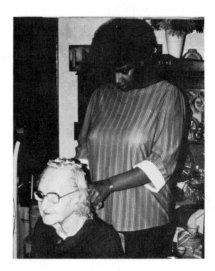

This nurse's aide helps an elderly resident with her hair care. Many nursing home residents need assistance with such basic health care.

Despite the tremendous growth of the industry and the government's financial support, studies have shown that nursing homes are generally small-scale operations administered on a profit basis. They are often understaffed.[27]

Nursing homes are classified as either (1) a skilled nursing facility or (2) an intermediate care facility. In a skilled nursing home, nursing services and rehabilitative care are available twenty-four hours a day. Patients who cannot function without medical supervision, or those undergoing long-term convalescence that necessitates nursing care or rehabilitative therapy, are usually placed in skilled nursing facilities. Individuals needing a special diet may receive special assistance in such a facility. Residents in a skilled nursing home often require and receive assistance in dressing, bathing, mobility, and elimination.

The patients who need supervised nursing care but have some ability to care for themselves may be placed in an intermediate care facility. Here they may receive medical care in addition to assistance in basic living activities such as bathing and eating. These facilities also provide rehabilitative therapy. This type of facility does not have round-the-clock medical care, however.

A third type of nursing home facility offers residential board and personal care for the elderly. These are retirement communities. These facilities do not provide regular twenty-four hour medical services since the residents do not have illnesses or disabilities that require ongoing care. However, the elderly individual does receive assistance in walking, dressing, or bathing in a protected living environment. When necessary the resident is also assisted in eating.

Some nursing homes are exclusively for people who are mentally retarded. These facilities, however, are licensed as residential nursing homes.

Until the 1960s, most mentally impaired elderly were placed in state or local mental hospitals for care and treatment. However, in the past two decades, nursing home services for the mentally impaired senior citizens have replaced the hospital as the psychiatric care center. In the early 1970s nursing home placement of the mentally impaired increased over 100 percent.[28] The two principal reasons for this change are economics and humanitarianism. Patients receive better nursing services and rehabilitative care in nursing homes than they do in large public mental health hospitals. Placing the mentally impaired person in the community where relatives and friends can provide social support has also contributed to the nursing home influx.

Placing an individual in a nursing home can be very expensive. The average cost of nursing home care usually exceeds a thousand dollars per month.[29] This is the cost of board, room, and general care; medical services are extra. The long-term nature of nursing home care compounds the cost factor for many families. Approximately one-half of the cost of nursing home care is paid by Medicaid.[30]

Many Americans regard long-term institutionalization as a last resort and usually approach it with varying degrees of "apprehension, guilt and revulsion."[31] These negative feelings may pertain to the physical characteristics of the nursing home. They may also be due to the nature of the staff. Numerous problems inherent in nursing home care also contribute to such feelings. Common problems include infrequent and brief physician visits, usually by someone untrained in geriatric medicine; understaffed nursing services; and lack of social workers, psychologists, and/or mental health workers with experience and knowledge in geriatric patient care.

Institutionalization is frequently used to relieve the burden on families due to the lack of any alternatives. The need for alternatives to long-term institutional care for the elderly stems not only from a physical and emotional level, but also from financial constraints.

Alternatives to Long-Term Care

Respite Care

In order to relieve the family of the necessity for institutionalization of the elderly and also of the need for twenty-four-hour care, there are several alternatives available. One area being developed that provides planned, short-term care is referred to as respite care.[32] This type of care provides periodic relief to the family, and makes available expanded health supportive services such as food preparation and shopping as well as supervision of the older person as needed. Unfortunately these services are not reimbursed by Medicare and most private insurance.

A type of respite care is the adult day-care center. Day-care services for the elderly began in England in the late 1950s. The elderly person is dropped off at the center several times a week. He or she is picked up after a designated period of time and returned home for the evening. Day care emphasizes health maintenance, health promotion, health restoration, and rehabilitation of physical problems. The services provided in such a facility are made available by physicians, occupational therapists, social workers, physical therapists, and nursing personnel. This provides an opportunity for certain rehabilitation and other health maintenance care to be obtained in an outpatient basis. It also provides time for the family to be relieved of the continual care of the elderly person.

A problem associated with the adult day care is that the medical costs are not covered by Medicare and only a few states cover such costs in their Medicaid programs.

Another form of adult day care emphasizes socialization and activity rather than physical health care and rehabilitation. The senior citizen center offers the opportunity for the elderly to socialize, learn new roles, maintain and develop involvement in the community, and gain a sense of usefulness and dignity. The elderly come to the center where they may have contact with other community agencies providing health screenings.

Home Health Care

Perhaps the most popular alternative to long-term institutional nursing home care for the elderly is the home health care program, where medical care and related services are provided in the home of the patient. A sick or partially disabled senior citizen should not always assume that they must enter a residential nursing home following illness and hospitalization. Thus, there is increasing interest in home health care for the elderly in this country.

Services that can be provided in the home include basic nursing care, rehabilitative therapy, nutritional assistance, home health aide services, and counseling. The health care specialists come to the home on a regular basis to provide these services. The physician is responsible for prescribing the medical treatment that the individual will need at home. Treatment may include medication, skilled nursing care, and physical, occupational, speech, and/or hearing therapy. The nurse is responsible for determining the type of nursing care needed to carry out the plan established by the physician.

There is evidence that patients respond to therapy more quickly in their own homes than in residential nursing homes. Studies have also shown that health improves more with patients involved in home-based care programs than those in nursing homes.[33] The patient is more relaxed at home around familiar and comfortable surroundings. As a result,

A double-amputee lifts himself from his bed into his wheelchair using a special hoist. This individual is one of many patients in the hospital-based home care program at the Boston VA Medical Center.

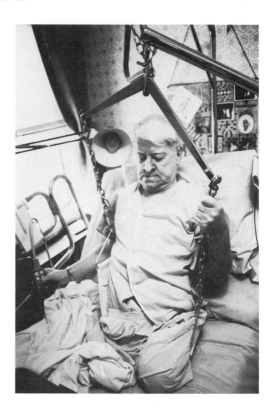

there is greater motivation to follow instructions. The psychological benefit to the individual also contributes to rehabilitation.

Home health care is provided by public health departments, hospitals, and some private agencies. Regardless of which type of home health agency a person chooses, the initial step in developing a home care plan rests with the physician.

Home health care is of interest to the government and private health insurance agencies as one approach to controlling hospital costs. Home health care is less expensive than extended hospitalization. However, before the concept of home health care is widely accepted, it will be necessary for hospitalization insurance, both private and Medicare and Medicaid, to extend coverage for the services.

Many community health projects support the preparation of geriatric nurse practitioners to improve nursing within the long-term care field. These projects also support the coordination of services offered by community health agencies to improve home care for the elderly.

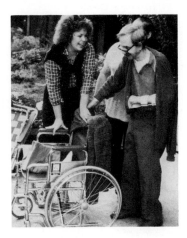

Medicare does not reimburse the costs of personal services such as general household services, assistance with dressing, bathing, meal preparation, and shopping. Medicare rarely provides for long-term care for chronic conditions in the home. It provides only for care when one is confined at home due to injury or illness. To be eligible for home health care services reimbursed by Medicare, one must have been hospitalized for three consecutive days for the same illness, have documented evidence that they are considered homebound, and the patient must need skilled nursing services, physical therapy, speech therapy, or other types of therapy. A plan of treatment must be established by the physician and recertified every sixty days.[34]

An offshoot of home health care is the community-based service. This service includes clinic screenings, adult day-care centers, day hospitals, and senior citizen centers. This program makes available certain health and social services during the day while the individual still resides in the home.

The adult day-care facility is not widely available in the United States, though for over twenty years, this form of health care has been available in England and in other European countries. Adult day-care facilities may be rehabilitative in nature or focus upon a specific type of health problem. The adult day-care facility should be encouraged in the United States, too, so that the elderly can receive the needed health care but still live at home among relatives and friends or on their own.

Two models of adult day-care centers exist. The day hospital has a strong health care orientation.[35] Physical rehabilitation is the primary goal of these centers. Most day hospitals are closely associated with health care institutions and usually the patients have been released from inpatient status.

The second model of adult day-care centers does not provide rehabilitative care but focuses on social services, nutrition, and social activities. Participants in these settings have fewer diagnosed medical problems and are less dependent on help.

A main reason for the failure of this approach to elderly care to take hold in the United States is the fact that most health insurance, particularly Medicare and Medicaid, will only reimburse expenses when they are provided in an institutional setting. Home health care costs have been paid for the most part only after release from an inpatient facility. Unless a person has been hospitalized, there is little financial assistance available for adult day care.

Aging — The Future

The demand for services for the elderly will increase in the future. This is due partially to the fact that the number of elderly will grow in the years ahead. In the near future, the next twenty to thirty years, the elderly will have greater expectations of services than has been the case in the past. Most of today's younger generation have had educational opportunities, health services, and other services that many in the present elderly population did not have. This younger generation also has had greater financial freedom than previous generations. As this population group grows older and begins to experience

The elderly population will continue to increase in the next quarter century. Thus, senior citizens must be recognized as an active and valuable sector of the nation's communities.

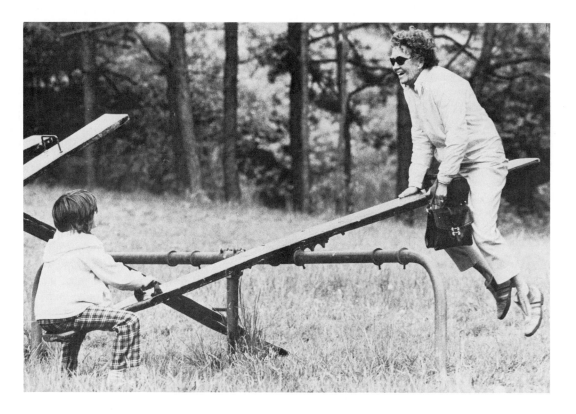

the problems of chronic illnesses and the need for certain health and social services, expectations will rise as well. This expectation will be complicated by the trend for such services to become more costly each year. Increased medical care costs, hospital expenses, and the economic expenditures needed for institutional care negatively affect both the present and future senior citizen.

The elderly population in the early twenty-first century will be more highly educated and politically aware than previous generations. As a result, the problems and needs of the elderly will receive greater interest, attention, and concern in the years ahead. The elderly population will be a force that cannot be shunned by politicians, economists, and society. "Gray power" is a force that will definitely be heard in the future.

The American society must accept the role of the elderly. It is important that we realize that the elderly need not be isolated from society in the institutional setting, but instead must be included as a vital figure in the life of the family as well as the community. The elderly should be encouraged to remain useful in their later years. This can be accomplished in numerous ways: as foster grandparents, helping in child day-care centers, and other similar programs. Senior citizens might even be encouraged to continue in their professions at reduced levels of involvement as they grow older.

Summary

A number of medical advances in the past century have lengthened the life span of many people in the United States. This, accompanied by other factors, has contributed to a growth in the number of people living past the age of sixty-five. Today over 11 percent of the American population is over sixty-five, and it is projected that this figure will surpass 20 percent in the next forty years.

There is no one point at which a person automatically becomes elderly. The Social Security legislation passed in 1935, retirement policies, and American culture have all influenced the establishment of the age of sixty-five as the point at which people are classified as elderly. However, many people, both historical and contemporary, live very productive years beyond sixty-five.

In spite of the general improvement in the health of Americans, health problems continue to plague the senior citizen. Chronic and degenerative diseases are a major health care problem for most elderly. The various chronic diseases, such as arthritis, cancer, and cardiovascular diseases, are usually long-term and have no known cures. As a result, the elderly patient must adapt to pain, debilitation, and unending medication.

Other elderly health problems are inadequate nutrition and a variety of physiological changes that occur in old age. Bone structure changes, metabolic performance is affected, and dietary patterns change. In addition, a variety of social problems have an impact on the health status of the elderly. Independence is greatly reduced. Transportation modes are limited so the individual is forced to rely upon others for mobility. Adequate, safe, and affordable housing is another problem for many senior citizens.

The very nature of elderly illnesses results in long-term care. About 5 percent of the elderly reside in long-term health care facilities. The principal long-term care facility is the nursing home. Nursing homes are classified as either skilled or intermediate nursing care facilities. In the skilled nursing home, the patient can receive medical care on a twenty-four-hour-a-day basis. Medical care is also available in an intermediate care facility. However, the patient placed in this facility is capable of tending to personal needs.

There are several alternatives to long-term institutional care for the elderly. Respite care provides a place where certain services can be made available to the elderly on a daily outpatient basis. The individual can live with family and friends, yet can receive needed care.

Another alternative to the long-term care institution is health care provided in the home. In these situations, the provider comes to the home and gives medical care, therapy, or rehabilitative assistance in the familiar setting of the patient's home. This approach has been the object of great attention. In order for alternative elderly care programs to become more widely accepted and used, it is important that costs for these services be covered by third-party insurers, such as private health insurance companies, Medicare, and Medicaid.

Discussion Questions

1. What factors have contributed to the increased longevity of people in the past century?

2. In your opinion, when does old age begin?

3. Discuss the various considerations that must be considered by a person thinking about retiring.

4. Discuss the effect of economics on the health and well-being of the elderly.

5. In what ways do chronic illnesses affect the quality of elderly life?

6. Why are senior citizens often malnourished?

7. What are the risk factors associated with osteoporosis?

8. What happens to the human body physiologically that results in the condition known as osteoporosis?

9. Discuss some of the housing problems faced by the elderly.

10. Explain the cause, the signs, and the symptoms of Alzheimer's disease.

11. What has been learned from research in the past few years about Alzheimer's disease?

12. What are the different kinds of long-term health care facilities?

13. Identify some alternatives to long-term institutionalization of the elderly.

14. What is provided for in a home health care program?

15. What changes need to be made, in your opinion, to improve the availability of care for the elderly in the institutional setting?

Suggested Readings

Allen, Lindsay, H. "Calcium and Osteoporosis." *Nutrition Today* 21, no. 3 (May/June, 1986): 6–10.

Arie, Tom. "The Future for the Elderly." *Journal of the American Geriatrics Society* 29, no. 12 (December, 1981): 557–62.

Beal, Virginia A. "Nutrition in the Later Years." *Medical Times* 114, no. 10, (October, 1986): 35–44.

Branch, Laurence G. "Health Practices and Incident Disability Among the Elderly." *American Journal of Public Health* 75, no. 12 (December, 1985): 1436–39.

Cohen, Gene D., ed. "Mental Health and Aging: Clinical Programs, Problems, and Practice." *Hospital and Community Psychiatry* 33, no. 2 (February, 1982): 101–50.

Corolli, Connie H. "Osteoporosis: Significance, Risk Factors and Treatment." *The Nurse Practitioner* 11, no. 9 (September, 1986): 16–35.

Cowart, Marie E. "Policy Issues: Financial Reimbursement for Home Care." *Family and Community Health* 8, no. 2 (August, 1985): 1–10.

DePaoli, T., and Zenk-Jones, P. "Medicare Reimbursement in Home Care." *The American Journal of Occupational Therapy* 38, no. 11 (November, 1984): 739–42.

Department of Health and Human Services, Public Health Service. *Changes . . . Research on Aging and the Aged.* NIH Publication No. 81–85. Washington, D.C.: U.S. Government Printing Office, (1980).

Douglas, Kaaren C., and Hosokowa, Michael C. "Better Health for Elderly Patients." *Medical Times* 114, no. 10, (October, 1986): 52–60.

Greenfield, Carol A. "Improving Elderly Access to Health Care Information." *Business and Health* 3, no. 7 (June, 1986): 26–30.

Ham, R. "Alternatives to Institutionalization." *American Family Physician* 21, no. 7 (July, 1980): 95–100.

Hasselkus, Betty, and Brown, Margaret. "Respite Care for Community Elderly." *American Journal of Occupational Therapy* 37, no. 2 (February, 1983): 83–87.

Kane, R. L., and Kane, R. A. "Alternatives to Institutional Care of the Elderly: Beyond the Dichotomy." *The Gerontologist* 20, no. 3 (1980): 249–59.

Krause, D. "Institutional Living for the Elderly in Denmark: A Model for the United States." *Aging* (September/October, 1981): 29–38.

Piano, Lois A. "Adult Day Care: A New Ambulatory Care Alternative." *Nursing* 16, no. 8 (August, 1986): 60–62.

Smith, Dorothy L. "Patient Education: Tuning in to the Needs of the Elderly." *Medical Times* 114, no. 10 (October, 1986): 27–31.

Wan, Thomas T. H. "Use of Health Services by the Elderly in Low-Income Communities." *Milbank Memorial Fund Quarterly/Health and Society* 60, no. 1 (1982): 82–107.

Waxman, Howard M. "Community Mental Health Care for the Elderly—a Look at the Obstacles." *Public Health Reports* 101, no. 3 (May/June, 1986): 294–300.

Yeo, G., and McGann, L. "Utilization by Family Physicians of Support Services for Elderly Patients." *The Journal of Family Practice* 22, no. 5 (1986): 431–34.

Endnotes

1. National Institute on Aging, *Special Report on Aging, 1983.* Washington, D.C.: U.S. Government Printing Office, 1984.

2. Department of Health and Human Services, Public Health Service. *National Institute on Aging,* NIH Publication No. 83–1129 (July, 1983): 15.

3. Posner, Barbara M. *Nutrition and the Elderly.* Lexington, Ky.: D. C. Heath and Co., 1979.

4. Wolf, Colleen A. "Oral Health Care of the Elderly." *Ohio's Health* 34, no. 1 (1982): 11.

5. Department of Health and Human Services, Public Health Service, National Institute on Aging, *Age Pages* (November, 1985): 66.

6. National Safety Council, *Accident Facts, 1986 Edition.* Chicago, Ill.: National Safety Council: 6.

7. Surgeon General's Report on Health Promotion and Disease Prevention. *Healthy People.* Washington, D.C.: U.S. Government Printing Office, 1979: 372.

8. United States Senate Special Committee on Aging. *Developments in Aging, 1976.* Washington, D.C.: U.S. Government Office (1976).

9. President's Commission on Mental Health. *Report to the President.* Washington, D.C.: U.S. Government Printing Office, 1978.

10. Department of Health and Human Services, Public Health Service. *Changes . . . Research on Aging and the Aged.* NIH Publication No. 81–85 (October, 1980).

11. Surgeon General's Report. *Healthy People,* 375.

12. Hovaguimian, Theodore. "Mental Health in Old Age." *World Health* (February/March, 1982): 31.

13. The subject of community mental health centers is discussed at length in chapter 12.

14. Gaitz, Charles M., and Varner, Roy V. "Principles of Mental Health for Elderly Inpatients." *Hospital and Community Psychiatry* 33, no. 2 (February, 1982): 132.

15. Pavkov, Janet. "Suicide and the Elderly." *Ohio's Health* 34, no. 1 (1982): 21.

16. Department of Health and Human Services, *Special Report on Aging, 1980.* Washington, D.C.: U.S. Government Printing Office, 1980: 17.

17. Department of Health and Human Services, Public Health Service, National Institutes of Health, *Q & A: Alzheimer's Disease.* NIH Publication 85–1646 (May, 1985).

18. Department of Health and Human Services, Public Health Service. *Changes . . . Research on Aging and the Aged.*

19. Department of Health and Human Services, *Special Report on Aging, 1980.*

20. Emr, Marian. "Senility: The Outlook is Bright." *World Health* (February/March, 1982): 14.

21. U.S. Senate Commitee on Finance, *The Social Security Act and Related Laws.* Washington, D.C.: U.S. Government Printing Office (December, 1978).

22. Surgeon General's Report, *Healthy People,* 268.

23. Freece, Debbie. "Issues Relating to Long-Term Care Placement." *Ohio's Health* 34, no. 2 (February, 1982): 5.

24. Ham, R. "Alternatives to Institutionalization." *American Family Physician* 21, no. 7 (July, 1980): 95–100.

25. Freece, "Long-Term Care," 5.

26. Williams, Stephen J., and Torrens, Paul R. *Introduction to Health Services.* New York: John Wiley and Sons, 1980: 172.

27. Ibid., 172.

28. Watson, Wilbur H. *Aging and Social Behavior,* Monterey, Calif.: Wadsworth Health Sciences Division, 1982: 325.

29. Williams and Torrens, *Health Services,* 172.

30. U.S. National Center for Health Statistics, *Charges for Care and Sources of Payment for Residents in Nursing Homes, Series 13.* Washington, D.C.: U.S. Government Printing Office, 1977.

31. Krause, D. "Institutional Living for the Elderly in Denmark: A Model for the United States." *Aging* (September/October, 1981): 29–38.

32. Hasselkus, Betty, and Brown, Margaret. "Respite Care for Community Elderly." *The American Journal of Occupational Therapy* 37, no. 2 (February, 1983): 83–87.

33. Mitchell, J. B. "Patient Outcomes in Alternative Long-Term Care Settings." *Medical Care* 16, no. 6 (1978): 439–52.

34. DePaoli, T., and Zenk-Jones, P. "Medicare Reimbursement in Home Care." *The American Journal of Occupational Therapy* 38, no. 11 (November, 1984): 739–42.

35. Burris, K. C. "Recommending Adult Day Care Centers." *Nursing and Health Care* 2, no. 8 (October, 1981): 437–41.

18

Substances of Abuse: Drugs, Alcohol, and Tobacco

The people of the United States use drugs extensively. In many instances, there is a definite purpose and value for such use; drugs have numerous medicinal purposes. Medications may be either prescribed drugs or nonprescription medications. Over 1.4 billion prescriptions are filled each year by pharmacists in the United States. In addition, more than $6 billion are spent each year on nonprescription medications.[1] Thus it is obvious why the United States is often termed a drug-taking society.

All too often, however, drugs are used to satisfy underlying psychological needs. There are substances that cause alterations in the mood and psyche of an individual. With habitual use of these substances, the person can become dependent either physiologically or psychologically. Without careful control the individual may feel it is impossible to meet the responsibilities of a day without the use of a drug.

It is this unnecessary use of alcohol, tobacco, and other drugs of abuse that causes problems in society. As such this drug overuse has become important in community health programming. The extent of the problem is highlighted by the economic costs, the number of deaths caused by use of these mood-modifying substances, and the upheaval or disturbance of family and personal social structures.

It is doubtful that a totally drug-abstinent society is possible, or even desirable. A more realistic goal is for controlled, responsible use of chemicals. The behavioral patterns of drug abuse must be curtailed and eventually eliminated. Drug use, as it negatively affects the health and well-being of others, must be abolished. This is an important challenge for community health in the years ahead.

Drugs of Abuse

Drug use and abuse are community health issues that the medical community cannot deal with in isolation. Though there certainly are medical and health considerations associated with drug abuse, many community agencies and services are also extensively involved in any comprehensive community drug abuse program. In addition to medical personnel, the behavioral scientist, the educational expert, and social and vocational rehabilitators are important in planning activities to help the drug abuser.

In many communities, drug programs are usually a component of community mental health or alcohol programs, due to federal mental health legislation that included support for alcoholism and drug abuse programming. However, because of the unique requirements for drug abuse treatment, autonomy is important. Drug abuse should be more than just a small part of community mental health programming.

Illicit use of drugs has always been a part of society. However, most communities have viewed it as a serious problem only since the 1960s. Prior to that, drug abuse was usually perceived to be a problem for social outcasts who were living in poor, slum conditions and who were not considered part of the mainstream of community life.

As drug use and abuse have increased, their growth has extended beyond the boundaries of race, geography, and socioeconomics. Though it is very difficult to ascertain the cost of drug abuse, it has been estimated that the cost exceeds $10 billion a year, and there is speculation that this figure is an underestimate. Though abuse of drugs is found in all ages, significant use of drugs for nonmedical purposes decreases with age. Most drug abuse is found among adolescents and young adults, those in the eighteen- to twenty-five-year-old age group.

Why People Abuse Drugs

Why do people abuse drugs? What has accounted for the serious increase of drug abuse in the United States? A number of social factors are associated with the misuse of drugs in society. Drug misuse often begins during adolescence or the early college years, a period when peer pressure is most significant. At these ages young people tend to adopt the behavioral patterns of their peers. Peer pressure, because of its inherent power, is one of the major influences leading to drug use.

Taking drugs has become a part of normal living in many households. Alcohol consumption is considered a natural activity in the lives of many people, and people in the United States consume hundreds of thousands of over-the-counter and prescription drugs each year. These drug consumption models have an effect upon young people. As young people see adults taking a drink or "popping pills" for such problems as headaches, inability to sleep, or to help them relax, it seems only natural to seek drugs as a solution to their problems as well. Thus adults must realize the relationship between their drug and alcohol use and their children's behavior.

Young people use drugs, particularly marijuana, as a display of their alienation from authority. They see their parents and other authority figures using alcohol and other drugs to "get through the day." For the young person marijuana is the drug of choice for relaxation or to release stress and pressure. They see no reason why marijuana use is not acceptable behavior for them if alcohol use is the "norm" for adults. As a matter of fact they often resent adult opposition to their drug use behavior and consider parental and authority figures' opposition to their drug use patterns as hypocritical.

Drug use is often a way to satisfy certain sociological and psychological problems. It may be the means for gaining support, respect, and meaning from a social group or an individual. When a person is unable to find meaning in life or personal identity in socially approved activities, the alternative is often drug use.

Such behavior is often accompanied by apathy and decline in school or work performance. This is referred to as the "amotivational syndrome." The person cannot find success or interest in sports, clubs, or academic achievement, so, in turn, becomes involved in drug abuse. It is still unknown, however, whether drug use causes the syndrome or whether the syndrome is a forerunner of drug use.

The extent of fatalities resulting from drug abuse cannot be measured precisely because such fatalities are often categorized as "unknown," or "accidental," or are listed as an "overdose." Nevertheless, it has been estimated that each year there are seven to eight thousand deaths and 275 to 300 thousand medical emergencies related to drug abuse.[2] Narcotics account for most of these drug-related deaths. More recently cocaine use has resulted in many fatalities. Often, deaths are caused by the use of more than one drug, or polydrug use.

Commonly Abused Drugs

Several drugs are considered drugs of abuse. The most commonly abused drugs are: alcohol, hallucinogenic drugs, marijuana, nicotine, opiates, sedatives, and stimulants.

Alcohol

Alcohol consumption is a multibillion-dollar-a-year business in the United States. Approximately 70 percent of the American population drink alcoholic beverages.

Drinking in America is a social phenomenon. Alcoholic beverages are advertised extensively on television, the radio, and in print. This advertising portrays drinking as being normal, socially acceptable, and healthy. Many people feel it is inappropriate to have a party or gathering without serving alcoholic beverages. Mention a New Year's Eve party or a wedding reception, and most people picture an affair where various alcoholic drinks will be served. A significant amount of business is also transacted over cocktails, so many businesses and corporations budget large amounts of money for entertaining and social functions that usually involve alcohol consumption.

Most people drink socially and are able to control their level of liquor consumption. But the problem of alcohol misuse in those who do not know their "limit" has become a major social problem and as such is an important public health problem.

There are a number of problems related to alcohol use. Of increasing concern are the alcohol-related birth defects, the most common of which is Fetal Alcohol Syndrome. There is a definite association between the alcohol consumption of pregnant women and birth defects in newborn infants. It is unknown how much alcohol must be consumed before the syndrome develops, but it is known that

Millions of Americans consider alcohol consumption an important part of socialization. Alcoholic beverages are served at such social functions as parties, receptions, and business luncheons.

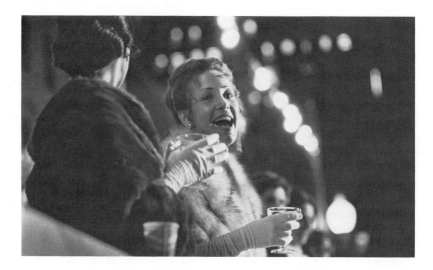

a variety of physiological abnormalities and mental retardation occur when the pregnant woman is a moderate-to-heavy drinker.[3]

Heavy drinking is associated with increased risks of cancer of several parts of the body: the tongue, mouth, larynx, and the liver. Alcohol consumption has also been associated with deterioration of the heart muscle, diminished cardiac output and the decreased ability of the heart muscle to contract. In fact, alcohol consumption is considered one of the major factors of cardiovascular disease.

Malnutrition is also linked to alcohol consumption. Alcohol is high in "empty" calories. The individual who drinks moderately to heavily often is deficient in vitamins and other essential nutrients needed for bodily functions.

One of the main organs affected by alcohol is the liver. An inflammation of the liver is known as *cirrhosis,* the seventh leading cause of death in the United States. It is almost always associated with alcohol consumption.

Alcohol consumption also results in accidental death and injury. Statistics indicate that over eighty thousand deaths a year are due to alcohol use.[4] Over half of these are the result of motor vehicle accidents involving intoxicated drivers.

Hallucinogenic Drugs

Several drugs create illusions in the mind of the user. These drugs alter perception, thought, and mood when taken in even very small amounts.[5] The user may see objects change color, shape, and appearance. In addition, different sights and sounds may be seen and heard. *Synesthesia,* crossing of sense responses—hearing colors and seeing sounds—may occur.[6] Hallucinogenic drugs also produce a variety of physiological and psychological effects.

The best-known hallucinogenic drugs are lysergic acid dethylamine (LSD) and mescaline (peyote). Other drugs that produce hallucinations, disorientation, and other mind-altering patterns are psilocybin, DMT (dimethyltryptamine), and PCP.

LSD has received the most attention of the hallucinogenic drugs, probably because it causes many serious physiological and psychological problems. It has been shown that LSD use impairs intellectual processes.[7] Prolonged psychosis and neurosis have also resulted from the use of this drug.[8]

Much of the concern over LSD is generated by the effect it has on chromosomes. Studies have shown chromosome breakdown in human white blood cells and in the fetus exposed to LSD.[9] Extensive research in this area continues in an effort to find more definite relationships.

Mescaline is an alkaloid found in the peyote cactus. Peyote is especially interesting because Native Americans have the legal sanction to use its derivative, mescaline, in religious ceremonies. The Native Americans believe that the visual hallucinations that occur with its use are a way of communicating with the spirits.[10]

Marijuana

After alcohol and cigarettes, marijuana is the third most frequently used drug in the United States. This drug has been used in various cultures for centuries in religious ceremonies and in important social celebrations. Today, though, marijuana is an illegal drug in most parts of the world.

Marijuana use has been a part of various cultures in the United States for decades. In the early part of the twentieth century many professional musicians were known to use this drug. However, the use of marijuana among the general "main-line" population first became a problem in the United States during the 1960s when it was heavily used by the counter-culture population. In the past two decades, the use of marijuana has increased and expanded to people of all social, economic, and cultural groups, not just the young. Though marijuana can be chewed, it is usually smoked in the form of marijuana cigarettes. The cigarettes contain a low potency level of the drug.

Despite this diffusion of marijuana use, it is still found principally among adolescents and young adults. The highest usage rates are found in the eighteen- to twenty-five-year age group. Marijuana use is increasing in a younger age group—among teenagers. As many as one-third of the high school seniors who use marijuana admitted that they began using the drug in ninth grade or earlier.[11] Marijuana usage, however, declines with age.

Marijuana is derived from the Indian hemp plant *Cannabis Sativa*. The flowering tops and leaves of this plant are dried, crushed, and then rolled into cigarettes. Marijuana cigarettes, known as "joints" or "reefers," are smoked by inhaling deeply into the lungs. The deep inhalation increases the amount of absorption of the active ingredient that causes the euphoric effects. This psychoactive ingredient in marijuana is *tetrahydrocannabinol* (THC).

The psychoactive effect upon an individual depends on the depth of the smoke inhalation, the strength (concentration) of THC, and the extent to which an individual has used the drug. Reactions to marijuana often include feelings of anxiety, depression, fatigue, nausea, and dizziness. Other noted physiological effects include an increase in pulse rate and blood pressure, dryness of the throat and mouth, and reddening of the whites of the eyes. Further intoxication can affect motor skills, reflexes, behavior, vision, and memory. In addition, sensitivity to pain has been noted among marijuana users.

Marijuana use has a depressant effect upon motor skills. As a result, motor vehicle operation and complex psychomotor performance are impaired, as they are when an individual is under the influence of alcohol. Habitual marijuana users tend to have more accidents than nonusers. This problem is compounded by the fact that marijuana is commonly used in conjunction with alcohol. The combined effect results in greater impairment than that which would result from the use of either alone.[12] There is sufficient evidence to recommend that marijuana users not drive while under the influence of the drug, just as they should not drive while intoxicated with alcohol.

Though the evidence is inconclusive, there seems to be a relationship between biological health and marijuana use. There have been reported instances of impairment of the body's natural defense system against disease among marijuana smokers. However, other reports contradict this.[13]

Another relationship involves the effect of marijuana use on reproduction. The drug decreases the number and mobility of sperm among males who use marijuana on a regular basis. Also, abnormal chromosomes have been noted among marijuana users. Both of these concerns, however, are subject to difference of opinion.[14]

Marijuana affects short-term memory, leading to impairment of intellectual performance.[15] Though this impairment varies according to the dose of the drug, the individual's level of motivation, and other variables, it does have definite implications for young people of school age.

Marijuana use has been an extremely controversial issue. Some contend that the drug is no more dangerous than alcohol. Thus, they argue, it should be legalized so its use is free from the stigma of drug abuse. Others believe that marijuana must be banned from society and its users must be punished. Between these two poles are a spectrum of opinions as to how society should cope with the problem of marijuana use.

It is interesting to note that marijuana has been used in medical treatment. It has been effective in the treatment of glaucoma and there have been instances where it has been used to help control nausea and vomiting in cancer chemotherapy patients. Marijuana dilates the bronchial tubes so some medical personnel working with asthma patients have suggested that it might be helpful in treating this respiratory condition.

Nicotine

Nicotine is a central nervous system stimulant that is present in the tobacco leaf and so is inhaled into the body when a person smokes cigarettes. Though nicotine is partially destroyed by the burning cigarette, as much as one-third passes into the body unchanged in the inhaled smoke.[16] Nicotine increases respiratory and heart rates as well as the blood pressure of a cigarette smoker. The stimulant has also been known to increase peristalsis of the intestines.[17]

Smoking has been called the ". . . single most important preventable cause of death and disease."[18] The Surgeon General, in a report of the health effects of smoking, said in 1982 that smoking is the most important public health issue of our time.[19]

Many health problems are associated with cigarette smoking, including cardiovascular disease, chronic bronchitis, emphysema, and cancer. Respiratory infections and stomach ulcers are also linked to cigarette smoking. Nearly a third of all cancer deaths in the United States are related to smoking; it is the major cause of lung cancer and contributes to cancer of the bladder, kidney, and pancreas.[20]

The single most effective way to reduce hazards of smoking continues to be that of quitting entirely.

Source: *The Health Consequences of Smoking. The Changing Cigarette: A Report of the Surgeon General* (1981): vi.

Opiates

The opiates are drugs derived from opium. These drugs, the opium alkaloids, are narcotics. Opium in its derivatives includes codeine (a prescription drug), morphine (a prescription drug), and heroin (an illegal drug). Narcotics have a depressant effect on the central nervous system, so are used for pain relief by producing drowsiness and sleep. Codeine is often prescribed as a cough suppressant; morphine as a pain reliever. When used in moderation, there are few side effects of codeine and little risk of addiction.[21]

Morphine, used as a pain killer and as an anesthetic, is more addictive. When used over a long period of time with increasing dosage, a person becomes psychologically and physically dependent upon the drug. An individual develops a tolerance to the drug, and consequently, larger doses are required to achieve the desired effect. This leads to physical dependency.

Heroin is considered to be the most seriously abused drug. Because of its adverse effect on users, it is illegal in the United States. The use of heroin causes a euphoric or pleasurable sensation for most users.

Heroin can be used in several forms. It is most frequently mixed with a liquid and injected directly into the vein, a practice called *mainlining*. This intravenous injection results in the most rapid and most euphoric sensation. Heroin may also be taken orally or inhaled. In both of these procedures, the euphoric effect is often not as strong and the effect is more delayed than when injected.

The danger of overdose that will result in death or physical disability is always present. Often the drug user is unaware of the exact strength or dosage of the heroin and so uses too much. Unless emergency help is available to assist the abuser through the overdose crisis, serious consequences may occur.

Heroin use can indirectly cause disease, especially hepatitis. Hepatitis develops when contaminated drug paraphernalia is used to inject the heroin into the bloodstream.

Addiction to heroin can result if there is continued use of the drug. An addicted individual finds it extremely difficult to break this reliance on heroin. The process of detoxification, described later in this chapter, can be both painful and difficult.

Heroin is very costly in terms of both physiological and social problems. For example, malnutrition is often found among heroin users. All too often the individual using heroin is unemployed so resorts to crime in order to support the habit. Any incoming money is applied directly to heroin purchase, not to the purchase of nutritious food.

Since the use, possession, and sale of heroin are illegal in this country, a user can only obtain the drug through illegal and black market sellers. This practice creates many serious social problems. The quality of the purchased heroin often is questionable, both in terms of strength and purity. Purchasing "bad" heroin may result in overdose, disease, or other problems.

Sedatives

Drugs that cause depressant effects on the central nervous system and upon the various physiological processes of the body are known as sedatives. Sedatives are prescribed for a variety of medical purposes. Certain sedatives are used in treatment of the psychotic mental patient. The antipsychotic drugs alleviate pain, fear, delusions, and tensions in the psychotic patient.

Thousands of sedatives are used daily to help people to relax, to encourage sleep, and to relieve nervous conditions. More prescriptions are written for tranquilizers than for any other drug in the United States.[22] This reliance upon tranquilizers to "make it through the day" provokes a variety of problems. For example, young people who see their parents using tranquilizers use this behavior as justification for their own use of drugs for pleasure.

Physiologically, the use of tranquilizers to induce sleep can have a detrimental effect upon the normal sleep pattern. The induced sleep is not as sound or complete as when these drugs are not used.

Sedative abuse refers to (1) the increasing reliance upon the drug or (2) to overdose, either accidental or intentional. Overdose reduces the body's physiological functioning and can cause death. If the respiratory functioning becomes depressed to the point where breathing stops, the individual is likely to suffer long-term impairment or death. Sedatives are the major prescription drugs used by people in the United States in attempts to commit suicide.[23] When combined with alcohol, serious depressing effects occur.

Stimulants

Central nervous system stimulants are also heavily used in the United States. Stimulants are used by dieters to lose weight, students at exam time, and long-distance truck drivers to keep awake. Because of their extensive use and despite their medicinal benefits, stimulants are frequently abused.

The abuse of stimulants begins innocently enough. Often the individual begins to take amphetamines (stimulants) for a specific medical purpose. The euphoric feeling produced becomes increasingly desirable. As a result, the user increases the dosage in order to obtain even greater effects from the drug. Physical dependence does not occur, but the psychological dependence necessitates progressively greater doses of the drug. The mental depression that follows a high is avoided by taking another round of the given drug.

Cocaine Probably the fastest growing drug abuse problem in the United States today is the use of cocaine. The use of this stimulant in recent years has increased dramatically. Whereas there were only about 5 percent of the United States population who had ever used cocaine in the late 1970s, by the mid-1980s nearly 20 percent reported having tried the drug. It is estimated that there are more than twenty million users of this drug at the present time. It is considered to be the drug of choice for millions of adults and school-age children. In the past, cocaine use was found most prevalently among entertainers, professional athletes, and wealthy businessmen. However, today it is widely used by middle, working class people.

Cocaine is an alkaloid extracted from the leaves of the coca plant found in parts of South America. In the late 1800s cocaine was thought to be a miracle drug having medicinal values.

Cocaine is usually taken by snorting—sniffing or inhaling through the nostrils—and free-basing (smoking). In either case, the effect of the drug on the central nervous system is immediate. Smoking, or free-basing, of cocaine results in quicker, more intense, euphoric, and addictive effect. It is usually smoked in a glass waterpipe using a lighter as a heat source. Cocaine is also smoked in cigarettes.

Upon inhalation of the smoke, cocaine is absorbed in the lungs directly into the circulatory system. It is transmitted to the brain as quickly as ten seconds. Hence instantaneous euphoria is attained. This is followed by a rebound dysphoria (crash), with intense craving for another euphoric state.

Cocaine increases the respiratory rate, the heart rate, and blood pressure. It can interrupt the normal electrical impulse conrol of the heart resulting in a sudden onset of seizures and cardiac arrest. In addition, it causes an acceleration of many other of the body physiological functions. This produces restlessness, euphoria, excitement, and an inability to relax. Serious overdose reactions often occur. These include such respiratory problems as chest congestion, chronic cough, wheezing, and the development of black phlegm. Following the "highs" produced by the drug, depresssion, anxiety, and other psychological problems occur.

Cocaine is not physiologically addicting, but psychological dependence does result and is as demanding as if there were physical dependency. Psychological effects include irritability, violent behavior, depression, the presence of hallucinations, and short temper. The individual using cocaine must cope with depression as well as sleep and appetite disturbances.

The cocaine user is often in need of the support of a substance abuse treatment program. Initial hospitalization is often needed to disrupt the compulsive use habit. Total abstinence is difficult to achieve, often requiring extensive rehabilitative care including counseling.

A new, smokable form of cocaine that has received much attention in the mid-1980s is "crack." Crack is extracted in a simple procedure using sodium bicarbonate (baking soda), heat, and water. It is easily manufactured and extremely addictive. This form of cocaine is called "crack" because of a "crackling" sound that is produced when it is being heated. It is sold as tiny "rocks" for under twenty dollars. It is cheap, readily available, and desired by the users because of its highly addictive feature. For the drug dealer "crack" provides extremely high profits, it is much easier to handle, and the addictive feature assures continuing need by the users.

Caffeine The most widely ingested central nervous system stimulant in America is caffeine. Caffeine is found in a number of drinks consumed by the American public: cola drinks, tea, over-the-counter preparations, and most specifically, coffee. Caffeine stimulates the cortex of the brain where breathing, the thought processes, and other vital function activities of the body are controlled. Greater sensitivity to stimuli, wakefulness, and better physical functioning result from use of this drug.

The widespread use of caffeine has raised concerns for various population groups. At particular risk are young people, cardiac patients, the elderly, and pregnant women. Educational efforts must be made to inform the public of the potential dangers of too much caffeine and to encourage its reduction in the diet.

Treatment and Rehabilitation

Treatment of drug abusers was not a public health concern until the early part of the twentieth century. At that time, treatment was a medical procedure conducted by private physicians. Since drug addiction was considered a physical disease that could be cured by gradual withdrawal, there was little concern for the psychological and sociological aspects of drug use. For this reason, care was provided in a quiet manner by the individual's private physician with as little public attention as possible.

With passage of the Harrison Narcotic Act in 1914, the availability of certain drugs, the opiates and cocaine, became restricted to the medical professionals. Physicians and dentists had access to these drugs only for use in their professional practice. This legal restriction led to the development of an illegal drug market. As with many other social issues, illegal markets compound problems, usually by introducing crime and skyrocketing costs. Since drug abuse was considered a felony, the prisons became populated with drug addicts.

In response to these problems, the federal government established two drug abuse treatment hospitals in the 1930s, in Lexington, Kentucky, and in Fort Worth, Texas. Here drug addicts underwent withdrawal measures. Unfortunately, though, the withdrawal was only temporary. A large number of patients in these facilities reverted to drug abuse after their release.

Until the early 1950s, these two facilities were the only major drug abuse treatment facilities in the United States. But as drug abuse increased during the 1950s and 1960s, several drug treatment programs were developed. At the present time, treatment for drug dependency is effective only for opiate addiction and alcohol. There is no chemotherapy for treating the abuse of amphetamines, barbiturates, and hallucinogens.

Therapeutic Communities

Residential programs, called *therapeutic communities,* have become important in drug abuse treatment. These programs attempt to effect behavioral change, leading to a reduction in drug use.

The first therapeutic community program for drug addicts, Synanon, was founded in 1959. The residential therapy concept instituted there involves a group of individuals living and working together while striving to solve their drug abuse problems. The psychological dimension of drug abuse is emphasized using group therapy, group interaction, and mutual support activities. The principles of behavior modification are the foundation of the program of the therapeutic community. Because this frequently demands small-group participation, residential therapeutic programs are only somewhat successful. They are limited in the number of individuals that can be treated.

The value of residential treatment centers is that the individual can receive social support during the rehabilitative process. Social and medical professionals help the patient to gradually work his or her way back into the community setting. The patient is still able to "lean" on the support of the residential center during this time.

Therapeutic community programs require individuals to remain in the program for varying periods of time. In some instances, this may be for months, and it is not unusual to find an individual involved in such a program for several years. It is for this reason that the operation of a therapeutic community can become a very expensive form of treatment. Many drug users do not have the financial resources to continue the treatment until they are "cured."

Methadone Maintenance Treatment Programs

The primary method of treating heroin use is through the methadone maintenance treatment programs. These programs were developed in the 1960s by Doctors Dole and Nyswander of Rockefeller University. These researchers noted that methadone, a synthetic narcotic drug, could serve as a substitute, or a blocking agent, for heroin and morphine to ease the pain of withdrawal.

Methadone maintenance treatment programs are found in many communities throughout the country. In this drug therapy, the drug user is stabilized with daily doses of methadone, taken orally either in tablet form or mixed with orange juice.

These programs can be conducted on an outpatient basis and so are much less costly than other treatment programs that require inpatient care. Even though the patient does not have to be hospitalized, it is necessary to return to the treatment center daily for methadone maintenance. As long as the individual takes the methadone on a daily basis, the craving for heroin does not occur. Methadone creates a "blocking effect" to the euphoria created by the opiate drug. The dependence is then shifted from heroin and morphine to methadone.

Because the long-term cure rate is not good, addicts must be kept on methadone maintenance for years. The ultimate goal of methadone maintenance treatment programs should be complete detoxification, a drug-free state. Unfortunately, these programs have not been successful in total detoxification.

Federal regulations require methadone maintenance programs to provide services other than administering methadone. Group therapy, vocational training, and social services must be a part of the treatment program, too. Thus, the needs of the total person are met. The individual's craving for heroin is relieved by the methadone, and the psychological and sociological needs are met through involvement in the additional services.

Hospitalization

Considered to be the least effective form of treatment, hospitalization is also the most expensive, as the patient is usually treated over a long period of time. When hospitals have been used for drug treatment, the relapse rate after release has been very high. Because of this lack of success in treating drug abuse, the federal hospitals in Fort Worth and Lexington are closed to drug patients today.

Emergency room services at the hospital are used when an individual is experiencing a drug crisis. But after the crisis passes, the patient is released and often does not receive the rehabilitative treatment needed. If there are associated health needs in addition to the drug dependency, it is likely that hospital inpatient care will be necessary. However, this inpatient care does not include treatment for the drug abuse problem itself.

Drug-Free Outpatient Services

Another approach to drug treatment offers drug-free services on an outpatient basis. In this approach, group or individual psychotherapy is usually provided, as are counseling, health services, and vocational and educational training. Some detoxification measures are taken, but the program centers more upon group support for a drug-free life-style. This approach, though somewhat successful for the young drug experimenter, is of less value to the addict. The outpatient nature of this program places the drug addict back into the community with no support mechanisms to withstand the social and personal pressures that forced the drug use originally.

Detoxification

The process whereby a person who is physically dependent upon a drug is gradually withdrawn from the drug is known as detoxification. The goal of detoxification is to provide a safe withdrawal by administering decreasing doses of the drug. Detoxification is necessary in order to prevent pain, discomfort, and other related problems created by abrupt termination of drug usage.

In a drug detoxification program (which should be joined voluntarily) the patient receives enough of the substitute drug to suppress severe withdrawal symptoms. Usually a long-acting drug is substituted for the short-acting drug of addiction. For example, methadone is substituted for heroin, phenobarbital is substituted for short-acting barbiturates, and valium and librium are substituted for alcohol.[24]

Detoxification must be part of an integrated long-term treatment program because besides removal from drug dependency, the treatment attempts to resolve the underlying social and psychological factors that led to the drug abuse. This social and psychological rehabilitation requires effective counseling, positive education, and the support of the community.

Drug rehabilitation services are provided in most residential treatment centers. At these facilities, the individual receives professional, social, and medical help to gradually reenter community life.

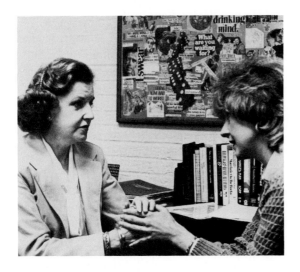

Multimodality Approach

Most recently, treatment and rehabilitation programs for drug abusers have used a multimodality approach. The need for prevention, treatment, education, and rehabilitation must be met in one drug treatment program that integrates these services. For example, a treatment program may include the use of methadone maintenance, detoxification, inpatient drug-free treatment, outpatient services, and a therapeutic community. The patient may be transferred from one type of program to another as the need arises. Some suggest that the multimodality approach may be the most effective method of treating abuse within the local community.

Alcoholism

For many people the term alcoholism evokes thoughts of poorly clothed, dirty, unemployed, transient men found on the skid rows of large urban communities. The stereotyped picture is often a homeless, lonely person who has spent years moving about, drowning loneliness in drink.

With the growing alcohol consumption in American society, alcoholism has taken on larger dimensions. Today most alcoholics are people who cannot control their intake of liquor, yet who are still employed and able to live an outwardly reasonable life-style. When confronted with the accusation of being alcoholics, they will almost always deny having a drinking problem.

Due to society's negative attitude toward the alcoholic, family members and close associates of an alcoholic often will not take measures to assist the individual until the condition has become obvious. These support people often do not understand the problem and therefore refuse to talk about it.

The Disease

Is alcoholism a disease or is it the result of a weakened personality? For many years the alcoholic was considered a deviate who simply could not, or would not, control the amount of alcohol consumed. This alcohol intake often led to intoxication or to nonsocial behavior. For many people, this problem had moral dimensions. The drunk was often put in jail; the alcoholic was hidden from society by family and friends; and certain groups taught that the problem was the result of evil or sin. There was relatively little success in the few attempts to rehabilitate the alcoholic.

Since the 1950s, the American Medical Association has considered alcoholism a disease, a deviation from normal health and well-being. Today most rehabilitation programs are based on the disease theory of alcoholism rather than the personality deviation theory.

Exactly what causes alcoholism is unknown. No chemical in alcoholic beverages, nor metabolic, physiological, or genetic defects in individuals have been identified that cause alcoholism. Research has examined hormone deficiencies, allergic reactions, and body metabolism as possible causes of alcoholism. In spite of such extensive efforts to find a cause, "The nature of the addictive process, the developmental sequence of events and the central nervous system alterations which define the condition of alcohol addiction are unknown. . . . The development of approaches to these very basic questions constitutes perhaps the major challenge to the biological scientist concerned with addiction."[25]

Today, most professionals treat alcoholism as a chronic disease. The alcoholic can never be cured, but can be treated and the disease arrested. With appropriate care and treatment, the alcoholic can resume a happy, healthy, and productive life-style. This is not an easy task, however. The person must completely refrain from the use of any alcoholic beverage. Failure to do so only precipitates a renewed problem with alcohol.

Alcoholism is a progressive disease in that the person's condition deteriorates without appropriate care. Physiological processes are affected, mental health is impaired, and social relationships deteriorate. Without proper care, alcoholism can eventually result in death.

A serious problem with alcoholism is that the alcoholic often is not aware of the problem. This may be the failure to admit to the condition, but it is more likely the result of the physiological effects of alcohol on the body. Alcohol depresses the neurological system and often an alcoholic does not remember anything related to the drinking episode. Since the problem usually is not recognized in the early stages by those who could treat the problem, the diagnosis of alcoholism occurs at an advanced stage. The patient is then unable to control personal drinking, organic damage has begun, and social relationships are endangered.

Treatment

Unfortunately, in the case of alcoholism, the individual is in need of medical treatment but fails to voluntarily obtain the care. This often leads to forced medical care, a process known as *intervention*. Intervention is a method of obtaining help for the alcoholic before it is physiologically too late to reverse the problem or before death occurs. People who care about the alcoholic seek treatment for the person. If necessary, the alcoholic is forced to enter a treatment program. Once in the program, it is hoped that the individual will recognize the problem and then take action to solve the problem. Intervention is usually only effective if more than one person is willing to help.

Three different steps in the treatment of alcoholism have been described:[26]

1. Management of episodes of intoxication to overcome the immediate effects of excess alcohol
2. Correcting the chronic health problems associated with alcoholism
3. Change in the alcoholic's behavior so as to discontinue the drinking patterns

Treatment of alcoholism is a complex process involving time, patience, professional competence, and the understanding of friends and relatives. The process begins with detoxification. Through medical supervision, the alcoholic is taken off alcohol and other mood-modifying chemicals, a procedure that is best accomplished in a general hospital. This is often a very difficult time for the patient.

In the past, general hospitals have not offered long-term inpatient care for alcoholism treatment. Most inpatient alcoholism treatment was conducted in state mental hospitals. If such care was available in the general hospital, it was usually quite costly. This denied treatment to those who could not afford it. As a result, the alcoholic was treated in the emergency department for related injuries, then discharged to other agencies, such as the jail or mental hospital, in order to sober up.

Even though state mental hospitals and community mental health centers still provide extensive alcoholic care, the American Medical Association and the American Hospital Association now recommend that alcoholic patients be treated in the general hospital. Hospitals now are developing treatment programs for the alcoholic. Such services involve programmatic activities for the family and associates. Another part of the treatment process involves educational measures to inform the alcoholic, family, and friends about the disease. These efforts provide information about how alcoholic beverages affect the body. Group therapy allows the patient to interact with others who have faced the same problems. Therapy sessions help the patient to understand and accept the disease, as well as to prepare for reentry into the community when the inpatient part of the treatment is completed. The patient must be prepared for problems that will occur when he or she returns home, to his or her job, and to social settings. Usually an alcoholic patient faces personal, family, and financial problems created by the drinking problem, all of which need therapeutic attention before release from the treatment center.

When hospital treatment ends, recovery from alcoholism becomes a lifetime process. The recovering alcoholic must from that time on take measures to stay well. This extremely difficult task usually requires the understanding, concern, and support of family, friends, and associates. The education, counseling, and therapy assistance family members receive during the treatment phase help them to assist the patient in abstaining from drink.

Most communities have several organizations that help the recovering alcoholic. These agencies, usually staffed by nonmedical personnel, aid the patient in adjusting to the new life-style of a recovering alcoholic. Possibly the best-known agency is Alcoholics Anonymous.

Alcoholics Anonymous (AA) is a voluntary fellowship of recovering alcoholics who come together to help each other stay away from alcohol. Before becoming involved in AA, a person must recognize a lack of control over alcohol and desire assistance from a therapeutic group.

Another organization modeled after Alcoholics Anonymous is Al-Anon. This organization is for relatives of alcoholic patients. The spouse or other relative is able to learn from the experience of others how to cope with the situation. Alateen is a similar organization for the teenage children of alcoholics.

In addition to these organizations, community professionals are available to counsel the alcoholic and his or her family. Clergy are often called upon for counseling. Public health nurses, vocational rehabilitation counselors, and parole officers have also received special training to assist the alcoholic. The key to successful alcoholic rehabilitation is recognition and use of these available resources in the community.

A number of government agencies have alcohol treatment programs. The Veterans Administration hospital system conducts the largest alcohol treatment program in the country. Veterans receive this care free of charge. Other programs are sponsored by various state and local government authorities.

Industry has shown increasing interest in the establishment of alcohol treatment programs. The first industrial alcohol treatment programs were established in the 1940s. Since then, hundreds of companies have developed similar programs. These industrial alcoholic rehabilitation programs are designed for early recovery from alcohol misuse. Usually such efforts are quite effective.

Tobacco Use

Smoking and Health

For many years, there was no clear association between smoking and disease. It was not until 1964, with the publication of the first *Surgeon General's Report on Smoking and Health,* that clear associations between smoking and specific diseases were noted. The report by the Surgeon General's Advisory Committee identified an association of lung cancer, emphysema, coronary artery disease, and chronic bronchitis with cigarette smoking.

A second *Surgeon General's Report on Smoking and Health* was released in 1979. This report updated the data on smoking in the United States and provided a foundation for the establishment of an antismoking campaign established by the Department of Health, Education and Welfare (HEW). Cigarette smoking was designated "Public Health Enemy Number One" by the federal government. Since that time, additional reports have been issued, more than one a year, each focusing upon some aspect of the hazards related to cigarette smoking. The various publications have reported links between cigarette smoking and cancer, particularly lung cancer; the close relationship between smoking and cardiovascular disease; the relationship between smoking and chronic obstructive lung disease; plus a variety of other matters.

Resolution by the American Medical Association Concerning Smoking, 1985

1. Call for a smoke-free society by the year 2000
2. Call for a complete ban on all advertising of cigarettes and smokeless tobacco products
3. Support for a minimum age of twenty-one for the purchasing of tobacco products
4. Ban on all vending machine sales of tobacco
5. Require a fifth warning label on chewing tobacco and snuff

Since the publication of the first report, many people have quit smoking and the proportion of adult smokers has declined from about 42 percent in 1965 to close to 30 percent today.[27] Though cigarette smoking has declined, there are still an estimated 320,000 deaths each year related to smoking.[28] Smoking rates for males have declined more rapidly than for females. However, the gap between male and female smoking is narrowing.[29] The fact that the percentage of smokers in all groups has declined does not eliminate smoking as a major community health concern.

Women of childbearing age should seriously consider the hazards of cigarette smoking. Women who smoke and use oral birth control pills have a 10 percent greater chance of having a heart attack or other cardiovascular diseases than those who do not smoke. There is also evidence that maternal smoking can have an effect on the fetus and on childbirth. Frequently children of smoking women are born prematurely or with birth defects. The risk of spontaneous abortion, fetal death, and infant death is also greater among smoking mothers.[30]

In spite of strong evidence linking cigarette smoking to various diseases, there still exists a strong opposition to antismoking programs and strategies. Tobacco is a multimillion-dollar agricultural business in several southeastern states and efforts to reduce the level of tobacco use have posed a serious economic threat to people living in these localities.

Tobacco Companies Diversify

In recent years the various tobacco manufacturing companies have diversified their businesses by purchasing or buying major financial interests in a broad range of other companies and corporations. For example, the Philip Morris Company purchased the General Foods Corporation for $5.75 billion. This meant that the Post Cereal line of Grape Nuts, Honeycomb, Alpha Bits, Sugar Crisp, and Fruit and Fiber is now owned by a tobacco company. Other products of the General Foods Corporation included Maxwell House Coffee, Sanka Coffee, Brim Coffee, Kool Aid, Oscar Mayer meats, Minute Rice, Tang, Log Cabin syrups and a variety of other products. Philip Morris had already purchased the Miller High Life Beer, Lowenbrau, 7-Up, and Meister Brau lines. The extent to which diversification has taken place can be seen by looking at the chart on the adjoining page.

TOBACCO INDUSTRY CONGLOMERATES—
Status Report on Diversification in the Tobacco Industry
1986
representative products

Tobacco Manufacturer (conglomerate owner or affiliate)	Tobacco Brands	Other Products
PHILIP MORRIS, INCORPORATED	Marlboro, Merit, Benson & Hedges, Players, Virginia Slims, Parliament	Miller Brewing Company (Miller High Life, Lite Beer from Miller, Meister Brau, Lowenbrau, Magnum Malt Liquor), The Seven-Up Company (7-up, Diet 7-up, Like Cola), General Foods Corporation (Post Cereals: Grape Nuts, Post Raisin Bran, 40% Bran Flakes, Post Toasties, Fruit & Fibre, Honeycomb, Alpha Bits, Pebbles, Sugar Crisp, Smurfberry Crunch, etc.; Maxwell House coffees, Sanka coffees, Yuban coffees, Jello Products, D-zerta gelatins, Kool Aid, Crystal Light, Country Time, Oscar Mayer Meats, Louis Rich Turkey products, Log Cabin syrups, Good Seasons dressings, Entenmann's bakery, Cool Whip, Stove Top Stuffings, Minute Rice, Birds Eye frozen foods, Tang, Shake n Bake, Ronzoni pasta), Mission Viejo Realty Group
R. J. REYNOLDS TOBACCO COMPANY (R. J. REYNOLDS INDUSTRIES)	Camel, Winston, Salem, Sterling, Bright, Doral, More, Century, Now, Vantage, Winchester, Ritz, Prince Albert, Carter Hall, Madiera Gold	Kentucky Fried Chicken, Canada Dry, Delmonte, Chun King oriental foods, Hawaiian Punch, Morton Frozen Foods, Nabisco Brands (Premium saltines, Ritz crackers, Wheat Thins, Triscuit, etc. Oreo cookies, Planters Nuts, Blue Bonnet margarine, Baby Ruth & Butterfingers candy bars, Life Savers roll candy, Care Free sugarless gum, etc.), Patio Mexican foods, Snap-E-Tom, Milk Mate, A-1 Steak Sauce, Escoffier Sauces, Grey Poupon, Ortega Mexican food, My-T-Fine, Brer Rabbit molasses, College Inn, Vermont Maid, Heublein (Arrow Cordials, Black Velvet, Cuervo, Don Q Rum, Irish Mist, Jose Cuervo, Popov, Smirnoff, The Club Cocktails, Yukon Jack, Inglenook wines, Napa Valley wines, Harvey's Bristol Creme, Lancer Vin Rose)
BROWN & WILLIAMSON TOBACCO (div. B.A.T. Industries) (British American Tobacco) (Canadian affiliate, Imasco)	Kool, Barclay, Belair, Viceroy, Richland 25's	Marshall Field & Company, Gimbels Department Stores, Saks Fifth Avenue, Kohl's Department Stores, Appleton Papers, Yardley, Imasco (Imperial Tobacco, Hardee's Restaurants, People's Drug, Shoppers Drug Mart, Burger Chef, Embassy Cleaners)
LIGGETT GROUP (Liggett & Myers Tobacco) (div. Grand Metropolitan, P.L.C.)	Chesterfield, L & M, Lark, Eve, many ''generic'' cigarettes sold in USA, Pinkerton Tobacco Company (Red Man Chew)	Carlsberg Beer, Alpo Dog Food, Diversified Products (gym equipment), Children's World, Inc., Intercontinental Hotels Corp., International Distillers & Vintners (J & B Scotch, Gilbey's Gin, Bombay Gin, Bailey's Original Irish Cream, Grand Marnier, Absolut Vodka)
LORILLARD (div. Loews Corp.)	Newport, Satin, Kent, Triumph, Kent Golden Lights, True, Old Gold, Max, Beech-nut Chewing Tobacco	CNA Financial (Continental Casualty Corporation and its insurance and financial affiliates), General Finance Corporation, Loews Hotels, Loews Theatres, Bulova Watch Company
AMERICAN TOBACCO COMPANY (div. American Brands, Inc.)	Lucky Strike, Pall Mall, Carlton, and Tareyton cigarettes; Half and Half, and Bourbon Blend smoking tobaccos; La Corona, Antonio y Cleopatra, Roi Tan, and Grenadiers cigars	Franklin Life Insurance Company, Southland Life Insurance, Pinkertons, Inc., Master Lock Company, Swingline Office Supplies, James B. Beam Distillery, Sunshine Biscuits, Wilson-Jones Office Forms, Acme Visible Office Supplies, Titleist and Acushnet golf products, Andrew Jergens Company
U. S. TOBACCO COMPANY	Skoal, Skoal Bandits, Copenhagen, Borkum Riff, Amphora, Perfecto Garcia	Chateau Ste. Michelle wines, Zig Zag cigarette papers, Cedar King pencils, Dr. Grabow pipes
CULBRO, INC.	General Cigar Co. (Garcia y Vega, White Owl, Robt. Burns, Corina, Wm. Penn, Tiparillo, Tijuana Smalls, London Dock, Kentucky Club), Helme Tobacco Company (Gold River, Mail Pouch, Silver Creek, Redwood, Chatanooga Chew)	Snacktime Company (Golden Pop, Chesty Potato Chips, Pepitos, Snack Time), Imperial Nurseries

NOTE: Sources: Company annual reports (1984 or 1985) and news releases. Based on latest available information.

Prepared by: William J. Bailey, MPH

Not only has the tobacco industry lobbied political bodies to put a stop to antismoking programs, but major advertising campaigns have been designed to show the pleasures of smoking.

Not only should concern be expressed for the person who smokes, but there is evidence that those who live and/or work around smoking may be at danger for certain problems. For example, it has been noted that children of smoking parents have more respiratory diseases such as bronchitis and pneumonia. There is a possibility that lung cancer may be caused by passive inhalation of smoke by nonsmokers. Women who are nonsmokers but whose husbands are smokers have shown an increased incidence of lung cancer. The matter of passive effects of smoking, or *sidestream smoke,* as many refer to it, is receiving an increasing amount of research.

Smoking Cessation Programs

Different programs have been developed to help people stop smoking. Several educational programs make use of the mass media. These programs include public interest statements that focus upon high-risk groups, including pregnant women, teenagers, and workers in potentially dangerous environments.

The American Cancer Society and the American Lung Association have smoking cessation programs. The American Lung Association introduced a program in 1981 entitled *Freedom From Smoking.* This program is based upon extensive research, development, and evaluation, and encourages ongoing support activities for the individual. It is designed to free cigarette smokers of the habit in as short a period of time as twenty days, primarily through behavior modification. It incorporates ways to improve eating habits, to reduce stress, and to assert feelings. The material employed is very attractive and seems positive in its approach and appearance. Other programs have been developed by industry and other private groups.

Most people who quit smoking seem to have some motivation to do so. Four factors have been identified as being of major importance in smoking

cessation: (1) concern about some health problem, (2) to set an example for others, (3) a desire for self-control, and (4) aesthetic reasons.[31]

Smokeless Tobacco

The increasing concern related to smoking and its effects on health has led many individuals to turn to the use of smokeless tobacco. Smokeless tobacco has been promoted by the tobacco industry as a safe alternative to smoking. An estimated twenty-two million people in the United States use smokeless tobacco.[32] Sales of smokeless tobacco have increased more than 10 percent each year in the past decade with annual sales now being nearly one billion dollars.[33]

Smokeless tobacco has been used throughout the history of this country. However, major concern in recent years is the increasing use by young adults, women, and school-age children. It has not been uncommon to find children in elementary and junior high schools "chewing" tobacco.

Smokeless tobacco is available in two basic types, as snuff (powdered tobacco) and as chewing tobacco. In the United States there are three main types of chewing tobacco: (1) loose leaf, (2) plug tobacco, and (3) twist. Snuff is powdered tobacco that can be made from finely cut tobacco leaves.

With this increase in use of smokeless tobacco have come increasing concerns about its effect on health. An increase in the incidence of oral cancer, particularly cancers of the cheek and gums, has been noted among users. Oral cancers usually appear at the site most in contact with the tobacco. Snuff users have been shown to be 4.2 times more likely to develop oral cancer and are fifty times at greater risk for gum cancer than nonusers.[34] Increased dental problems are found among users of smokeless tobacco with greater gum recession and advanced periodontal destruction of the tissue of the mouth. Smokeless tobacco users are two to three times more likely to lose their teeth.

Smokeless tobacco may be more addictive than cigarette smoking. Nicotine is absorbed more slowly than is the case in cigarettes. As a result the nicotine levels are higher than among smokers.[35]

Recognition of the health hazards of use of smokeless tobacco has led to legislation directed toward reducing the use, particularly among younger children and teenagers. In 1985, Massachusetts became the first state to enact legislation requiring that warning labels be placed on all smokeless tobacco products. In 1986, the United States Congress passed legislation that barred television and radio advertising of smokeless tobacco products.[36] This legislation required that, as of 1987, health warnings must be placed on smokeless tobacco cans. The warnings indicate that use of the product may cause oral cancer, gum disease, and tooth loss. The consumer is also warned that smokeless tobacco is not a safe alternative to cigarette smoking. The Department of Health and Human Services was to establish and conduct education programs to warn the public of the dangers of the use of this product.

Public Policy

Legal Control of Drug Abuse

Legal action involving drug usage is to prevent or minimize the use of drugs that impair health and well-being. If a substance results in abnormal behavior that affects the individual and society, legal action is appropriate.

Since the early years of this century, there have been several federal laws designed to control narcotic drugs. The Narcotic Drugs Import and Export Act prohibited the import of narcotic drugs except for use in certain medical and scientific environments. The Harrison Narcotic Act established regulations for the control of narcotic drugs within the country.

In 1970 Congress passed the Comprehensive Drug Abuse Prevention and Control Act, better known as the Controlled Substances Act.[37] It repealed and superseded other federal drug laws, particularly the Harrison Narcotic Act. This new federal law was designed to control the distribution of all stimulants, depressants, and other abused drugs.

The Controlled Substances Act established five different classifications, or schedules, of drugs. Every drug is classified from I to V depending upon its potential for abuse, its acceptability for medical use, and its potential for causing physical or psychological dependency.

Drugs with high abuse potential and for which there is no current medical use are classified in Schedule I. Heroin and marijuana are two drugs in this classification. All drugs in Schedule I are illegal and penalties for sale, use, and possession have been established.

Drugs classified in Schedule II have a high potential for abuse, but they are also acceptable for certain medical purposes. Morphine and codeine are examples of drugs in this classification. A characteristic of these drugs is that, when abused, they can result in severe physical or psychological dependence. A prescription for a drug in this schedule can only be written by typewriter or with indelible ink and must be signed by the physician. The law forbids refill of a prescription of a Schedule II drug.

Comprehensive Drug Abuse Prevention and Control Act (Controlled Substance Act)

Class

I	High Abuse Potential	Heroin, Marijuana
	No Medical Use	
II	High Abuse Potential	Morphine, Codeine
	Some Medical Uses	
III	Less Abuse Potential	Prescription Cannot Be Refilled More Than
	Medical Use with Written or Oral	Five Times
	Prescription	
IV	Low Abuse Potential	Prescriptions May Not Be Refilled More
	Accepted Medical Use	Than Six Months After Date of Original
V	Low Abuse Potential	Over-the-Counter Drugs

Schedule III drugs have abuse potential less than those in Schedules I and II. Use of these drugs leads to high psychological dependence or low physical dependence. Drugs in this classification have medical use and may be obtained with either a written or an oral prescription. They may not be refilled more than five times per each prescription.

Drugs with a low abuse potential and recognized as having an accepted medical use are classified in Schedule IV. Use of these drugs may lead to limited physical or psychological dependence. These drugs, most often tranquilizers, may be prescribed either in writing or orally and are limited to no more than five refills. They may not be refilled more than six months after the date of the original prescription.

Drugs that can be sold without a prescription are described in Schedule V. They have a low potential for both physical and psychological abuse. The drugs in this classification are often referred to as the "over-the-counter" drugs.

The Controlled Substances Act set specific penalties for illegal possession, manufacture, distribution, and use of the drugs. The penalities include both

fines and imprisonment; penalties for selling drugs to minors are greater than those for distribution of drugs to persons over the age of eighteen.

Additional legislation and regulatory action have occurred at the state and local levels in attempts to further reduce the incidence of drug abuse. In particular, states and local communities have passed laws and ordinances designed to control the paraphernalia used by the drug abuser. For example, the possession of hypodermic needles that can be used to inject a drug are illegal in some localities. An individual having such a needle can be arrested and fined or sentenced to a jail term. Pipes and other gadgets that are used to smoke a drug are controlled by such laws, too. There is significant difference from one locality to another in what is legal, as well as in what is considered a felony or a misdemeanor.

The control of drug use has put a great deal of responsibility on law enforcement agencies. At the federal level, personnel of the Department of Justice and Immigration authorities are responsible for controlling the importation of illegal drugs into the United States. State and local law enforcement agencies use a variety of tactics and techniques to

War on Drugs

Much has been said and written in the mid-1980s about a "War on Drugs." Politicians, including the nation's president, have spoken out concerning actions needed to reduce the drug problem. The mass media have presented various options directed toward improving this problem.

Toward whom should this "war on drugs" be directed? The user? The seller? The importer of the drugs? The peasant in a Third World nation growing the coca leaves that become cocaine? What procedures should be taken? How is such a "war" going to be financed?

Such questions have increasingly brought the issue of drug abuse into the political spectrum.

Law enforcement has been the principal measure in the past to control drug use. Local and state law enforcement agencies, along with the United States Drug Enforcement Administration, have carried out drug busts, made arrests, and attempted to stop the flow of drugs into our communities.

Some believe that increased public drug education programs can be an effective activity in this "war." However, it must be pointed out that there is little evidence that school drug education programs have been effective in halting the increase in drug usage. Whether mass media appeals to not use drugs by popular personalities are effective is open to question.

Military operations have been used. In 1986 the United States military conducted operations in Bolivia designed to destroy cocaine laboratories, confiscate equipment used in drug manufacturing, and damage jungle airstrips used by drug manufacturers. In Bolivia eighty thousand acres of coca are grown. The leaves of these plants are chewed and brewed as tea by Indian tribes living in the Andes. Doubt exists as to how effective military might is in winning a "war on drugs."

What priorities need to be established in countering the increasing use of drugs in American society? How would you relegate resources—financial, personnel, media, etc.—to be most effective in this campaign?

---

apprehend drug sellers as well as users: search and seizure, surveillance, undercover investigation, and the use of informers.[38]

In 1986 federal legislation designed to reduce the spread of drug abuse was passed by Congress and signed into law by the president that greatly increased federal funding and also expanded public policy initiatives.[39] Stronger law enforcement measures to control drug use were included in this legislation. Penalties for trafficking in substance abuse were greatly increased, both in terms of prison sentences and fines. Expanded efforts in drug treatment programs and drug education programs in the schools were a part of this legislation. Funding was increased for the military to provide surveillance of illegal drug traffic into the United States from other nations, particularly from Latin America. The bill also permitted trade sanctions and the withholding of bank aid from nations who fail to cooperate with the United States in international drug control efforts.

Alcohol

There is no clear resolution to the problem of alcohol abuse. In the past, many laws were passed to eliminate the excessive use of alcoholic beverages. Early in American history, in 1619, a law was passed in the Virginia Colony which decreed that ". . . any person found drunk for the first time was to be reproved privately by the minister; the second time publicly; the third time to 'lye in halter' for 12 hours and pay a fine."[40]

In the early 1800s, the temperance movement was started and gained momentum in the United States. Originally the goal of this movement was to encourage moderation in drinking, but through the years the meaning of temperance shifted from moderation to total abstinence. At the beginning of the twentieth century, increased public demand led to total prohibition of alcoholic beverages.

In 1919 the United States tried to solve the problems of alcohol use with passage of the Eighteenth Amendment to the Constitution. This amendment made it illegal to manufacture or sell alcoholic beverages. This period of national prohibition extended from 1920 to 1933, when the Eighteenth Amendment was repealed.

Many problems arose during Prohibition. By most standards, the effort was not successful. No other measures have been successful in reducing the problems of alcohol consumption since the Eighteenth Amendment was rescinded.

Nevertheless, efforts need to be taken to reduce the many emotional, social, and economic problems resulting from drinking. This includes the drinking problems of the vast majority of Americans, not just those of alcoholics. One report suggested several measures that, if made public policy, would reduce some of the problems associated with the use of alcohol:[41]

1. Place a series of higher taxes on alcoholic beverages. This would raise the cost of drinking and hopefully reduce liquor consumption in the nation.

2. Develop effective community-wide educational programs. Such programs would be designed for people of all ages.

3. Disallow tax deductions on alcoholic beverages bought as part of business-related meals. Extensive alcohol consumption frequently occurs in connection with business affairs.

4. Greater and more strict enforcement of drunk driving laws are needed. This movement would raise the legal age for drinking in many states.

Alcohol was one of the fifteen areas identified by the office of the Surgeon General in 1979 for which objectives for the nation were established.[42] One of the alcohol-related objectives was to reduce the proportion of the population considered heavy drinkers. Activities directed at all levels of the population have been designed, with specific consideration for young adults and teenagers.

Of particular concern during the 1980s has been the carnage on the highways resulting from drunken driving. Several movements designed to curtail drunken driving have arisen in recent years. The efforts of these movements have led to the establishment of a variety of regulations and legislation being passed by state legislators and local authorities.

The catalyst for this movement has been such voluntary groups as Mothers Against Drunk Driving (MADD) and Students Against Drunk Driving (SADD). In a number of states penalties for driving while under the influence of alcohol have been stiffened. In addition, various local ordinances now hold those persons liable who provide minors with alcoholic beverages.

Federal and state courts have made drunken driving more costly for bartenders, tavern owners, and businesses, as well as private party hosts. In 1984 the New Jersey Supreme Court ruled that a host could be held liable if he or she served liquor to a guest and that person caused injuries to others in an automobile accident. Other courts have extended liability to employers who provide liquor at a party or picnic, to bartenders and tavern owners, and to wholesale vendors. There have been increasing numbers of civil suits with jury verdicts resulting in increased concern about driving and drinking.

In an attempt to help employees in the restaurant business to cope with their responsibilities relating to consumption of alcoholic beverages, the Educational Institute of the American Hotel and Motel Association has developed an educational program for those who serve alcoholic beverages entitled *Serving Alcohol with Care*.[43] Concern over alcohol-related traffic accidents is the basic motivation behind the development of this program. The program informs the student about liability laws which apply to servers of alcoholic beverages and provides suggestions to help prevent intoxication.

It is illegal to serve alcoholic beverages to a minor—under age twenty-one in most states. In many states it is illegal for a liquor licensee to serve alcoholic beverages to an intoxicated person.[44] A number of states have established third-party liability referred to as *Dram Shop Acts*. These laws hold that bartenders, servers, and bar owners can be held liable if they sell alcoholic beverages to an intoxicated person who later causes injury to a third person.[45] These laws have been changing in recent years.

Mass media advertising of alcoholic beverages is big business. It accounts for over $700 million of income for the mass media each year. Many have questioned the appropriateness of advertising alcoholic beverages and at the same time having legislation which prohibits advertising of tobacco products. It has been suggested that short of a total ban on alcoholic beverage advertising, legislation should be passed that would require that broadcast time with messages about the health effects and the risks of alcohol use should match the time allotted for alcohol advertising.[46] When one realizes the tremendous effect of mass media advertising and the dangers of alcohol use and driving, such measures would seem to be reasonable considerations.

Concerted efforts to reduce alcohol consumption, bring about more positive behavior in the social use of alcohol, and reducing the advertising of the alcohol industry have not occurred in the United States. These measures must be addressed in our society, either individually or as a part of public policy, if the problems associated with alcohol abuse are to be reduced. Failure to do so will only result in increased problems in the community health field.

Smoking

Legislative Action

In 1970, cigarette advertising was banned from television and radio. The tobacco industry could no longer advertise its products over the airwaves. Federal legislation also mandated that all packs of cigarettes must contain warnings that read, "Warning: the Surgeon General has determined that cigarette smoking is dangerous to your health."

In 1984 Congress passed legislation which mandated that these warnings should be expanded, be more precise, and be more disease-specific as to the actual effects of cigarette smoking on health.[47] Four warnings now appear on a rotating basis.

Smoking causes lung cancer, heart disease, emphysema, and may complicate pregnancy.

Quitting smoking greatly reduces serious health risks.

Smoking by pregnant women may result in fetal injury, premature births, and low birth weight.

Cigarette smoke contains carbon monoxide.

The same legislation that expanded the warnings required that cigarette companies must disclose to the Department of Health and Human Services a complete list of all chemicals and other ingredients added to cigarettes during the manufacturing process. A new federal agency council was established to oversee government and private educational and research efforts regarding health hazards of smoking.

Nonsmoker Rights

For many years, little consideration was given to the nonsmokers who had to endure cigarette or cigar smoke in rooms, restaurants, airplanes, and other public locations. Often, the smoke was more than just a nuisance. For some people, this passive smoking was not only discomforting but even a hazard to health. Yet not until the 1970s were any major efforts made to protect nonsmokers.

Nonsmoker rights have become an important policy issue because it has been shown that measurable levels of nicotine enter the bloodstream of nonsmokers exposed to tobacco smoke. Breathing air polluted by tobacco smoke on a regular basis can result in unsafe levels of carbon monoxide. Asthma, respiratory infections, and certain allergic conditions may be agitated.

Three movements—(1) the consumer movement, (2) the environmental pollution movement, and (3) the individual rights movement—have led to legislation and regulatory measures for the prohibition of smoking in certain localities. The state of Arizona was the first state to prohibit smoking in public places with legislation passed in 1973.[48] Thirty-nine states now have enacted laws restricting smoking for the purpose of protecting nonsmokers. These laws vary, but they usually prohibit smoking in general office space, lobbies, restrooms, elevators, libraries, conference rooms, and classrooms. Usually the smoker can smoke in his or her private office.

Increasingly, nonsmoking areas are now found in many public buildings, rooms, and facilities. Nearly a hundred municipalities now have ordinances that ban smoking in city offices, civic buildings, and in a variety of different workplaces. For example, in 1984 the voters of San Francisco approved a proposition that requires every public gathering place and workplace to have separate areas for smokers and nonsmokers. Any complaint by a nonsmoker is enough to require separate facilities.[49] A 1986 ordinance passed in Denver requires that employers must provide a smoke-free worksite if a majority of workers request such an arrangement.

In 1986, the United States Army established a regulation that prohibits smoking in enclosed public spaces, such as auditoriums, conference rooms, dining halls, and military vehicles. One base commander went so far as to prohibit smoking for all basic recruits.

Smoking was of great enough concern that the Surgeon General in 1980 identified it as one of fifteen health problems that need special attention in the decade of the eighties. A number of smoking goals were set for achievement by the year 1990.[50]

> "We're moving toward a smoke-free society by the year 2000."—U.S. Surgeon General, C. Everett Koop, 1986.

Price-Support Program

The federal government has supported the tobacco-growing industry with the tobacco price-support program. This program, like other agricultural price-support programs, guarantees the farmer a certain price for a product. In the case of the tobacco farmer, if the tobacco fails to bring a certain determined price guaranteed by the federal government, federal subsidies will be paid to assure a given income.

Public health officials and some legislators believe that federal price support of tobacco should be terminated. In their view it is paradoxical and inconsistent to fund a product (tobacco growing) through price supports while developing and funding programs that deal with the detrimental effects of smoking. It seems reasonable then, from a health perspective, that governmental price-support programs for the tobacco industry should be eliminated. However, because of the economic importance of tobacco farming in several southeastern states and because of the tax revenues obtained from the sales of cigarettes and other tobacco products throughout the nation, legislation that would eliminate tobacco price supports has not yet been approved.

Selected National Objectives for Smoking by the Year 1990

1. Proportion of adults who smoke should be reduced to below 25 percent.
2. Proportion of teenagers who smoke should be reduced to below 6 percent.
3. Proportion of adult population that are aware that smoking is a major factor for heart disease should be increased to 85 percent.
4. Proportion of workers provided with a smoking cessation program at work or in the community should be at least 35 percent.
5. All states should have laws that prohibit smoking in enclosed public places.

Source: U.S. Department of Health and Human Services, *Promoting Health, Preventing Disease: Objectives for the Nation.* Washington, D.C.: U.S. Government Printing Office, (Fall, 1980).

Summary

A number of drugs are widely abused in America. Drugs of abuse include alcohol, hallucinogenic drugs, marijuana, nicotine, opiates, sedatives, and stimulants. Cocaine has increasingly become the drug of choice of a large segment of the American population. The extent of abuse differs, depending upon age, race, economic status, and geographical location. For all substances, federal, state, and local agencies have taken measures attempting to control abuse and related problems.

Various treatment and rehabilitation programs for drug abusers are found throughout the country. Residential therapeutic communities, methadone maintenance treatment programs, hospitals, drug-free services provided on an outpatient basis, and multimodality programs are the most common drug rehabilitation programs. There are benefits, as well as deficiencies, in all drug treatment and rehabilitation programs. Unfortunately the percentage of totally rehabilitated drug abusers is relatively low.

Alcohol consumption is a common behavioral pattern for a majority of Americans. Responsible drinking is a socially acceptable activity in much of modern civilization. The majority of people in the United States drink socially and can control their level of consumption. Nevertheless, there are a variety of problems associated with alcohol use, including economics, physiological matters causing certain diseases and health problems, accidents, and alcoholism.

Alcoholism is a disease requiring special attention, care, and treatment. The alcoholic is often unaware of the condition that has progressively affected him or her. Treatment of alcoholism includes, in addition to medical attention, group and individual therapy. The family and friends of the alcoholic must also be involved in any effective rehabilitative effort.

Tobacco use is another major concern in the United States. Habitual use of tobacco can result in a number of health problems. A relationship exists between cigarette smoking and cancer, chronic bronchitis, and emphysema. With increasing concern about cigarette smoking, many people are turning to the use of smokeless tobacco. The relationship between smokeless tobacco and oral cancer and dental problems is causing many to warn about the dangers of use of tobacco in any form. Concern about the negative health effects of cigarette smoking has led to the development of smoking cessation programs conducted by voluntary agencies and industry, as well as public health departments.

Legal regulatory controls and law enforcement have played important roles in the control of use and sale of illegal drugs. In 1970, federal legislation was passed that provides a framework for classifying drugs as illegal or legal for restricted medical purposes. In addition, this legislation set penalties for illegal use, possession, or sale of illegal drugs. Legislation passed in 1986 has increased the efforts of government to control the problem of expanded substance abuse.

Many fatalities and long-term injuries result from drunken driving. Public policy initiatives have focused upon reducing the incidences of driving while intoxicated. Responsibility must be faced by those providing the alcoholic beverage in many situations and localities.

Throughout the country many jurisdictions have passed laws and ordinances designed to protect against the effects of the smoking individual. In an attempt to reduce the incidence of cigarette smoking, federal legislation has been implemented to expand the number and types of warnings to be placed on cigarette packages.

Discussion Questions

1. Explain why drug abuse treatment and rehabilitation programs are often found to be a part of community mental health programming.
2. What are some social and psychological reasons found for involvement in substance abuse?
3. Explain how hallucinogenic drugs affect one's behavior.
4. What are some of the physiological effects of marijuana on the human body?
5. Explain some of the long-term effects of marijuana on the chronic user.
6. What is meant by decriminalization of marijuana?
7. What is cocaine and how is it taken by the drug user?
8. Explain some of the reasons that "crack" has become a serious problem in the United States.
9. Discuss some of the issues involving methadone maintenance treatment programs.
10. What is the basic concept underlying detoxification for drug abuse?
11. Explain the various provisions of the Comprehensive Drug Abuse Prevention and Control Act of 1970.
12. What kinds of measures were implemented as a result of the legislation passed by Congress in 1986 directed at the "war on drugs?"
13. How extensive is alcohol use in the United States?
14. Is alcoholism a disease? Give reasons for your answer.
15. What is intervention as it relates to alcoholism?
16. Should there be legislation outlawing the use of alcohol? Defend your answer.
17. Discuss the issue of third-party liability in relation to drunken driving?
18. Do you agree that smoking is the "single most important preventable cause of death and disease?" Why or why not?

19. What are some measures that you feel should be taken to reduce cigarette smoking in our nation?

20. What have been some of the factors contributing to an increase in the use of smokeless tobacco in the mid-1980s?

21. Explain some of the negative ways in which the use of smokeless tobacco can affect one's health.

22. Do you support the elimination of price-support subsidies for tobacco? Why or why not?

23. Explain some of the principles underlying the most effective programs of smoking cessation.

24. Should taxes be increased on alcoholic beverages and cigarettes? Why?

25. Has the nonsmokers' rights movement been a positive movement? Defend your answer.

Suggested Readings

Botvin, Gilbert J. "Substance Abuse Prevention Research: Recent Developments and Future Directions." *Journal of School Health* 56, no. 9, (November, 1986): 369–74.

Chandler, William V. "Banishing Tobacco: Nonsmokers Demand Clean Air." *The Futurist* XX, no. 3 (May/June, 1986): 9–15.

Conolly, Gregory N., and others. "The Reemergence of Smokeless Tobacco." *New England Journal of Medicine* 314, (April 17, 1986): 1020–27.

Consensus Conference. "Health Applications of Smokeless Tobacco Use." *Journal of the American Medical Association* 255, no. 8 (February 28, 1986): 1038–44.

Cullen, Joseph W., and others. "Health Consequences of Using Smokeless Tobacco: Summary of the Advisory Committee's Report to the Surgeon General." *Public Health Reports* 101, no. 4 (July/August, 1986): 355–73.

Duda, Marty. "Snuffing Out the Use of Smokeless Tobacco." *The Physician and Sportsmedicine* 13, no. 10 (October, 1985): 171–75.

"Gum to Help You Stop Smoking." *Consumer Reports* 49, no. 8 (August, 1984): 434–35.

Kelleher, Maureen E.; MacMurray, Bruce K.; and Shapiro, Thomas M., eds. *Drugs and Society: A Critical Reader.* Dubuque, Ia.: Kendall/Hunt Publishing Company, 1983.

Koop, C. Everett, Surgeon General. "The Campaign Against Smokeless Tobacco." *The New England Journal of Medicine* 314, no. 16 (April 17, 1986): 1042.

Liska, Ken. *Drugs and the Human Body: With Implications for Society.* New York: Macmillan Publishing Co., 1981.

McBay, A. J., and Owens, S. M. "Marijuana and Driving." In *NIDA, Research Monograph Series* no. 34, Washington, D.C.: U.S. Government Printing Office, 1981: 257–63.

Moore, Mark H., and Gerstein, Dean F. *Alcohol and Public Policy: Beyond the Shadow of Prohibition.* Washington, D.C.: National Research Council, National Academy Press, 1981.

Murray, David M. "Dissemination of Community Health Promotion Programs: The Fargo-Moorehead Heart Health Program." *Journal of School Health* 56, no. 9, (November, 1986): 375–81.

National Institute on Drug Abuse. Marijuana Research Findings: 1980. Research Monograph Series no. 31, Washington, D.C.: U.S. Government Printing Office, 1980.

Pinney, John M. "A Hidden Risk in Low Tars?" *American Lung Association Bulletin* 67, no. 5, (June/July, 1981): 5.

Polich, J. Michael. "Epidemiology of Alcohol Abuse in Military and Civilian Populations." *American Journal of Public Health* 71, no. 10 (October, 1981): 1125–32.

Schinke, Steven Paul, and others. "Smoking and Smokeless Tobacco Use Among Adolescents: Trends and Intervention Results." *Public Health Reports* 101, no. 4 (July/August, 1986): 373–78.

Shopland, Donald R. and Brown, Clarice. "Toward the 1990 Objectives for Smoking: Measuring the Progress with 1985 NHIS Data." *Public Health Reports* 102, no. 1 (January/February, 1987): 68–73.

"Smokeless Tobacco Use in the United States—Behavioral Risk Factor Surveillance System, 1986." *Morbidity and Mortality Weekly Report* 36, no. 22 (June 12, 1987): 337–40.

Weintraub, Jane A. and Burt, Brian A. "Periodontal Effects and Dental Caries Associated with Smokeless Tobacco Use." *Public Health Reports* 102, no. 1 (January/February, 1987): 30–35.

Williams, Allan F., and others. "Drugs in Fatally Injured Young Male Drivers." *Public Health Reports* 100, no. 1 (January/February, 1985): 19–25.

Endnotes

1. Tanner, Ogden. *The Prudent Use of Medicines.* Alexandria, Va.: Time-Life Books, 1981, 6–7.

2. Department of Health and Human Services. *Promoting Health/Preventing Diseases: Objectives for the Nation.* Washington, D.C.: U.S. Government Printing Office, 1980, 67.

3. These relationships were discussed in chapter 10.

4. Department of Health and Human Services. *Promoting Health.* 84.

5. Liska, Ken. *Drugs and the Human Body.* New York: Macmillan Publishing Co., 1981, 229.

6. Girdano, Dorothy Dusek, and Girdano, Daniel A. *Drugs—A Factual Account.* Menlo Park, Calif.: Addison-Wesley Publishing Company, 1976, 82.

7. Ibid., 81.

8. Ibid., 87.

9. Ibid., 88.

10. Ibid., 93.

11. National Institute on Drug Abuse. *Marijuana Research Findings: 1980, Research Monograph Services 31* (1980).

12. Ibid., 37.

13. Ibid., 23–25.

14. Ibid., 23–25.

15. Ibid., 15.

16. Liska, Ken. *Drugs and the Human Body.* 145.

17. Ibid., 146.

18. Department of Health and Human Services. *Promoting Health.* 61.

19. Department of Health and Human Services. *The Health Consequences of Smoking, The Changing Cigarette: A Report of the Surgeon General.* Washington, D.C.: U.S. Government Printing Office, 1981.

20. Ibid.

21. Tanner, Ogden. *Prudent Use.* 55.

22. Girdano and Girdano. *Drugs—A Factual Account.* 137.

23. Ibid., 140.

24. National Institute on Alcohol Abuse and Alcoholism. *Facts About Alcohol and Alcoholism.* (1976), 20.

25. Ibid., 24.

26. Department of Health and Human Services. *Promoting Health.* 61.

27. CDC. *Smoking and Health: A National Status Report.* Rockville, Md.: Public Health Service, 1986, DHHS Publ. No. (CDC) 87–8396.

28. Department of Health and Human Services. *The Health Consequences of Smoking for Women: A Report of the Surgeon General.* Washington, D.C.: U.S. Government Printing Office, 1980.

29. CDC. *Smoking and Health: A National Status Report.*

30. Ibid., 123.

31. Public Law 91–513 passed in 1970.

32. Council on Scientific Affairs. "Health Effects of Smokeless Tobacco." *Journal of the American Medical Association* 255, no. 8 (February 28, 1986): 1038–44.

33. National Institute of Health Consensus Development Conference on Smokeless Tobacco. "Health Implications of Smokeless Tobacco Use." *Public Health Reports* 101, no. 4 (July/August, 1986): 349.

34. Winn, D. M.; Blot, W. J.; Shy, C. M.; et al. "Snuff Dipping and Oral Cancer Among Women in the Southern U.S." *New England Journal of Medicine* 304, (March 26, 1981): 745–49.

35. Ibid., 172.

36. Comprehensive Smokeless Tobacco and Health Education Act, 1986, P. L. 99–257, 1986.

37. Duncan, David, and Gold, Robert. *Drugs and the Whole Person.* New York: Wiley and Sons, 1982, 168–69.

38. Liska. *Drugs and the Human Body.* 225.

39. Omnibus Drug Enforcement, Education, and Control Act, 1986.

40. Moore, Mark H., and Gerstein, Dean R. *Alcohol and Public Policy: Beyond the Shadow of Prohibition.* Washington, D.C.: National Research Council, National Academy Press, 1981.

41. Department of Health and Human Services. *Promoting Health.* 67–72.

42. Ibid., 61–66.

43. Educational Institute of the American Hotel and Motel Association. *Serving Alcohol with Care: A Manual for Servers.* East Lansing, Mich.: The Educational Institute (1985): 3.

44. Ibid., 4.

45. Ibid., 4.

46. American Public Health Association. *The Nation's Health* (September, 1985): 15.

47. The Comprehensive Smoking Education Act of 1984.

48. Koop, C. Everett. "A Society Free of Smoking by the Year 2000?" *World Health Forum* 7, no. 3 (1986): 226.

49. Ibid., 226.

50. Department of Health and Human Services. *Promoting Health/Preventing Disease: Objectives for the Nation.* Washington, D.C.: U.S. Government Printing Office, (1980): 68.

19

Occupational Safety and Health: Protection and Prevention at the Worksite

Approximately one hundred million Americans spend a portion of each day at work. The working conditions often have profound effects upon the health and well-being of these Americans. Some working conditions are much more dangerous than others: mining, construction, and heavy industrial settings are far more dangerous than offices, schools, and retail stores. Nevertheless, there is the potential for injury, exposure to health hazards, and stress-producing situations in every occupational setting.

Innumerable efforts have been made to improve working conditions, some instituted by industry and management, others as the result of union demands agreed to in the bargaining process. Often, however, it has been necessary for the government to pass legislation and to establish regulations to improve the health and safety of the workplace.

In spite of the far-reaching improvements in working conditions, accidents, exposure to harmful and toxic industrial agents, and disease-causing conditions still occur and exist too frequently in industrial settings. It has been estimated that the total cost to society of occupational injuries is more than $37 billion annually.[1] These costs are measured in terms of lost wages, increased insurance premiums, medical care, fire and destruction in the workplace, and administrative overhead.

Job-related accidents account for more than eleven thousand fatalities annually.[2] More than two million workers a year suffer some disabling injuries, the result of "on the job" accidents. An estimated eighty million work days are lost each year from work-related injuries.[3]

Health and the Workplace

Not only is it costly to industry and business, but occupation-related diseases negatively affect the work force. Governmental statistics indicate that an estimated three hundred thousand occupation-related diseases occur each year. This data amplifies the importance of improving the health and safety conditions of employees in the workplace.

Occupational health programs date back many years. An example of an early employee health program can be traced to 1894. In Dayton, Ohio, the National Cash Register Company introduced a program of morning and afternoon exercise breaks for the employees. This same company installed a gymnasium on the fourth floor for employee use in 1904, and in 1911 opened a 325-acre park for employees.[4]

Unfortunately, not all businesses and industries have been as progressive in employee health care as has National Cash Register. As a matter of fact, the working conditions of many have remained deplorable. For example, hundreds of coal miners still suffer serious respiratory diseases at a very early age, owing to inhalation of coal dust. Many times industry does not establish appropriate safety standards nor provide employee health care coverage until either mandated by legislation or negotiated with the union as part of the benefit package.

Several industrial developments have been designed through the years to protect the health and safety of employees. These developments include the addition of health and safety medical personnel to the payroll. Medical services in a clinic are found in some industrial settings, usually among the large companies with hundreds of employees. Smaller companies have to rely upon the services of a nurse for emergency care and leave the associated medical care to individual workers' private physicians.

A comprehensive occupational safety and health program includes environmental monitoring and safety review. Other occupational health activities include such health promotion and education activities as corporate fitness programs, employee stress management, nutrition and weight control education, smoking cessation programs, health counseling, and alcoholism and drug abuse rehabilitation.

Occupational health and safety programs should extend beyond the needs of the employees since the health of the employees, their families, job fulfillment, industrial production, and the community as a whole are all interrelated. Without question, this programming is a far-reaching community health program affecting many people.

The American Medical Association has suggested that the scope of occupational health programs include the following:[5]

1. Protect employees against health and safety hazards at work
2. Protect the general environment
3. Place workers in job capacities without endangering their health and safety or that of others
4. Assure adequate medical care and rehabilitation of the ill and injured
5. Encourage and assist in measures designed for personal health maintenance

Comprehensive Health Service Programs

Health problems are among the main causes for absenteeism from work. These problems may include physical and mental illnesses or they may be the result of accidents. A variety of personal habits, such as drinking, drug usage, stress, and other preventable problems, also result in absence from work.

Some businesses and industries require a preemployment health examination. These examinations eliminate job applicants who have disabilities or health problems that would prevent them from performing work duties. Such examinations also provide the company with baseline health information that can be used for reference in later years of employment. But such examinations are not required during employment. Less than half of the occupational work force are given periodic medical examinations while employed.[6]

Many companies do pay for a routine annual health examination. These examinations may be conducted by the industrial medical staff, in some instances by a group prepaid medical staff contracted by the industry, or by private, personal, or family physicians where the company provides payment.

The Occupational Safety and Health Administration (OSHA) has mandated that employees exposed in the workplace to certain toxic substances such as asbestos, benzene, and ethylene oxide must be provided with a medical screening program by their employers. It is mandated that the employee have a preplacement examination, a yearly medical examination, and a termination examination.[7] Though this provides for medical examinations for certain employees working with toxic agents, it does not mandate them for all workers.

From a humanitarian point of view, business and industry should provide health and safety programs for their employees. Unfortunately, it is often necessary to argue the cost benefits rather than the humanitarian reasons in support of such programs. If it can be shown that a specific health or safety activity has cost benefits, then there is greater likelihood that the activities will be implemented.

Clinical Services

Some companies and industries provide medical services for their employees. This may simply be an arrangement with local physicians to provide emergency care when accidents and injury occur. In these circumstances, any required medical care, services, or examinations are the responsibility of the individual employee's physician. But in other instances, larger companies will provide in-plant health clinics of varying sizes. Some industries operate comprehensive health maintenance organizations for employees, relatives, and, in a few cases, for community residents.

The clinical services include preemployment and periodic medical examinations. Laboratory services are also found in some occupational clinics. Most commonly, though, emergency care is provided. On occasion industries will have well-trained emergency medical personnel available, but in most instances, only the occupational nurse and a few first-aid supplies are provided.

Not all Americans work in factories and offices that have well-staffed occupational medical clinics. In fact, 70 percent of the labor force work in settings with less than five hundred employees where such facilities are too costly. These smaller companies usually have to refer injuries and medical problems to the private sector. Preventive health programs are minimal.

Occupational Health and Safety Personnel

Larger companies usually have a program, administered by a medical director, that employs occupational health and safety professionals. The four professionals most commonly found in occupational health and safety are (1) occupational physicians, (2) occupational nurses, (3) industrial hygienists, and (4) safety engineers.

Occupational Physicians The occupational physician is a medical doctor who services the medical needs of the worker in the occupational setting. The physician is familiar with the occupation-related diseases, both their causes and treatment. This individual usually serves as the medical director for the health program of a company, industry, or business.

Only the largest corporations employ physicians having knowledge, training, and experience in occupational medicine on a full-time basis. This knowledge and skill is usually obtained through experience on the job since very few medical schools provide instruction in occupational medicine.[8] Most companies unable to afford a full-time medical director employ a physician on a part-time, on-call, or consultative basis.

Occupational Health Nurses The occupational health nurse is a specialist having specific knowledge and skills that are different from the clinical nurse. This individual sees a fairly stable group of well people rather than the sick and disabled.

The occupational health nurse provides primary nursing care in the work place for injuries and illnesses, both work-related and nonoccupational. In addition, this nurse plans and administers nursing services for all company employees. This involves assisting with physical examinations, recording health histories, and collecting other data. The position may also involve providing immunizations, screening for health defects, or evaluating activities relating to the health status of the workers.[9]

Often when a health problem is noted, the occupational health nurse makes the appropriate referral to health care facilities in the community. This role as counselor also includes working with employees on health behavior and personal life-styles. Increasingly, the occupational nurse is involved in health promotion and disease prevention.

The occupational nurse must be knowledgeable about the harmful substances and working procedures to which the employees are exposed in the industrial environmental setting. He or she not only works to reduce such hazards but also is expected to educate employees about the hazards.

An example of the importance of educating employees about the unique health conditions that can develop in specific work settings relates to Raynaud's phenomenon.[10] A certain metal manufacturing process in which vibrating handtools are used was causing this syndrome. This condition of pain, numbness, and tingling in the hands, accompanied by a developing paleness of the fingertips, is reversible if caught in the early stages. It is estimated that approximately 1.2 million United States workers are at risk for Raynaud's phenomenon. In 1983 the National Institute of Occupational Safety and Health issued a recommendation that jobs be redesigned to minimize the use of vibrating handtools. It is easy to see the importance of education relating to this condition and how workers can learn to prevent it.

With the growing interest in health promotion and cost containment of medical expenditures by industries, there may be an increase of nurses employed in industrial settings. They will provide a broad range of educational services, including counseling and others that are beyond the traditional nursing role. In fact, the occupational nurse is often the only source of health information available to the employees and their families.

Industrial Hygienists The industrial hygienist deals with the environmental factors that may cause sickness and injury, or otherwise impair health. This individual is trained to survey and analyze the various chemical, physical, and biological agents that can affect the health of workers. Not only does the industrial hygienist assess hazardous agents; this individual is also responsible for control of these hazards in the workplace.

These tasks are complicated by the thousands of potentially hazardous agents. The *Registry of Toxic Effects of Chemical Substances,* published by the National Institute of Occupational Safety and Health, lists over twenty-five thousand chemicals that are found in industrial use. Every year some five hundred to one thousand new chemical compounds are produced in the United States to which the worker is exposed during the manufacturing, processing, and packaging processes.[11] Some of the more common compounds are pesticides, plastics, and hydrocarbons.

Many of these toxic agents cause industry-related diseases. These diseases result from dusts such as silica, asbestos, coal, and cotton. Other toxic agents include gases, fumes, and vapors. The industrial hygienist must also be familiar with the biologic agents that cause disease such as bacteria, viruses, metazoa, fungi, and rickettsia.

The industrial hygienist must make sure that federal exposure limits are not exceeded. Should the levels exceed the federal standards, it is necessary to remove the hazard, to substitute a less hazardous material into the manufacturing process, or to require the use of protective devices.

Ten Leading Work-Related Diseases and Injuries, United States

1. Occupational lung diseases
2. Musculoskeletal injuries
3. Occupational cancers (other than lung)
4. Amputations, fractures, eye loss, lacerations, traumatic deaths
5. Cardiovascular diseases

6. Diseases of reproduction
7. Neurotoxic disorders
8. Noise-induced hearing loss
9. Dermatological conditions
10. Psychological disorders

Source: National Institute of Occupational Safety and Health as reported in CDC, *Morbidity and Mortality Weekly Report* 32, no. 14 (April 15, 1983): 190

Safety Engineers The safety engineer is concerned with hazards in the workplace that can cause injury to workers. This person's responsibilities include the identification of potential hazards and the development of ways to control or eliminate them.

Accident and safety education programs are designed by this specialist. The focus of activities in the industrial setting is upon both accident prevention and the creation of a safer working environment. In recent years, since the passage of the Occupational Safety and Health Act, it has become a very difficult task to monitor all industrial safety regulations established by the federal government. But despite the difficulty, this remains the primary task of the safety engineer in the industrial setting.

Occupation-Related Diseases

Occupation-related diseases account for approximately one hundred thousand deaths annually with nearly four hundred thousand new cases developing every year.[12] Many work-related diseases develop only after long and continuous exposure to an environmental substance in the work setting. Sometimes these diseases develop as the result of a combined effect: exposure and smoking, drinking, or life-style.

Occupational disease surveillance has not been particularly effective. A congressional subcommittee concluded that occupational disease surveillance "... is ... 70 years behind (surveillance of) communicable disease."[13] There are numerous reasons why such surveillance is lacking. With workers being exposed to hundreds of different chemical, biological, and physical agents, it is extremely difficult to pinpoint specific disease-related causes. The Occupational Safety and Health Administration has established regulatory standards for only about five hundred agents of more than eight thousand potential exposure agents.[14] One can see the tremendous difficulty of being aware of all potential disease producing agents in the workplace.

Skin diseases account for the largest single group of occupational illnesses.[15] These result from exposure to manufacturing corrosive and irritating agents that cause dermatitis. Or they may be the result of an accident where a toxic substance came in contact with the skin and caused irritation, burning, or other damage. Dirt, too, causes skin problems for many. Skin disorders are found to be a very extensive problem among agricultural workers. Most skin diseases associated with the workplace can be prevented with protective clothing. Workers should be given gloves, shirts, and other clothing that will protect against the specific irritant. Proper emergency care should be followed when toxic agents are accidentally spilled on the skin. Workers should also be educated to clean their skin after exposure to dirt and other substances.

Programs have been designed to increase employee awareness of the toxicity of substances used in the workplace and to improve protective clothing

The coal miner is exposed to many hazards. Not only is the underground environment dangerous, but black lung disease, *pneumoconiosis*, has debilitated thousands of miners.

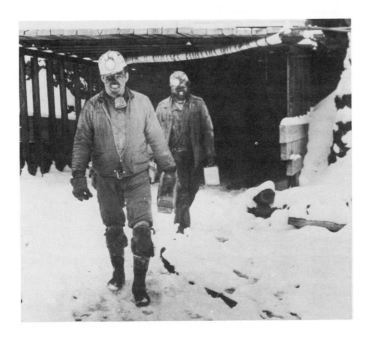

for workers. Not only has the National Institute of Occupational Safety and Health (NIOSH) been working to develop better protective clothing, but educational efforts to motivate employees to use such clothing have been developed and conducted.

A number of respiratory diseases are caused by exposure to substances in the workplace. Yet, proof that the work environment, not other factors, causes the problem is difficult to find. For example, asbestosis is found in a significant number of construction and shipyard workers who are exposed to asbestos. Asbestosis has a latent period of between ten and twenty years. Hence, its appearance in terms of symptoms may not appear for years after the individual has been exposed. Asbestos exposure causes extensive scarring of the lungs which gets worse even after the direct exposure ends.

Silicosis is prevalent among workers exposed to silica. This condition is found among workers in mines and foundries and among those individuals involved in glass, stone, and clay manufacturing.

Another respiratory disease known as byssinosis, or "brown lung," is noted among textile workers, particularly those in the cotton industry and in yarn manufacturing.

Pneumoconiosis, or "black lung disease," results from exposure to various dusts. This is most frequently found among coal miners who inhale coal dust. Black lung disease may be responsible for as many as four thousand deaths a year.[16]

Pneumoconiosis is not a curable condition. Like most of the other occupational respiratory diseases, measures can only be taken to help the person to adapt to the condition. The victim must learn to live with the lung impairment and make life-style adaptations to account for its debilitating effects.

Work-related back injuries create significant costs to industry. Back injuries are considered the number one source of absenteeism, accounting for approximately twenty-five million lost work days each year.[17] Most back problems are not the result of a single incident, but of improper use of the anatomical structure over a long period of time. Quite often these problems are the result of poor posture, inadequate exercise and activity, or change in body weight. If employees know about proper lifting and body carriage, the incidence of low back pain can be reduced.

Industrial health programs must not only inform employees about how to prevent low back pain, but measures must also be available to provide emergency care when a back injury occurs on the job. The occupational health personnel, particularly the nurse, need to work with the employee in rehabilitation efforts after a back injury.

Loud noise in the workplace has the potential for causing hearing loss among workers. Loud noise produces irreversible damage to the auditory system. The hair cells of the organ of Corti in the cochlea are destroyed by continued exposure to loud noises over a long period of time. Hearing loss is initially limited to the high frequencies, but over time, the hearing loss can affect all levels of hearing.

Noise-induced hearing loss occurs so gradually that it is likely a person will not be aware of the loss until permanent damage is done. For this reason, employees should undergo periodic hearing screening. Workers should be informed of the dangers associated with continual exposure to loud sounds, and they should be required to wear such noise-resistant devices as plugs or muffs.

The protection of workers' hearing has been important for centuries. As early as 600 B.C., a law was passed in ancient Greece barring metalwork hammering in populated areas because of the excessive noise.[18] In recent years, because of the Occupational Safety and Health Act, standards for noise exposure in the workplace have been specified. Presently, no worker should be exposed to a noise level above ninety decibels. Any time that workers are exposed to noise limits over eighty-five decibels, protective equipment must be worn and workers must submit to periodic hearing testing.

In addition to requiring workers to wear hearing protection devices, industry must also seek ways to limit the noise generation at the source. This may involve modifying the machine or instrument causing the noise.

The working environment is an excellent place to encourage preventive measures for the two major causes of death in the United States—heart disease and cancer. It has been estimated that United States industries lose more than 140 million work days due to heart disease each year. The cost to industry in terms of lost work days, disability payments, medical expenses, and substitute personnel is approximately $50 billion per year.[19] Educational programs, screening procedures, and facilities to encourage an active life-style are measures that the industrial and business world can take to help reduce the incidence of cardiovascular disease.

Smoking in the Workplace

There are numerous issues that arise in relation to the employee and smoking. Should employees be permitted to smoke while on the job? The secretary at his or her desk? The executive in a conference room? The individual on the assembly line?

A surgeon general's report stated that for the majority of American workers cigarette smoking is a greater cause of death and disability than is the workplace environment.[22]

The economic consequences of smoking can be noted as follows:[23]

1. Business loses $26 billion in productivity each year due to smoking.
2. Smokers are 50 percent more likely to take sick leave than nonsmokers.
3. Job-related accident rates are twice as high for smokers as nonsmokers.
4. Employers spend an average of $300 more in insurance claims each year for smokers than nonsmokers.

One person in four will get cancer. Several occupations have been closely linked with the occurrence of this disease.[20] For example, coal miners and rubber workers are prone to stomach cancer. Lung cancer has been noted in metal miners and foundry workers. Cancer of the mouth and pharynx is prevalent among textile workers and newspaper printing press operators.[21]

The occupational setting is an ideal place to inform adults about cancer. Occupational health programs should include cancer education and screening. For women employees, regular self-examinations for breast cancer and Pap tests for uterine cancer should be encouraged. For males, a proctoscopic examination for cancer of the colon and rectum should be performed annually after the age of forty. Any indication of respiratory congestion should be noted for the possibility of lung cancer. Surveillance of the worksite must be increased in the years ahead to identify specific relationships between the work environment and cancer, and measures must be expanded to inform employees of the dangers, signs and symptoms, and prevention of cancer.

Health Promotion Programs in the Workplace

In addition to providing the medical care facilities and surveillance of the work environment, industry and business have become more interested in health promotion. An increasing number of occupational health promotion programs have been established in recent years. Industry has realized a number of benefits from providing these programs, including reduced absenteeism, use of sick leave, illnesses, injuries, and disabilities. Such reductions result in more productive work and greater output. Employee benefits include improved health, feelings of well-being, and a more positive attitude. These benefits, in turn, affect the company, since the employees are motivated to do quality work on the job and productivity increases.

Through health promotion activities, business and industry can encourage its employees and their families to become more responsible for their health. The establishment of such activities and provision of corporate facilities assist employees in becoming more productive persons, both on and off the job. A physically fit person is most likely to be a mentally and socially well-adjusted individual.

The Kimberly-Clark Health Management Program offers a range of health promotion activities for employees, retirees, and their spouses. The program's goal is to reduce people's health risks, increase their productivity and energy, and to slow the rising cost of medical and hospital expenses.

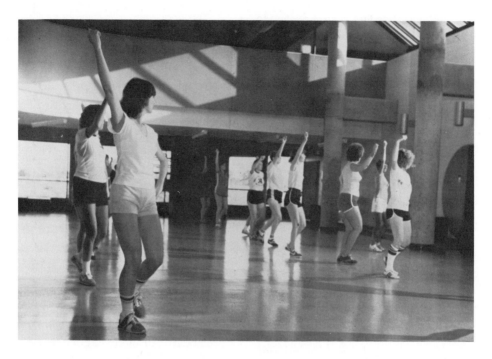

A number of health promotion activities are provided in the industrial health setting: fitness programs, alcohol and other substance abuse rehabilitation programs, hypertension and cardiovascular screening, stress management, weight control, smoking cessation, and health education.

Fitness

Many companies are developing physical fitness programs for their employees for a variety of reasons. With the cost of health care escalating rapidly, many businesses and industries are recognizing the potential cost benefits of health promotion measures. It is hoped that with the provision of health programs, the need for curative health services will be reduced. Because of this, more than four hundred major corporations now have exercise facilities.[24]

Mobil Oil, Exxon, Phillips Petroleum, Kimberly-Clark, and Rockwell International are examples of corporations that employ physical fitness directors. A professional organization known as the American Association of Fitness Directors in Business and Industry has been formed.[25]

Physical fitness programs range from highly structured workouts using fully equipped company facilities, to low profile walking and jogging programs using in-house facilities or grounds. Where companies do not have their own facilities, local health clubs, YMCAs, school gymnasiums, and other community resources have been used.

Such programs are important and often help to improve the employee attitude about the management of the company. As employees participate in a variety of fitness activities, they generally become better acquainted. The impersonal relationships so often present in industry will then be replaced by more personal relationships.

One industrial fitness program is the "Health Management Program" for salaried employees developed by the Kimberly-Clark Corporation in Neenah, Wisconsin.[26] This program, which emphasizes wellness, consists of a computer-analyzed medical history and health risk profile, multiphasic screening, physical examination, exercise testing and treadmill, and a health review. The company has an exercise facility where a variety of aerobic exercise programs are conducted. The goal of this program is to help employees maintain or improve their health. Employees are not only made aware of health risks and how to control them, but are encouraged to make positive changes in their life-style.

The Kimberly-Clark program is conducted in a company-owned facility. However, other industrial physical fitness programs for employees may be designed and conducted by community agencies. Urban YMCAs often schedule a fitness program for area business people during the lunch hour or before and after working hours. Some businesses send their employees to these fitness programs as an alternative to staffing and maintaining in-house programs.

Other fitness activities provided by industries include tennis lessons, bowling and golf leagues, and access to outdoor jogging paths on employer-owned land.

To encourage fitness program participation, some firms offer incentives to motivate employees. The Hospital Corporation of America in Nashville pays exercisers by the mile. Runners and walkers receive sixteen cents for each mile; bicyclers, four cents per mile; and swimmers, fifteen cents a mile.[27]

Alcohol, Chemical Abuse Treatment, and Smoking Cessation Programs

A growing number of industries and businesses offer alcohol and chemical abuse and alcoholism programs. As employee performance and output have been affected by the use of these substances, business has recognized a need to do something about the situation.

Alcoholism on the job causes a range of problems: lost time from work, additional medical expenses, workmen's compensation, as well as many safety and social problems. Thus, alcoholism affects both the employee and management.

The first employee alcoholism treatment programs were established in the early 1940s by the E. I. Dupont Company of Wilmington, Delaware, and the Eastman Kodak Company of Rochester, New York. Since then, a number of programs have been established that include not just the employees, but also family members.

With increasing use and abuse of drugs, it has been necessary to develop chemical abuse programs in addition to those dealing with alcoholism. Industry's alcohol and drug rehabilitation programs have proven to be successful. General Motors reported a savings of $9,878 in disability insurance benefits and 10,850 work hours that would have been lost from twenty-five alcoholic employees. In another General Motors drug and alcohol rehabilitation project that cost the company $11,114, a 49 percent decrease in lost employee hours, a 29 percent decrease in disability insurance benefits, and a 56 percent decrease in leaves of absence among 117 hourly workers were reported.[28] These returns justify such rehabilitation efforts.

Supervisors at the worksite and the occupational nurse learn to identify early indicators of alcohol and drug abuse. The first signs of such abuse include tardiness, sick time, long lunch hours, irritability, and declining quality of work.[29]

The major benefit to employers of treatment programs for problem drinkers is improved work attendance. Other benefits include reduced labor turnover, fewer job accidents, improved worker morale, and lower medical care costs.[30]

Approximately 15 percent of United States businesses have programs designed to help employees quit smoking.[31] It is estimated that smoking costs approximately $3 billion annually in lost wages.[32] Smoking contributes to a number of chronic diseases including lung cancer, emphysema, and chronic bronchitis.

Smoking cessation programs in industry and business are usually developed in cooperation with community agencies involved in similar programs. The American Lung Association, the American Cancer Society, and various other voluntary and private organizations have programs that are used by various companies.

Some companies have used economic incentives to encourage employees to stop smoking.[33] The employees are awarded cash bonuses for not smoking over a given period of time. Other incentives include a weekly bonus for not smoking while on the job. This uses group support and encouragement to help people stop smoking and also reduces nonsmoker exposure to the smoke. These bonuses are considered worth the cost in terms of a more healthy and productive employee, decreased group health insurance rates, and the reduced risk of debilitating respiratory illness which could result in long-term physical disability payments by management. On the other hand it is important to question the ethical nature of corporations using economic incentives for health promotion. An important issue that must be considered is whether the use of such incentives is in some ways coercive in nature. Also is such practice discriminatory? In reality nonsmokers are excluded from the opportunity to receive economic benefits simply because they do not have the negative health habit.

The most successful smoking cessation programs make use of group smoking withdrawal clinics and counseling on an individual basis.[34] These sessions make use of various behavioral modification strategies and permit the participant to draw on the experiences of others.

Hypertension Screening

A health problem that affects employees in all businesses and industry is high blood pressure (hypertension). As many as fifteen million working Americans have high blood pressure. This condition results in more than fifty-two million lost workdays a year.[35]

Many industries have incorporated blood pressure screening into their health promotion programs. The screening procedure often reveals employees with potential high blood pressure problems who may never have suspected there was a problem. In addition to the hypertension screening, information about high blood pressure, referral, and follow-up are necessary components of these programs. At risk individuals should be informed that hypertension can be treated through stress reduction, exercise, proper diet, and careful life-style monitoring. The employee may be referred to a private physician, a medical resource in the community, or an in-house program designed to reduce the hypertension.

Nutrition and Weight Control

The diet of millions of Americans results in a weight problem. Such eating patterns have a serious effect upon the well-being of employees and their productivity. Thus, industry has begun to develop nutritional awareness programs for employees.

Nutritional awareness can be encouraged in company cafeterias and dining facilities. Information about foods and diet can be displayed and food offerings can be modified to provide a nutritious diet.

Instruction about proper nutrition is an important part of the program. There is a significant amount of ignorance about the subject and about how to evaluate the many commercial diets on the market. Instructional programs and company publications can combat some of the ignorance about diet and nutrition.

Weight reduction and control programs in industry are usually components of a larger exercise and fitness program. Because of this, the emphasis

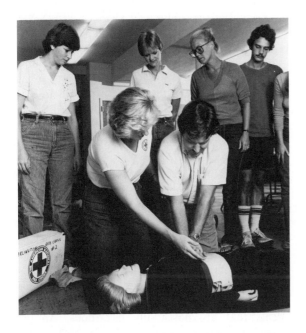

of industrial nutrition programs should be on general dietary guidelines. Specific diets should be prescribed in cooperation with the individual's physician. After the employer's physician has examined the individual, a registered dietitian or nutritionist can work with the person to provide an appropriate diet.

Stress Management

Stress is the cause of many work-related problems. Often the pressures of the job lead to emotional and physical problems. Symptoms of stress include emotional upset, cardiovascular problems, increased use of medication, abuse of alcohol and other drugs, or other chronic ailments.

Stress is a problem for employees in industry at both the management and labor levels. Since stress reduces the effectiveness of work capabilities, it has become increasingly important that industry and business develop programs in stress management.

These programs are designed to help individuals cope with the pressures of work, home, and their personal lives. Such programs include measures to help understand the need for relaxation as well as how to relax. Oftentimes this is accomplished with the use of counseling and biofeedback.

Health Education

If conducted through the workplace, health education can be a very effective means of promoting health and understanding about all of the previously mentioned health problems and concerns. Health education activities in the industrial setting include health counseling in connection with health examinations, safety and first-aid training classes, distribution of printed materials in employee newspapers, pamphlets, and posters, and the use of films.

The effectiveness of any health education activity depends upon a number of variables. The efforts should be directed toward the employee, as well as the employee's family, and must be designed to incorporate effective theories of adult learning. Industrial management wants assurance that the health education strategies will result in improved health behaviors that, in turn, will affect the productivity of the worker and, as a result, the productivity of the company. Experience has shown that health education is most effective when the employer demonstrates a sincere and continuing interest in the health of the employees and when employees are encouraged to participate in the planning and conducting of health education activities.[36]

Safety and the Workplace

In spite of the importance of occupational health measures, most emphasis in industrial health and safety has focused upon safety. This is partly because of the simplicity of identifying a cause-and-effect relationship in accidents. When an accident in the workplace occurs, it is obvious who is injured and what caused the incident. But if a disease is related to the workplace, it is often quite difficult to ascertain the specific disease-causing agent.

Industrial safety programs are the responsibility of both management and employees. Management is interested in maintaining a safe working environment so that productivity is not hindered or reduced. An accident may lead to the shutdown of the production line. It may mean that the time, money, and effort put into training a skilled worker is lost if the person is injured while on the job. All too often, however, even though management is interested in safety, it fails to pay for measures to improve the safety of the workplace. Frequently, only when forced to do so by law and worker demand are safety measures implemented.

Employees, particularly through the collective bargaining process, have been able to effect changes in the work setting. Safer working environments have resulted from negotiation, strikes, and legislation. Nevertheless, accidents are still too frequent in such industries as mining, construction, and agriculture. Continuing surveillance and effort by both management and labor are needed to improve the safety of such workplaces.

Occupational Safety and Health Act

The data collected on job-related accidents resulting in fatalities, work-related disabilities, and the extent of occupation-related diseases led to the congressional passage of the Occupational Safety and Health Act (OSHA) in 1970. This federal legislation had as its goal a safe and healthful working environment for all employed men and women.

This goal was to be achieved through several programs. The act created a National Institute for Occupational Safety and Health (NIOSH). NIOSH conducts health hazard evaluations when requested by either industry or by individual workers. These evaluations involve a number of health-related problems and safety issues.

After conducting the appropriate health hazard evaluations, NIOSH issues a report, including recommendations that must be followed. For instance, corrections in hazardous exposures may be required. The conclusions are based upon the NIOSH-established recommended levels of exposure standards.

It would be impossible to identify all of the health hazard evaluations conducted by NIOSH. But the following examples should indicate the types of requests for such evaluations.

Employees working at a public roadway were tested for exposure to carbon monoxide, lead, sulfuric acid, particulate matter, benezene, and noise.[37] Hospital employees were tested for exposure to elementary mercury. Employees in a battery manufacturing plant were tested for exposure to lead, arsenic, sulfuric acid, benezene, and several lesser-known chemicals.

In one request by several workers, a survey found overexposure to inorganic lead. Recommendations were presented on personal hygiene and for the installation of an exhaust system.

Often requests are made for health hazard evaluations where employees are experiencing certain signs and symptoms of illness. Such symptoms have included respiratory and gastrointestinal problems, headaches, nausea, and eye and throat irritation.

Research programs have been designed, conducted, and financed with respect to the numerous agents that are potentially hazardous. An outgrowth of such research was the establishment of specific exposure criteria for toxic materials and harmful physical agents in the workplace. The most obvious benefit of this research has been the determination of harmful levels of exposure by a specific agent and measures that are needed to control the hazard. Agents such as asbestos, beryllium, carbon monoxide, noise, lead, mercury, benezene, and arsenic have been identified by the National Institute for Occupational Safety and Health for study and recommendation.

Employees have the right to file a complaint with the Occupational Safety and Health Administration (OSHA), and request an inspection if they feel that working conditions are unsafe or unhealthful. The act protects employees who make such requests from discharge or discrimination by the employer. OSHA will not release names of employees who submit a complaint about working conditions.

The Occupational Safety and Health Administration conducts worksite inspections of hazardous conditions and substances. These inspections identify safety hazards and evaluate the level of conformity to specified standards. OSHA inspections are conducted by compliance officers who have been specifically trained in the regulations developed as a result of the act.

It is impossible for OSHA compliance officers to inspect all worksites on an annual basis. In reality, it is possible to inspect only about 3 percent of American businesses each year.[38] As a result, OSHA has established a system of inspection priorities. A number one priority is assigned to situations where there is imminent danger to the life or physical well-being of employees. A second priority is the inspection of a worksite where an accident resulted in death or the hospitalization of five or more employees. It is required by the law that whenever either of these situations occurs, OSHA must be informed within forty-eight hours. Employee complaints rank third in priority, and a fourth priority is random inspections.

OSHA inspections have created controversy. Many people oppose the inspections because OSHA compliance officers are often poorly prepared to understand the specific manufacturing process of a given industry. The penalty for failure to meet regulations is very "soft." For example, inspectors cannot give penalties for first-offense, nonserious violations unless they are able to cite ten or more specific violations.

Legal opposition to the inspections has been raised, too. The issue involves the legality of OSHA compliance officers' inspection of a business or industrial establishment without a search warrant. Even police authorities must have a warrant before they can search a private home or business establishment. This concern was taken as far as the Supreme Court in 1978. In the Barlow case, which originated in Idaho, the owner of a plumbing and electrical supply store refused to permit a compliance officer to enter his place of business. This issue went through the judicial system all the way to the Supreme Court. The Court supported the store owner's right to refuse admission of a warrantless OSHA inspector to private premises. As a result of this decision, there has been a significant reduction in the effectiveness of present inspection procedures.

Many other questions have been raised regarding whether the Occupational Safety and Health Act has achieved significant impact on employee health and safety. It is very difficult to learn from a review of statistics how effective this legislation has been. There has been a slight reduction in the number of fatalities in worksite accidents since the passage of the act. However, the incidences of disabling injuries have remained about the same. Even though standards have been established for a number of toxic and potentially dangerous agents, there are still many other hazardous agents in the work environment.

OSHA opponents feel that many of the regulations are arbitrary and often have little effect on the well-being of the employees. Without question, the act has resulted in additional administrative paperwork for businesses and industry. This, combined with the necessity to comply with measures mandated by the act, has increased costs. The increased costs have been passed on to the consumer and have contributed to inflation.

Supporters of OSHA point out that the private industrial sector has never been particularly effective in policing its own safety and health standards. Labor has been supportive of the Occupational Safety and Health Act and has opposed political efforts to eliminate the regulations or to radically change the act. Organized labor feels that the act ensures the rights of the working person and has built-in safeguards for better health and safety in the workplace.

Current political thinking is that the authority of OSHA must be reduced. Some believe it is inappropriate for the federal government to police private industry. Possibly the federal government should support useful health and safety research, but the monitoring and establishing of regulations should be accomplished by state and local government, not federal government. Business and management have been particularly supportive of these changes.

The form occupational safety and health legislation will take in the 1990s is unknown. The present federal government administration has required a cost-benefit analysis during the process of establishing health standards. With increasing opposition throughout the country to federal regulations and reduced federal budgets for occupational safety and health programs, it is likely that the shape of OSHA and NIOSH will change significantly in the future.

Summary

People are exposed to a variety of disease-causing agents and conditions, as well as accident situations, while at work. Though management and labor have attempted to reduce these problems, injury, death, and economic loss are still serious concerns in the American industrial and business world.

Occupation-related diseases often develop only after exposure to a substance over an extended period of time. Respiratory diseases, such as pneumoconiosis and asbestosis, cause the debilitation of thousands of workers. Work-related back injuries cause significant cost to industry. Skin diseases and damage to hearing due to continual exposure to loud noise over a long period of time are other health-related problems in the workplace.

A number of health and safety services have been provided in an effort to improve employee well-being. Some companies provide clinical health services for their workers. Through these services, employees are provided preemployment and periodic medical examinations; or they may receive emergency care or rehabilitative services.

Four categories of occupational health and safety personnel are found in the workplace. The occupational physician usually serves as medical director of the company's health program. Some physicians are employed by industry on a full-time basis and others on a part-time or consultant basis. Occupational health nurses provide primary nursing care at the industrial worksite. Other occupational health and safety personnel include the industrial hygienist and the safety engineer.

Industry and business have become increasingly involved in developing preventive health programs. The emphasis in these efforts is to improve the health and well-being of the employees. Such developments should result in greater employee productivity, better morale, and economic benefits for the company. Industrial preventive or promotional health includes programs for fitness, smoking cessation, alcoholism, drug and substance abuse, hypertension screening, nutrition and weight control, stress management, and health education.

Accidents and injuries are all too common at work. Accidents cause death, disability, and economic loss. Safety programs are varied, though widespread, throughout the industrial world.

In 1970 the United States Congress passed the Occupational Safety and Health Act. This legislation was established to provide for a safe and healthful working environment for all employed Americans. The act created a mechanism whereby numerous health and safety regulations were established. The Occupational Safety and Health Administration (OSHA) was established to monitor, inspect, and enforce federal health and safety regulations. In addition, the National Institute of Occupational Safety and Health (NIOSH) was established to conduct extensive research programs in occupational safety and health matters.

Discussion Questions

1. What should constitute the scope of an occupational health and safety program?
2. Identify some of the clinical services that are provided as part of an occupational health program.
3. Discuss some of the responsibilities that the occupational health nurse fulfills.
4. What is an industrial hygienist?
5. What are the roles of occupational physicians?
6. Explain the difference between a safety engineer and an industrial hygienist.
7. Explain how debilitation results from pneumoconiosis.
8. In what ways does the work-related environment cause different types of cancers?
9. Why are skin diseases a particular concern in the occupational setting?
10. Describe what might be included in a well-designed and executed industrial fitness program.
11. Why is alcoholism a problem in industry and business?
12. What kinds of stress management activities do local industries in your community conduct for employees?
13. What relationships should be encouraged between an industry's food service department and a program of nutrition and weight control?
14. Should employees who smoke cigarettes be permitted to smoke at the worksite? Discuss the reasons you have for your answer.
15. What are some of the provisions of the Occupational Safety and Health Act?
16. Describe some of the responsibilities of the OSHA compliance officer.
17. Describe some of the significant outcomes of the Barlow Decision made by the United States Supreme Court.
18. Do you believe that the Occupational Safety and Health Act should be strengthened or eliminated? Explain your answer.

Suggested Readings

Arnold, Helen. "Weight Off Permanently Program." *Occupational Health Nursing* (April, 1981): 23–26.

Banning, Margaret N. "The Occupational Health Nursing Puzzle." *Ohio Monitor* 59, no. 4 (April, 1986): 4–7.

Bennett, Diane, and Levy, Barry S. "Smoking Policies and Smoking Cessation Programs of Large Employers in Massachusetts." *American Journal of Public Health* 70, no. 6 (June, 1980): 629–31.

Bezold, Clement; Carlson, Rick J.; and Peck, Jonathan C. *The Future of Work and Health.* Auburn House Publishing Company (1985).

Dedmon, R. E., and others. "Employees as Health Educators: A Reality at Kimberly-Clark." *Occupational Health and Safety* 49, no. 4 (April, 1980): 18–24.

Fielding, Jonathan E. "Banning Worksite Smoking." *American Journal of Public Health* 76, no. 8 (August, 1986): 957–59.

Grzelka, Constance. "Smoking at Work: No Ifs, Ands, or Butts." *Health Link* 2, no. 1 (March, 1986): 39–41.

Kerr, Lorin E. "Occupational Health in the United States—the Next Decades." *American Journal of Public Health* 63, no. 5 (May, 1973): 381–85.

MacDonell, Frank J. "Alcoholism in the Workplace: Differential Diagnosis." *Occupational Health Nursing* 29, no. 3 (March, 1981): 14–16.

Massachusetts Medical Society. "Leading Work-Related Diseases and Injuries—United States." *Morbidity and Mortality Weekly Report* 35, no. 12 (March 28, 1986): 185–87.

Parkinson, Rebecca S. and Associates. *Managing Health Promotion in the Workplace.* Palo Alto, Calif.: Mayfield Publishing Company (1982).

Public Health Service. *The Health Consequences of Smoking: Cancer and Chronic Lung Disease in the Workplace.* Washington, D.C.: U.S. Government Printing Office (1985).

Schilling, Robert F., and others. "Smoking in the Workplace: Review of Critical Issues." *Public Health Reports* 100, no. 5 (September/October, 1985): 473–79.

Scrivner, Rose A. "Handling Stress Makes Dollars and Sense." *Occupational Health Nursing* 29, no. 3 (March, 1981): 17–18.

Sundin, David S., and others. "Occupational Hazard and Health Surveillance." *American Journal of Public Health* 76, no. 9 (September, 1986): 1083–84.

Tichy, Anna Mae. "Wellness, The Worker and the Nurse." *Occupational Health Nursing* 29, no. 2 (February, 1981): 21–23.

United States House of Representatives, Committee on Government Operations. *Occupational Illness Data Collection: Fragmented, Unreliable, and Seventy Years Behind Communicable Disease Surveillance.* Washington, D.C.: U.S. Government Printing Office (1984).

Zoloth, Stephen, and others. "Asbestos Disease Screening by Non-Specialists: Results of an Evaluation." *American Journal of Public Health* 76, no. 12 (December, 1986): 1392–95.

Endnotes

1. Data is from National Safety Council, *Accident Facts, 1986.* Chicago, Ill.: National Safety Council, 1986: 4.

2. Ibid. 3.

3. Ibid. 24.

4. Martin, Jack. "The Business Boom—Employee Fitness." *Nation's Business* (February, 1978): 68–73.

5. American Medical Association. "Scope, Objectives, and Functions of Occupational Health Programs." Chicago: American Medical Association, 1971.

6. Department of Health, Education, and Welfare. *Healthy People: The Surgeon General's Report on Health Promotion and Disease Prevention.* Washington, D.C.: U.S. Government Printing Office, 1979: 395.

7. *Federal Register.* June 20, 1986, 22612–790.

8. Department of HEW. *Healthy People.* 397.

9. Lee, Jane. *The New Nurse in Industry.* Washington, D.C.: U.S. Government Printing Office, 1978.

10. Banning, Margaret N. "The Occupational Health Nursing Puzzle." *Ohio Monitor* 59, no. 4 (April, 1986): 4–7.

11. Department of HEW. *Healthy People.* 390.

12. Department of Health and Human Services. *Promoting Health/Preventing Disease: Objectives for the Nation, Fall, 1980.* Washington, D.C.: U.S. Government Printing Office, 1980: 39.

13. U.S. House of Representatives, Committee on Government Operations. *Occupational Illness Data Collection: Fragmented, Unreliable, and Seventy Years Behind Communicable Disease Surveillance.* Washington, D.C.: U.S. Government Printing Office, 1984.

14. Sundin, David S., and others. "Occupational Hazard and Health Surveillance." *American Journal of Public Health* 76, no. 1 (September, 1986): 1083–84.

15. Department of Health and Human Services. *Promoting Health/Preventing Disease.* 39.

16. Ibid., 39.

17. Goldlberg, Henry M. "Diagnosis and Management of Low Back Pain." *Occupational Health and Safety* 49, no. 6 (June, 1980): 14.

18. Woodford, Charles M. "Noise-Induced Hearing Loss." *Occupational Health and Safety Physician* 50, no. 3 (March, 1981): 62.

19. Chenoweth, David. "Risk-Reduction Strategies Improve Industrial Completions." *Occupational Health and Safety Physician* 50, no. 4 (April, 1981): 22.

20. Department of HEW. *Healthy People.* 390–91.

21. Ibid., 390–91.

22. Public Health Service, *The Health Consequences of Smoking: Cancer and Chronic Lung Disease in the Workplace.* Washington D.C.: U.S. Government Printing Office, 1985.

23. Grzelka, Constance. "Smoking at Work: No Ifs, Ands, or Butts." *Health Link* 2, no. 1 (March, 1986) 39–41.

24. Hitchings, Bradley. "The Healthy Trend Toward Corporate Exercise Programs." *Business Week* (April 3, 1978): 91.

25. American Association of Fitness Directors in Business and Industry, 700 Anderson Hill Road, Purchase, New York.

26. "Kimberly-Clark Health Management Program Aimed at Prevention." *Occupational Health and Safety* 46, no. 6 (November/December, 1977): 25–27.

27. "As Companies Jump on Fitness Bandwagon." *U.S. News and World Report* (January 28, 1980): 36–39.

28. Chamber of Commerce of the United States. *How Business Can Protect Good Health for Employers and Their Families* Washington, D.C.: National Chamber Foundation, 1978: 13.

29. "Solving the Problem of the Drinking Worker." *Occupational Health and Safety* 48, no. 1 (January/February, 1970): 43.

30. Schramm, Carl J. "Measuring the Return on Program Costs: Evaluation of a Multi-Employer Alcoholism Treatment Program." *American Journal of Public Health* 67, no. 1 (January, 1977): 51.

31. Reported in *Occupational Safety and Health* (May, 1970): 31.

32. Bennett, Diane, and Levy, Barry S. "Smoking Policies and Smoking Cessation Programs of Large Employers in Massachusetts." *American Journal of Public Health* 70, no. 6 (June, 1980): 630.

33. Ibid., 630.

34. Thompson, E. L. "Smoking Education Programs, 1960–1976." *Public Health* 68 (1978): 250–57.

35. Penn, Ann C. "Finding the Silent Killer: High Blood Pressure." *Job Safety and Health* 4, no. 10 (October, 1976): 16–22.

36. Howe, Henry Forbush. "Organization and Operation of Occupational Health Program." *Journal of Occupational Medicine* 17, no. 6 (June, 1975): 367.

37. Examples presented in this section are taken from *Health Hazard Evaluation Summaries, May 1981,* publication of the National Institute of Occupational Safety and Health, Cincinnati, Ohio.

38. Bingham, Eula. "What OSHA Expects of Physicians Serving in the Industrial Community." *Journal of Occupational Medicine* 20, no. 12 (December, 1978): 818–19.

20

Violence: Interpersonal Actions Needing Community Health Services

Throughout the history of humankind, violence has had a major impact on people's lives. Death and debilitation resulting from natural phenomenon, warfare, and interpersonal violence have affected millions of individuals. Violence not only results in debilitation and death but it often leads to upheaval in the personal lives of those affected. Violence is more than physical injury. It may produce psychological problems with which the individual must cope. Violence is closely related to poverty, low socioeconomic status, and fear of enemies or destruction.

Natural occurrences such as earthquakes, eruption of volcanoes, tornadoes, hurricanes, and floods have been disruptive. In history we learn of the eruption of Mt. Vesuvius in 79 A.D. that totally destroyed Pompeii and Herculaneum. The loss of life for some 830,000 people in China in 1556 from earthquake may be the greatest incidence of destruction from natural violence.

More recently we are familiar with the destruction in 1985 by the volcano of Armero, Colombia, with the death of more than twenty thousand and the displacement of thousands of survivors. In the United States the explosion of Mt. St. Helens in the state of Washington in 1980 had great impact on the lives of many people. In 1976 nearly a quarter of a million people were reported to have been killed in an earthquake in interior China.

In 1985 an earthquake in Mexico City killed an estimated thirty thousand individuals and left thousands homeless. In one hospital that was destroyed by the earthquake, several hundred patients, physicians, nurses, and other employees were killed.

Damage, destruction, and upheaval resulting from natural causes will continue as long as life exists on earth. Humankind must learn to cope. There is need to develop earlier warning systems. People must learn to take cover when danger of an approaching tornado is present. They also must heed warnings to evacuate when conditions seem eminent for potentially damaging natural events.

The medical care and community health professions must learn more about care and treatment of those injured by such natural violence.

Agencies providing social services need to develop greater understanding of the emotional and psychological effects of exposure to such violence. Not only are relief services necessary at such time, but long-term assistance to the survivors becomes paramount.

Throughout history, warfare has been another form of violence that leads to death of combatants, as well as innocent civilians. Villages and homes are destroyed, fields are burned, and diseases occur. Families are disrupted by death or the necessity to evacuate. Throughout the world today millions of refugees are living in poverty due to warfare. Children are particularly affected by a lack of adequate resources such as health care, food, and shelter.

Interpersonal violence results from those actions between people on a more personal basis than warfare or natural events. It is this type of violence that is more commonly seen by community health personnel in the United States. Interpersonal violence may occur in a number of different settings, involving strangers as well as family members and close acquaintances.

Interpersonal Violence and Community Health

No one agency or discipline has total responsibility for solving problems related to interpersonal violence in our society. Current services for victims of abuse are fragmented and often inadequate. A number of different kinds of professionals become involved in working with the victims of violence as well as those responsible for violent actions. One agency may treat the physical injuries of the abused while another provides legal advice; another may provide shelter and council; yet others may provide financial help.

Often law enforcement personnel are the principal individuals to deal with acts of violence. The judicial system comes into play as charges are brought against the person who commits the act. Personnel in the various social service fields must provide help, assistance, and council to both the abused and abuser. Therefore, the need exists for a multidisciplinary approach to coping with the problems of interpersonal violence.

Objectives for 1990

1. Death rate from homicide among black males ages 15 to 24 should be reduced to below 60 per 100,000.
2. Suicide among people 15 to 24 should be below 11 per 100,000.
3. Injuries and deaths to children inflicted by abusing parents should be reduced by at least 25 percent.

Violence is an increasing concern within the field of community health. Health care personnel and other workers in the various fields of community health must learn how to prevent or deal with the many different kinds of abuse and violence. Health care providers often are required to respond to the physical wounds left by violence. Emergency room personnel in hospitals need to know how to help the victims of violence. They must be able to treat all forms of injuries associated with violence. Health care providers must know when to recognize the indicators of violent behavior. It is important that they learn how to diagnose potential abuse victims and help the victims deal with the psychological, emotional, and social stigma attached to the abusive situation.

Although the epidemiological model has been used in identifying etiological factors of abuse, a need exists for more reliable and valid data. Unfortunately, accurate data are unavailable since most interpersonal violence is greatly underreported. Health care personnel need to know what types of questions to ask, what physical and emotional signs to look for and how to help the victim recover from both the physical and emotional wounds.

The importance of including acts of violence in health promotion and disease prevention programming and planning was noted in the 1990 objectives for the nation. Specific objectives relating to homicide, child abuse, and suicide were included.[1]

The family is often perceived as that environment that is a safe haven for most individuals. Ideally, the home should be a place where love, understanding, and support can be found. However, violence within the family has become an increasing problem to society. In the past, familial problems usually were kept isolated from the public. With increased openness about such problems, child abuse, spouse abuse, and elder abuse have become major health and social concerns.

Child Abuse

One of the most rapidly developing social and community health problems in America today is child abuse. Some cases of child abuse are easily recognized: the small child with multiple bruises on the face or the infant with doughnut-shaped burns on the buttocks. On the other hand, there are numerous other more subtle forms of abuse that rarely come to the attention of authorities. This form of abuse may include verbal abuse, overly strict discipline, or poor supervision and negligence. All are factors that need the attention of personnel working in the fields of education, community health, and social work today.

Although the exact extent of child abuse is impossible to determine, government data estimates that somewhere between one and four million children suffer either physical abuse or neglect each year.

A serious type of physical abuse of children is burns. Often the abusing adult will put the child in scalding water or will place other hot substances against the child. Burns result in trauma, such as pain and infection.

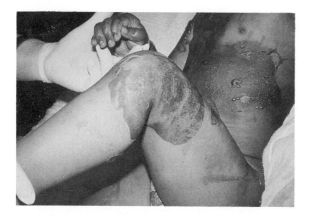

Many of these children experience long-term physical and emotional scarring or even die. It is estimated that two thousand to five thousand children die each year from child abuse.

Children who are abused are likely to be negatively affected by these experiences. Not only do they often come to accept the abusive actions as being normal behavior, but they often carry over such behavior into other relationships. Abused children are likely to strike, hit, or exhibit other abusive behavioral patterns in their relationships with schoolmates, brothers and sisters, and other acquaintances.

Forms of Abuse

The forms of abuse vary. The most prominent and identifiable is *physical abuse*. This type of abuse is manifested by the presence of bruises, lacerations, fractures, burns on various parts of the body, and in a variety of other ways. *Child neglect* is a more difficult problem to identify. Generally, neglect refers to failure by parents or guardians to provide the child with minimum needs such as food, health care, shelter, clothing, and other necessities. The third form of abuse is *sexual abuse;* another form is *emotional abuse.*

Physical Abuse

Younger children are more likely than older children to be physically abused. They may be beaten, kicked, thrown about, or handled in such a way that physical disability occurs. Bruises, wounds, burns, lacerations and abrasions, dental damage, and skeletal or head injuries are often indicators of physical abuse. Such mistreatment can lead to brain damage, mental retardation, or a variety of other psychological and emotional problems.

However, not all injuries resulting from physical abuse are noticeable immediately by medical or social agency personnel. Head injuries may be accompanied by hemorrhaging beneath the scalp and retinal hemorrhages or detachments in the eye. Internal injuries, such as rupture of interior organs, may result from hitting or kicking.

Child Neglect

Child neglect is a rather difficult problem with which to cope. Neglect takes on a variety of different patterns. Often neglect does not produce visible signs. The indications of child neglect usually occur over a period of time. During this time span the child is experiencing many emotionally disturbing relationships that have a negative impact on his or her growth and development. While neglect is found among all ages of children, most cases of adolescent abuse involve neglect rather than physical harm.[2]

Child neglect may take a number of different patterns. It may be neglect in the form of social isolation. The child is not permitted to socialize, to play, and to interact with children as is normal. Without the opportunity for social interaction while growing up the child will find it impossible to develop relationships with others in society. This often leads to many antisocial behaviors.

Neglect takes the form of failure to care for the physical needs of the child. This may be seen when the caretakers—parents or guardians—fail to provide adequate food, clothing, or hygienic measures. Lack of adequate nutrition and good hygiene can result in the development of chronic communicable diseases and illnesses. The child is unable to function in school due to the presence of fatigue, colds, restlessness, or other socially unapproved patterns.

The most common kind of physical abuse of children results from beatings using belts and extension cords. These injuries are often found over several parts of the body. This boy had belt and extension cord injuries over the back and the thigh. Extensive

medical care and social work assistance brought this individual back to normal health. The emotional scars of the beating lasted longer than the physical wounds.

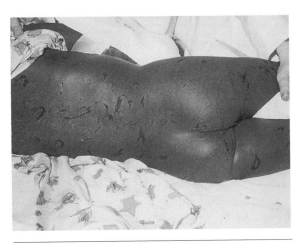

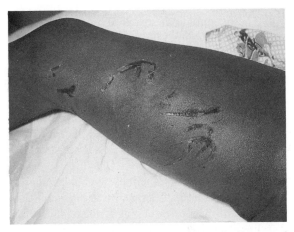

Placing lighted cigarettes against the skin is a form of physical abuse of children. Indications of this type of abuse are the presence of round marks with reddened skin.

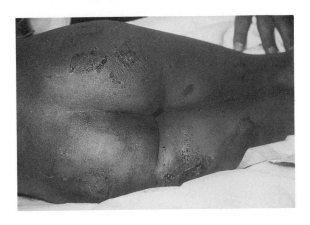

overcrowding in the home, or prolonged absence of one parent are common environmental factors associated with child neglect.

The child who has been neglected will often exhibit certain behavioral indicators such as falling asleep in school, poor achievement and attendance at school, chronic hunger or fatigue, a dull apathetic appearance, engaging in socially unacceptable behavioral practices, and the use of drugs, alcohol, and tobacco. Unfortunately, child neglect goes unnoticed for long periods of time. It may not be recognized by authorities who can be helpful to the child until some physical indicators are manifested or until emotional disturbances are noticed.

Sexual Abuse

Considerable concern has been directed at the problem of sexual abuse among school-age children. Victims of this type of abuse may be males or females of almost any age; however, adolescent females are particularly vulnerable. Sexual abuse, though occurring predominantly among adolescents, has even been reported among children of primary school age. This form of abuse is most likely initiated by a parent, guardian, or caretaker, usually a father or male relative; it is referred to by several different terms: incest, family sexual abuse, molestation, and child sexual victimization.

Child neglect in whatever form may be purposeful or circumstantial. It may result from the purposeful attempt to discipline the child. The parent may consider withholding food or other necessities a means of correcting the child. Neglectful behaviors may be the result of anger, distress, and frustration of the parent generated by the child's behavior. Neglect may also stem from environmental circumstances including long-term parental illness, poverty, or marital discord. Alcoholism,

Sexual abuse of children by family members means using a minor child for sexual stimulation of an adult or older child. Most cases involve genital manipulation, indecent exposure, and obscene language as well as vaginal intercourse and rape.

The magnitude of sexual abuse in the United States is uncertain. It is assumed that it is greatly underreported, leading to a lack of reliable incidence data. This underreporting of sexual abuse stems from the reluctance of most abused to follow through to prosecution. Statistics that are used in analyzing sexual abuse of children have been obtained primarily from court records. Because of the family connections, victims of sexual abuse seldom report it.

Sexual abuse causes serious psychological problems for the abused. Victims often suppress their feelings and memories of the incident. There are varying degrees of feelings of guilt, fear, anger, shame, physical pain, confusion, and depression. Often a decline in academic performance, increased involvement in substance abuse, and runaway behavior are seen in individuals who have been sexually abused.

A basic problem associated with sexual abuse is a violation of trust that the child has had in the family. The normal processes of child development have been disrupted. Commonly noted psychological effects of sexual abuse include the betrayal of trust, feelings of violation, and negative identity formation. Clinical studies also reveal a deep sense of low self-esteem among the abused.[3] These poor self-concepts are manifested in depression and withdrawal.

Problems with sexual attitudes and behavior often follow the incidences of child sexual abuse. For victims, sexual behavior often is manifested in either a total aversion to sex or in promiscuity.[4] Many individuals who have been molested sexually as children experience chronic sexual dysfunction as adults.

Unfortunately, child sexual abuse is often a hidden problem. A very small percentage of the abused see appropriate health or social service agencies. In 1984 amendments to the Federal Child Abuse Prevention and Treatment Act mandated that information about incest be disclosed to local child protective services agencies. As such the health profession must report children who have been identified as having been molested sexually by parents, guardians, or caretakers. These reports are to be made to the local police authorities or to the child protective services agency. As a result, health care workers, educational personnel, and social agency professionals should be trained to identify, collect, and document evidence of sexual molestation.

Emotional Abuse

This form of abuse usually involves continual degrading interactions with the individual child. The children who are constantly told that their actions are inappropriate, that they can never do something satisfactorily, or who have little feeling of success are emotionally abused. Parental behavior that is psychologically destructive to the child can be a very difficult problem.

A number of family social patterns often lead to this type of abuse. Such measures as ongoing friction in the home between the parents and the child, excessive drinking and argumentation by the parents, frequent marriages and/or broken homes, promiscuity and/or prostitution are commonly identified with emotional abuse. The child who is emotionally abused will manifest a variety of different behaviors such as hyperactivity, withdrawal, nervous skin disorders, psychosomatic disorders, and stuttering. Suicidal behavior, truancy, delinquency, and increase in substance abuse are often noted.

Causes of Child Abuse

The specific cause of child abuse or child neglect is too complex to identify. It is only possible to identify general characteristics of abusing parents. Various socioeconomic stresses affect abusing parents. Alcoholism and drug abuse are related to this problem, too. Many parents who have abused or neglected their children have a poor self-concept as well as possessing unrealistic expectations about the development of the child. Child abuse often results in situations where parents are in conflict over child

Social Factors that Account for Child Abuse

1. Pressure of single parenting, particularly among women
2. Economic and psychological stress created by poverty
3. A feeling of isolation from help and social control
4. Parents who were punished physically as children

Adapted from: United States Department of Health and Human Services, *The Status of Children, Youth, and Families.* Washington, D.C., 1979: 64.

custody and visitation in cases involving divorce and separation. Very young parents are more likely to be child abusers.

Child abusers often do not have realistic expectations about the behavior of their children. They fail to understand the normal needs and developmental patterns of children at various ages. They often believe in extreme discipline patterns. These individuals tend to overlook the cries for need, help, and attention that the child gives.

Many people have no training in parenting. Specific knowledge of child development would aid all parents, but especially those prone to child abuse. Community agencies, schools, churches, and community health agencies should provide educational opportunities for parents to learn effective parenting strategies.

Help for Child Abuse

Measures that can help reduce and/or prevent child abuse are necessary. In response to that need, programs and agencies have been established. In addition, legal mandates relating to child abuse have been passed in recent years.

A number of preventive measures are available in many communities to help both the abused and the abuser. The principal agency in most communities responding to child abuse and neglect is the Child Protective Services agency. Child Protective Services are usually found in city, county, or state departments of social welfare or social services. These agencies will evaluate reports of cases of child abuse and neglect and provide necessary services. Such services include foster home care, social worker counseling with the abusers, early childhood educational programs for maltreated children, and classes in parenting.

Telephone hot lines have been established where adults can call for assistance, counseling, and help when feelings are present that could result in abuse. Often the availability of someone to talk with at times of stress can prevent an abusive action. These hot lines have also been useful for children and adolescents following abuse. These services provide someone who can be trusted at a time of trauma.

Some child abuse agencies provide the service of caring for a child at times when stressful situations may be conducive to abusive actions. When a parent is under stress due to unemployment or during a bout with alcohol, it may be best for the child to be removed from the home for a period of time.

All fifty states plus Washington, D.C., have mandatory reporting regulations for child abuse. Under provisions of federal legislation passed in 1974, the Child Abuse Prevention and Treatment Act, state laws regarding child abuse must cover both mental and physical injury. Legal immunity must be granted to those who report abuse and neglect. Coverage of such state legislation must include all children under the age of eighteen. The Child Abuse Prevention and Treatment Act provided funds for states to develop and implement programs to protect children. It also created the National Center on Child Abuse and Neglect, an agency within the Department of Health and Human Services, which serves as a clearinghouse on programs relating to child abuse and neglect.

Though there are some differences in the specific legislative mandates from one state to another, most require that individuals working with children who have been abused must report such incidents to appropriate authorities. School personnel, social workers, and health and medical personnel are the most likely individuals who have access to early warning signs of child abuse. In spite of concern by many professionals who wish not to become involved in these cases, it is felt that such state child abuse laws have been helpful. At the very least, they have led to increased public awareness concerning the magnitude of this problem.

Despite legislation mandating the report of suspected abuse, many instances of abuse are never recognized by school authorities, police, medical professionals, or community authorities. Many times it is not until a child is severely injured or even killed that the case comes to the attention of the legal and social authorities in a community. Many community health workers who have direct contact with families are the first to suspect or identify abuse and neglect.

Another very positive program has been group support of parents who have abused their children. This self-help organization, known as Parents Anonymous, assists parents in solving this problem. Through the process of group dynamics and interaction, parents gain self-esteem, and social isolation is reduced. These activities help parents to overcome the problems that led to their abusive action.

Spouse Abuse

Domestic or family violence is a very difficult problem to cope with in American society. When the matter of domestic violence or spouse abuse is considered, usually the problem involves situations where the male takes abusive action against the female. Though there are increasing reports of females abusing males, the typical pattern is for the woman to be the victim. Wife abuse occurs among all ages and is found within all social groups. Women who are most likely to be abused are very young teenage wives, women who are pregnant, and those with small children.

The extent to which spouse abuse occurs in the United States is very difficult to ascertain. It has been estimated that half of American families experience some form of violence.[5] Spouse abuse occurs at least once in two-thirds of all marriages. Half of those men who do beat their wives do so three or more times a year.[6] As many as 20 percent of the adult population may be involved in spouse abuse.[7]

In spite of the statistics, there is little doubt that spouse abuse is greatly underreported. The abused often refuse to report due to fear, guilt, and/or shame. Embarrassment also keeps many abused individuals from reporting the incidents. Often the abused have a sense of low self-esteem and lack a support system. For some individuals the abusing situation is perceived to be normal behavior.

Spouse abuse often is referred to as the "battered wife syndrome." This syndrome usually takes one of three different forms: (1) physical abuse, (2) psychological abuse, and (3) sexual abuse. The battered wife syndrome may be the outgrowth of any intimate male-female relationship; it is not limited to legal husbands.

Physical abuse occurs when there is a physical and/or verbal dominance by the abuser over the abused. It usually involves actions such as slapping, hitting, and kicking the victim. It also may involve shoving the person into something or down stairs. Physical abuse may also include the use of a dangerous weapon such as a gun, knife, or bat. This kind of abuse arouses a deep sense of fear in the abused. Often the first evidence of abuse involves bruises, fractures, and lacerations. The abused woman is hesitant to talk about the injuries. She may present some rather vague complaints and explanations as to why and how the injuries occurred.

Psychological abuse is different in that the indicators are not as readily observable as they are in cases of physical abuse. Threats made by the abuser may occur over a long period of time. This creates an atmosphere of fear. In other cases the woman may not be permitted appropriate social interaction. The male may not permit the female to socialize with certain groups, often where other males are part of the social activity. The male may isolate his wife, or lover, from her friends and relatives.

Every individual, male and female, has certain emotional needs. Abuse may occur when the abuser fails to meet the emotional needs of the spouse. Psychological abuse tends to weaken the support system of the abused. This individual, usually the female, becomes more docile and is forced to depend more upon the spouse. There is a destruction of the woman's self-worth and the creation of deep dependency needs of the woman upon the man. Independence is destroyed.

Sexual abuse of women by husbands or long-term lovers is a significant problem. Such abuse involves intercourse characterized by force, by threat of force, or by an inability of the woman to consent. Spouse abuse often is reported in the form of deviant sexual acts and marital rape, which occurs when the male forces the wife to have intercourse against her will. There has been some question as to whether rape can occur in a husband-wife relationship. However, in recent years marital rape has had legal definition and is now punishable by law in some states.

All too often the abused female develops a "learned helplessness."[8] The woman believes that she has no power to change her life and that no one can help her. In her thinking she has lost control over her life. Guilt often develops and she comes to blame herself for the abusive situation. A similar pattern is noted in an enforced loyalty to the aggressor; the female exaggerates her husband's good qualities.

Men who are most likely to abuse women usually have serious personal adjustment problems. They may be jealous and insecure, which leads to the various actions of social isolation and psychological abuse that are commonly seen. Males who do not trust their wives are often abusive. Men who are unable to become emotionally intimate with their wives tend to become abusive. It has been shown that many male abusers have been abused themselves as children and came from families where there was spouse abuse. Further, males are at increased risk for spouse abuse when there is a high level of alcohol use. As a result, these males exhibit signs of depression and psychosis.

It is difficult for the abused female to leave the situation in which she finds herself. There are a number of risks involved in any escape attempt, not the least of which is fear and guilt. The insecurity found in most abused females adds to the difficulty to escape the situation.

In an attempt to help the battered woman, or abused male, laws are needed and community services are necessary. Presently forty-three states as well as Washington, D.C., have laws that allow battered women to receive civil protection independent of domestic relation proceedings.[9] A victim does not have to file for divorce or separation in order to receive protection under the law.

Community shelters and protective environments for the abused female need to be available. Spouse abuse agencies should provide economic, social, health, legal, and mental health services.[10] When a woman is in danger of being abused, there should be a place where protection can be sought, where the abused will be understood, where help can be provided, and where the woman can reside until the conditions are acceptable for her to return to her home. It is important that a woman victim be helped as much as possible by a female advocate.

Elder Abuse

Abuse and neglect of the elderly have become major concerns in recent years. As with child and spouse abuse, the extent of elder abuse is unknown. This is because many instances are never reported. Victims of abuse may attempt to hide the fact that they have been abused. Furthermore, many types of elder abuse behaviors are difficult to categorize.

It is estimated that between 500,000 and 2.5 million senior citizens are victims of abuse and neglect each year.[11] Possibly as many as one in ten citizens over the age of 65 experiences some type of abuse. This type of abuse is found among all groups: racial, social, ethnic, and religious. The abusers in most instances are relatives or caregivers. The victim of elder abuse is often dependent upon the abuser for physical and emotional needs. This is especially the case following the death of a spouse.

The abusers in most instances are relatives or caregivers of the individual. Daughters and sons of the victims are found to be the most frequent abusers. Daughters tend to be more involved in psychological abuse and neglect, while the sons are more likely to use physical abuse.[12] Often the abuser is experiencing many family problems of his or her own. It may be a period of time when the abuser is experiencing financial problems due to the demands of his or her own children. Having the added burden of an elderly relative makes for a very difficult situation which leads to both active and passive abuse.

Types of Abuse

Elder abuse takes several different forms. It may be physical abuse, neglect, psychological abuse, exploitation, and maltreatment. Often several or all of these forms may be present in a given case.

Possibly the easiest type of abuse to identify is physical abuse, which is the direct infliction of physical injury to the individual. This type of abusive action usually results in injuries, welts, sprains, fractures, and lacerations. It may take the form of beating, hitting, slapping, pushing, shaking, or other direct physical contact. All too often the elderly are unable to react, and out of helplessness appropriate medical attention and care are not obtained.

Neglect of the elderly can take many different forms. Neglect is considered a lack of attention and/or confinement of the individual. Neglect often is not malicious but passive. Since the person may not request help and assistance or feels that to do so would inconvenience others, the needed care is unavailable. An individual who is immobile may lie in one spot long enough to cause bed sores. Failure to provide necessary treatment and services to maintain health and well-being, such as failure to give needed medication, is a common practice among senior citizens. Active neglect is seen in situations where the caregiver withholds a basic need. Withholding nutrition or fluids, medicine, personal care, or clothing and supervision are associated with this type of abuse. Individuals who are malnourished, or dehydrated, have urine burns or other ulcers and sores, or have an unkempt appearance can be suspect of neglect.

Elder abuse often takes the form of neglect. When the person is disabled and unable to move without help serious decubitus ulcers often develop where the body is in contact with the bed for long periods of time. Such ulcers often become infected and serious related problems result.

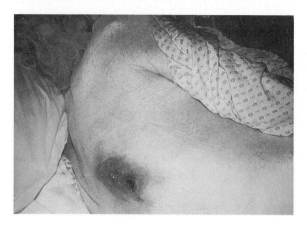

Situations that involve threats and produce fear create psychological abuse. Where there is a withholding of affection and where social isolation is permitted, psychological abuse occurs. Intimidation in the form of verbal abuse (shouting or scolding) and nonverbal abuse (silence, threats of abandonment or institutionalization) is commonly noted. Verbal abuse may include name calling, insults, threats, and humiliation. Individuals experiencing this type of abuse would appear passive, fearful, and have a low sense of self-esteem. They are often withdrawn, passive, and depressed; out of fear, they may appear to be helpless. Psychological abuse can be very devastating to the individual. Unfortunately, it is very difficult to obtain evidence against the abusers in these situations.

Exploitation, another form of psychological abuse, is taking advantage of the resources of the elderly person. This usually involves the dishonest misappropriation of money or property. This type of abuse may be seen when a senior citizen is overcharged for needed home repairs, necessary purchases, health care, or funeral costs. There are instances where the family members or caretakers will withhold pension or insurance checks and use the money for their own purposes. This kind of theft

When neglect has occurred, an individual may develop decubitus ulcers over many parts of the body. This patient came to the attention of the medical staff of a hospital when the patient was brought in from a skilled nursing facility. Ulcers covered (a) the hip and (b) the heels, as well as other parts of the body. Infection of the wounds led to the death of this patient.

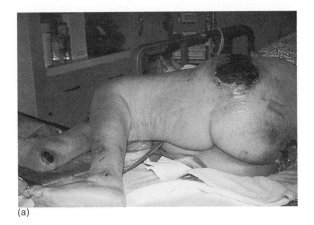

(a)

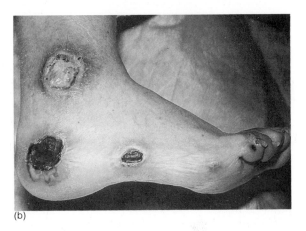

(b)

is particularly unfortunate in that the elderly person may not be able to respond. Forcing the elderly person to sign over power of attorney or forcing a change of will are other examples of exploitation. When one's possessions are missing or known resources are not available to cover costs for food, clothes, housing, and other necessities of life, exploitation can be suspected.

Intervention Needs

There is a growing need for intervention services to help the elderly. Those individuals whose professional responsibilities bring them into contact with the elderly, such as medical care providers, social workers, and criminal justice personnel, need to be better prepared to detect, assess, and provide treatment for elder abuse victims.[13]

There are numerous indicators of abuse. For example, when a discrepancy exists between the injury, related history and explanation by the victim and/or others, abuse may be suspected. Other possible abuse indications may be evidence of untreated injuries, multiple injuries of varying stages of healing, and the presence of injuries on areas of the body which are normally covered by clothing.

Services such as emergency shelters and therapeutical care are necessary. Counseling is important. Home help services, day-care centers, and alternative housing services can be developed in many communities to help the elderly. In addition to services for the elderly, relief for the caretaker is essential. If such caretaker services were available, the potential abuser could obtain assistance during periods of crisis and stress.

Accompanying increased concern regarding elder abuse has come increased recognition of the need for legislation. Today forty-one states have some type of statutes for adult protection. The major provision of these laws is that they require reporting of elder abuse. However, differences exist regarding who is required to report such abuse. In most instances medical and health personnel have such obligations along with members of the clergy.

The various laws define what kinds of abuse are to be reported. Unfortunately, a type of abuse that is reportable in one state may not be reportable in another. In addition, each state specifies to which agency a report of elder abuse is to be made; state and local departments of social services, the state attorney general's office, county probation departments, and county welfare departments are some examples.

Injuries to the Feet: The Result of a Fall or Abuse?

Often hospital medical and social service staff are faced with contradictory stories concerning the cause of bruises and injuries of elderly individuals brought to the emergency department. All too often the explanations given do not seem appropriate for the type of injuries seen by these professionals.

The explanation given by family members who brought this individual to the municipal hospital was that the 79-year-old woman had fallen and hurt her feet. It seemed odd that the extensive injuries were on both the top and the bottom of both feet. Fur-

ther examination revealed bruises on the thighs, the torso, and the arms. All indicated evidence of physical abuse.

What is, or should be, the role of the emergency room physician in such a case? The emergency room nurse? The hospital social worker? The law enforcement personnel?

Why is it necessary that medical centers develop team approaches to working with the increasing problem of elder abuse in this country?

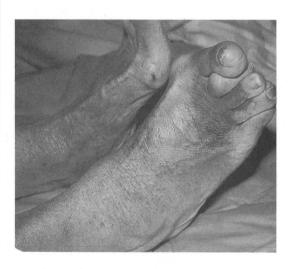
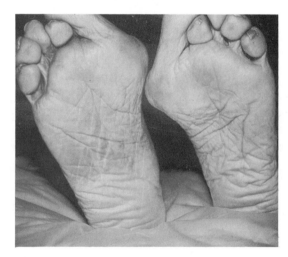

Because of the variance from state to state, there is a need for comprehensive federal legislation relating to elder abuse. Medical personnel who work with the elderly need to be made more aware of the signs and symptoms of this kind of violence. Emergency trauma physicians, emergency nurses, and social workers are often at the forefront in identifying potential abuse cases.

The problems related to elder abuse likely will continue to increase in the years ahead. With an increasing percentage of the population in the United States over sixty-five, greater numbers will impact this problem. Historically, the rights of the elderly have received little attention. With increased concern over the rights of this population group, the incidence of elder abuse will necessitate quality care facilities, improved legislation, and better preventive measures.

Rape

An act of violence involving sex or attempted sex without the consent of the victim is rape. This action is also referred to as sexual assault, which has been defined as "nonconsensual sexual behavior, including stranger, acquaintance, and spousal assaults against either male or female victims."[14]

Incidence statistics regarding rape vary as have those for other types of abuse. It is estimated that one in ten rapes are reported to the authorities. Further estimates have been made that as many as one in four females and one in eight males are victimized sometime in their lives.

Rape occurs in all levels of society, with most rapes being planned. Often the sexual assault takes place in the home of the victim. Sometimes the rapist forces entry and other times the individual is known by the victim and permits entry, not expecting the possibility of assault. Offenders typically rape more than once.

Often rape occurs by an acquaintance of the victim. These occurrences take place among individuals who are known to each other as friends. They may be having a "dating" relationship. At some point in the relationship the male forces the female against her will to engage in sexual acts as part of the dating relationship. This form of rape has come to be known as *date rape.*

Although most people think of the female as the typical victim, rape of males also occurs. Male rape is usually more violent and often involves gang rape.

Rape takes a serious toll on its victims: physiologically, emotionally, and mentally. It usually has a profound and prolonged impact on the victim. The crisis resulting from sexual assault can be divided into two phases: (1) the initial experience, the confrontation, or the acute phase and (2) the long-term effect or reorganization phase. The initial crisis necessitates encouraging the victim to seek medical treatment following the assault. It must be remembered that during this period the victim often experiences personal shock and trauma. There is a need for the medical care provider to be gentle and tactful. Some have recommended that, in the case of rape of a female, it is wise to have available the services of a female physician. It is essential that the medical examination be accomplished in private. Rape victims are usually given antibiotics during the examination to prevent sexually transmitted diseases. Pelvic examinations provide evidence that rape has taken place. However, such an examination is effective only for a short period of time as sperm and semen will only be found for about seventy-two hours. Other physical injuries, bruises, and cuts must also be treated at this time.

Although rape is a violation of one's physical person, the resulting emotional and psychological factors can require long-term care. Emotional reactions of the victim such as shock, disbelief, confusion, and fear are often found among rape victims. In an effort to help the victim overcome these problems, counseling is required.

Following the physical care, effective social counseling services can be most helpful. The victim should be referred to a local rape counseling service. The individual will need to express and work through the various feelings of anger, fear, hurt, and mistrust that usually follow such an assault.

Rape is a legal crime. Health care providers are required to report to law enforcement authorities all criminally caused injuries. In any case involving sexual assault, the medical personnel must be careful in the collection and transfer of specimens that may be used in legal documentation. Health care providers need appropriate education in helping the victim of sexual assault.

All too often the offender is never punished for the act of sexual assault. This may be the result of overburdened court schedules, improperly gathered evidence, or the failure of the victim to testify against the rapist. The importance of stricter punishment for the act of rape was noted in a summary statement of the Surgeon General's Workshop on Violence and Public Health in 1985:[15]

". . . the criminal justice system should clearly recognize sexual assault as a serious violent crime; that sanctions, including incarceration, should be imposed upon assailants commensurate with the devastating impact of the crime upon their victims; and that treatment to prevent future criminal behavior be part of sentencing wherever possible."

Suicide

Suicide is a major problem of violence. On one hand, we are confronted with behavior that demands our understanding, concern, and help. On the other hand, suicide is a topic about which most people in the United States would rather not talk. For many there are misunderstandings, numerous misconceptions, and even fear of the topic of suicide.

It is difficult getting an accurate indication as to how widespread the incidence of suicide is in American society. The National Center for Health Statistics reports that over twenty-eight thousand persons a year commit suicide.[16] However, the American Association of Suicidology has estimated that approximately fifty thousand persons commit suicide annually in the United States. Both statistics may be greatly underestimated. Many suicides will never be reported as such. They will be identified as accidental death or be listed as death from some other cause. What is known is that suicide rates are increasing among all age groups and racial groups, regardless of economic status and sex.

Though suicide occurs in all population groups, it is of particular concern for the teen population and young adults. It is known that suicide is the second leading cause of death among adolescents, with as many as five thousand successful suicides a year. Suicide rates in the past fifteen years among the 15- to 24-year age group have increased 37.5 percent. The major population involved in this rise has been white males.[17]

For many it seems difficult to understand why a person in the prime of life should desire to take his or her life. The youth during these years experience numerous conflicts that seem to be insurmountable. Such pressures may be financial or social—the loss of an important relationship, a feeling of isolation from and by their parents, and pressures concerning academic performance and a sense of not belonging.

Attempted suicide is often a cry for help. Those working in school settings, health agencies, family care agencies, and other community settings must become aware of the various warning signs of the potential suicide. Numerous signs have been identified of potential suicidal behavior. One indication of potential suicide is that the individual tends to take actions directed toward the cessation of living. This is noticed as the individual cuts himself or herself off from some important portion of life. Often noticed is the failure to expose oneself to situations which in some way may be painful, either physically or emotionally. This may be seen in the student who is increasingly absent from classes or the employee who fails to perform at work as previously.

Another sign in a case of potential suicide is depression. Depression may have developed over the long-term or it can have very short onset. Depression may manifest itself in feelings of sadness, by tears, diminished interest in life, and feelings of failure.

Physical signs of suicidal tendency may be seen in sleep disturbance, an unkempt appearance, and agitation. Problems with weight are often noticed among the suicidal behavior. This may take the form of excessive or compulsive eating.

Another phenomenon that is often noticed is that the suicide victim may have spent time in putting personal affairs in order. This may take the form of paying outstanding bills or taking out a will. It can involve making plans and arrangements for one's funeral. It has been noted that in some instances the suicide victim says "good-bye" to certain people. It is quite common at this time for the individual to give away things that have been particularly meaningful, such as money, a prized picture, or something simply of personal value.

The act of suicide may include several different practices. Males tend to use more violent measures. The firearm is the chief suicide method used among males, with hanging second. Females tend to use more passive measures, such as medicines or poisons. Slitting wrists is another, more violent procedure used by females.

There is great need in the United States for personnel and facilities which can provide assistance to potential suicide victims and counsel to the relatives and friends of suicide victims. Professionals involved in community health, medicine, schools, or social agencies must become aware of the many factors associated with suicide and be equipped to help those in need.

Suicide prevention and crisis intervention centers can be found in many communities throughout the United States. These centers provide a place where the individual can get emergency help in times of suicidal crises. The basic purpose of suicide prevention centers is to stop individuals from carrying out plans to kill themselves. These centers provide twenty-four-hour calling service, which gives the individual in crisis someone to talk with. It provides opportunity to arrange professional help, medical care, or other desired assistance.

Volunteers often play an important role in a suicide prevention or crisis intervention center. This person often is the "first line of defense." A call is made and the individual on the phone, often a volunteer, will listen, talk, and refer the patient as needed. The volunteer needs to be sensitive and show understanding to the individual in crisis.

Homicide

The eleventh leading cause of death in the United States is homicide. Approximately 24,000 individuals die at the hands of another person annually, resulting in 690,000 potential years of lost life.[18] The greatest number of homicides occur among the young, minorities, and males; the homicide rate is four times greater for men than women.

Homicides are committed by knifings, beatings, strangulations, and firearms. Two out of every three homicides are the result of firearm use. Increased possession of weapons in American society has aggravated the problem.

Several factors are related to homicide and aggravated assaults. Drug dealing is a leading factor. Arguments over money, "turf" in the drug dealership, and other factors all too often end in shootings, stabbings, and beatings.

Robbery is another important factor. When individuals are unemployed, there is a high risk factor of robbing people or institutions. All too often the robbery ends in a homicide.

Homicides also occur when people are involved in arguments and disputes. Nearly half occur where the victim and perpetrator are known or related to each other. It is estimated that less than 15 percent of all homicides occur between strangers. In the remaining third the relationship is unknown.[19]

Alcohol is a factor in a great number of homicides. Alcohol increases the likelihood of risk taking and provocative behavior. Inhibitions often are lessened, leading to irrational and nonnormal behavior. Alcohol presence is common in the blood of a high percentage of homicide victims.

The homicide rate is six times greater among black males, between the ages of 15 and 24, than among the nonblack population.[20] It is the leading cause of death for black males in this age group. Numerous socioeconomic factors have been identified that account for this. Unemployment, with accompanying stresses that lead to robbery and alcohol and drug usage, is possibly the leading factor.

The Surgeon General's Task Force on Violence and Public Health addressed a number of the issues related to homicide.[21] This task force recommended specific actions that need to be implemented in communities across the nation. One recommendation stated that services should be available in communities to help both the relatives and associates of victims of homicide and aggravated assault, as well as the individuals themselves. Development of victim assistance programs was given high priority.[22]

Numerous agencies and organizations in communities throughout the country can play important roles. In addition to the health care profession and community health organizations, religious organizations, educational institutions, and criminal justice agencies can develop appropriate activities.

If any improvement in the problem of homicide and aggravated assault is to occur, efforts must take place to meet the underlying causes and risk factors associated with the problem. This will mean actions in the socioeconomic dimension as well as a serious rethinking of the need for some type of control of the weapons that are used in such assaults.

Gun Control Legislation: Yes or No?

A major controversial issue in the United States for more than twenty years has centered around gun control legislation. Should the federal government or state governments pass legislation that would ban the ownership of firearms? Particular concern is expressed about the possession of handguns.

Americans own some ninety million firearms. More than thirty thousand people are killed each year by guns. Although a number of these fatalities occur each year to individuals involved in accidents while hunting, a major percentage of these deaths occur in homicides and suicides. One-third of all homicides and suicides are committed with firearms, resulting in death to over twenty thousand individuals annually.

Thousands of innocent poeple are killed each year at the hand of another by the use of guns. It may be a star basketball player near his school in Illinois, the supervisor of several employees in Oklahoma, or a drug-related death in New York. Regardless of the circumstances, firearm violence results in the loss of many years of potential life productivity in the United States. It is estimated that more than 1.2 million years of potential life are lost annually due to suicides and homicides.[23]

Evidence is quite strong that in nations with bans on the possession of firearms the incidences of homicide are significantly lower. For instance, more than ten thousand homicides occur annually in the United States due to the use of firearms, while in Japan, which prohibits firearm possession, there were less than fifty homicides by firearms in 1980.[24] The same conclusion can be reached by comparing United States homicide statistics with Canada and various European nations that have firearm ban legislation.

Support for gun control legislation seems to expand after the assassination, or attempted assassination, of a leading public personality. This was seen in the 1960s with the assassinations of the Rev. Martin Luther King, of President John F. Kennedy, and his brother, Robert F. Kennedy. In the 1970s the attempted assassination of President Gerald Ford and the same action in the 1980s against President Ronald Reagan focused attention on the need for gun control legislation.

On the other hand, there is regularly strong opposition against any type of firearm control in the United States. Many people point out the constitutional right that all citizens have to own and have possession of firearms. Nationally, a leading lobby effort against gun control has been led by the National Rifle Association. This association has been instrumental in arguing against such legislation.

Declaring that there is little use for handguns other than as directed toward other humans, in 1985 the Surgeon General's Workshop on Violence and Public Health published a call for a ban on the sale, manufacture, importation, and possession of handguns.[25] The report called for criminal penalties against individuals who are in possession of any firearm where alcohol is sold or served. Alcohol consumption, firearm possession, and related interpersonal violence are very serious problems.

Summary

Violence has been a part of human existence since the beginning of time. Although natural occurrences have killed and maimed millions, it is interpersonal violence which must be understood and controlled by man. Numerous agencies and organizations play important roles in providing services to the victims of violence as well as to those who commit the violence. A need exists to encourage the cooperation and integration of services of these different agencies.

Interpersonal violence includes child abuse, spouse abuse, and elder abuse. Each victim can be abused physically and emotionally. Physical abuse is probably the most easily identifiable. Neglect is less identifiable but may be just as serious. Emotional or psychological abuse often is an accumulation of years of actions and attitudes that lead to feelings of unimportance and low self-esteem for the victim.

Sexual abuse is a tragic form of violence. The incidence of child sexual abuse has increased significantly in recent years, with a majority of victims offended by relatives or acquaintances. Rape is another form of sexual abuse. Though a majority of instances of rape occur to women, male rape is increasing.

Numerous reasons can be identified for abuse. The abused, as well as the abusers, need the help of various professionals. Legislation at both the national and state levels now makes it mandatory that when there is evidence of abuse, caretakers must report it. The particular agencies to whom reports must be filed differ from one jurisdiction to another. However, all health care workers, educational personnel, social workers, religious leaders, and others involved in community work must be aware of their responsibilities.

Probably the ultimate tragedy of interpersonal violence is aggravated assault and homicide. Numerous causes for this type of violence can be identified. Though homicide occurs to all age and racial groups, it is a particular problem for young, nonwhite, minority populations. Within the black 15- to 24-year age group, homicide is the leading cause of death.

The issue of gun control in the United States has been a controversial matter for many years. There is no question that a majority of homicides and many suicides result from the use of firearms. Suicide, while not interpersonal violence in the strict sense, does result in the loss of life and accompanying loss of productive life years.

The importance for action in health promotion and disease prevention programming and planning related to violence was set forth in 1979 when the federal government identified several specific objectives to be achieved by the year 1990 related to homicide, child abuse, and suicide. A multidisciplinary approach to program development is needed where the various factors associated with violence, such as poverty, social isolation, stress, and socioeconomic problems are addressed.

Discussion Questions

1. Why should the matter of interpersonal violence be a programmatic concern to the field of community health?

2. Discuss and differentiate the various types of child abuse.

3. What are some of the long-term effects of sexual abuse on children?

4. Identify some of the factors that tend to contribute to child abuse.

5. Discuss the various legislative provisions for reporting child abuse. What are the provisions in your particular state?

6. Why is it difficult to obtain accurate data on the incidence of any type of abuse: child abuse, spouse abuse, and elder abuse?

7. Discuss some of the different forms that spouse abuse takes.

8. Identify some of the preventive measures that can be taken to reduce the likelihood of abuse.

9. What are some unique factors of elder abuse that do not relate to either child or spouse abuse?

10. It is stated that "rape is a legal crime." Discuss the ramifications of this statement.

11. Identify some of the signs and indications of potential suicidal behavior.

12. What are the significance and value of suicide prevention and crisis intervention centers?

13. Identify some of the risk factors related to homicides.

14. Why is homicide a particular problem among the young, nonwhite, minority population in the United States?

15. Discuss some of the controversy over gun control legislation.

Suggested Readings

Alexander, Greg R., and others. "Firearm-Related Fatalities: An Epidemiologic Assessment of Violent Death." *American Journal of Public Health* 75, no. 2, (February, 1985): 165–68.

Bhatia, Subhash C.; Khan, Mujeeb H.; and Sharma, Arum. "Suicide Risk: Evaluation and Management." *American Family Physician* 34, no. 3 (September, 1986): 169–74.

Blair, Kathryn. "The Battered Woman: Is She a Silent Victim?" *Nurse Practitioner* 11, no. 6 (June, 1986): 38–47.

Boulette, Teresa Ramirez, and Anderson, Susan M. "Mind Control and the Battering of Women." *Community Mental Health Journal* 21, no. 2 (Summer, 1985): 109–18.

Burgess, Ann W. "Resisting Rape Without Getting Killed." *American Journal of Nursing* 85, no. 9 (September, 1985): 947–48.

Cron, Ted. "The Surgeon General's Workshop on Violence and Public Health: Review of the Recommendations." *Public Health Review* 101, no. 1 (January/February, 1986): 8–14.

Fulmer, Terry, and Wetle, Terrie. "Elder Abuse: Screening and Intervention." *The Nurse Practitioner* 11, no. 5 (May, 1986): 33–38.

Goodman, R., and others. "Alcohol Use and Interpersonal Violence: Alcohol Detected in Homicide Victims." *American Journal of Public Health* 76, no. 2 (February, 1986): 144–49.

Herman, Judith, and others. "Long-Term Effects of Incestuous Abuse in Childhood." *American Journal of Psychiatry* 143, no. 10 (October, 1986): 1293–96.

Matlaw, Jane R., and Mayer, Jane B. "Elder Abuse: Ethical and Practical Dilemmas for Social Work." *Health and Social Work* 11, no. 2 (Spring, 1986): 85–93.

Payne, Jennie S., and others. "Helping the Abused Woman." *Nursing* 16, no. 9 (September, 1986): 53.

Phillips, Linda R., and Rempusheski, Veronica F. "A Decision-Making Model for Diagnosing and Intervening in Elder Abuse and Neglect." *Nursing Research* 34, no. 3 (May/June, 1985): 134–39.

Rosenberg, Mark L. "Surveillance for Suicide, Homicide, and Domestic Violence: Strengths, Weaknesses, and Issues." *Public Health Reports* 100, no. 6 (November/December, 1985): 593–95.

Rosenburg, Marcia S. "Rape Crisis Syndrome." *Medical Aspects of Human Sexuality* 20, no. 3 (March, 1986): 65–71.

Salend, Elyse, and others. "Elder Abuse Reporting: Limitations of Statutes." *The Gerontologist* 24, no. 1 (1984): 61–69.

Strange, Cheri. "An Overview of Incest in Current American Society." *The Prenatal Journal* 9, no. 4 (Fall, 1986).

Stever, J., and Austin, E. "Family Abuse of the Elderly." *Journal of the American Geriatric Society* 28 (1980): 372–76.

Surgeon General's Workshop on Violence and Public Health: Report. DHHS Publication No. HRS-D-MC, 86–1, (May, 1986).

Endnotes

1. Department of Health and Human Services. *Promoting Health, Preventing Disease: Objectives for the Nation.* Washington, D.C.: U.S. Government Printing Office, Fall, 1980: 85.

2. *The Status of Children, Youth, and Families.* Washington, D.C.: U.S. Government Printing Office, 1979: 111.

3. Strange, Cheri. "An Overview of Incest in Current American Society." *The Prenatal Journal* 9, no. 4 (Fall, 1986): 8.

4. Ibid., 8.

5. Blair, Kathryn. "The Battered Woman: Is She a Silent Victim?" *Nurse Practitioner* 11, no. 6 (June, 1986): 38.

6. Department of Health and Human Services. *Surgeon General's Workshop on Violence and Public Health: Report.* DHHS Publication No. HRS–D–MC 86–1, (May, 1986): 12.

7. Ibid., 12.

8. Blair, Kathryn. "The Battered Woman." 40.

9. Ibid., 44.

10. Department of Health and Human Services. *Surgeon General's Workshop.* 73.

11. Matlaw, Jane R., and Mayer, Jane B. "Elder Abuse: Ethical and Practical Dilemmas for Social Work." *Health and Social Work* 11, no. 2 (Spring, 1986): 85.

12. Mildenberger, C., and Wessman, H. "Abuse and Neglect of Elderly Persons by Family Members." *Physical Therapy* 66 (April, 1986): 537.

13. Department of Health and Human Services. *Surgeon General's Workshop.* 64.

14. Ibid., 69.

15. Ibid., 70.

16. Centers for Disease Control. Annual Summary 1984: Reported Morbidity and Mortality in the United States. *Morbidity and Mortality Weekly Report* 33, 54 (March, 1986): 114.

17. Ibid., 116.

18. Department of Health and Human Services. *Surgeon General's Workshop.* 11.

19. Rosenberg, Mark L. "Surveillance for Suicide, Homicide, and Domestic Violence: Strengths, Weaknesses, and Issues." *Public Health Reports* 100, no. 6 (November/December, 1985): 593–95.

20. Centers for Disease Control. Annual Summary 1984: 91.

21. Department of Health and Human Services. *Surgeon General's Workshop.* 49–54.

22. Ibid.

23. Centers for Disease Control. Annual Summary 1984: 120.

24. Department of Health and Human Services. *Surgeon General's Workshop.* 16.

25. Ibid., 53.

Epilogue: You . . . and Community Health

Each person reading this book has specific health needs, problems, interests, and concerns. Your skill in coping with your individual health is dependent on a number of variables, including economic considerations, individual values, personal knowledge, and background.

However, no one lives in a vacuum unaffected by the world and the environment. Throughout our daily activities we interact within numerous "communities." But for the most part, the focus of our concern for health is on self. We seek health care for ourselves and our families. In much of America this is accomplished through the private, fee-for-service model of health care. We do not give community health serious thought unless we cannot cope with our own health problems.

With increased urbanization, rising health care costs, and greater mobility and social concern, the fact that each of us is a part of several "communities of solution" to specific health problems necessitates a clear understanding of community health. Community health is not just providing programs for the poor or the underprivileged. Nor is it the establishment of programs funded and operated by government for the provision of health care. Community health must be viewed in terms other than curative medicine. Preventive medicine and primary health care are seen today as important foundations of the health status of our communities and individuals within those settings. Community health should include various dynamics focusing upon wellness promotion that results in good health for all.

Community health is also more than disease control and ensuring a sanitary environment as was once the case. It is no longer a discipline based solely upon the foundations created by biomedical research and development, though these are still important and necessary. Medicine and health care have long been associated with the physical sciences.

Health and wellness increasingly are recognized as having social dynamics. This means that the social sciences will play important roles in improving the health status and behavior of citizens in our communities. The dimensions of political involvement, economics, and cultural awareness as they relate to health and wellness must be understood.

Community health is a dynamic, changing discipline which is influenced by not only the findings of biomedical research but, more importantly, by the social sciences. Nowhere is this more obvious than in the political spectrum. The swing of political philosophy toward a government-programmed, semi-regulated, and funded provision of health care services in the 1960s and 1970s brought significant attention to community health. It caused many to speak of the need for a national health insurance or a national health care system. The "rights" of all people to receive preventive and curative health care were viewed as a foundation for such national programs.

With a feeling that the programs of the 1960s and 1970s were ineffective in eradicating many problems, the political philosophy changed in the early 1980s. The new political philosophy suggested that health, economic, and other problems could best be resolved by the private sector rather than by the government. The result was reduced federal spending. Many regulations that had been established by governmental agencies were abolished or reduced.

The political thinking left a huge vacuum for many community health professionals, as well as many consumers. The nation had become so accustomed to government support and so oriented to governmental programming and regulation that alternatives were hard to identify. Thus, many in the field of community health reacted negatively to the government action and did not think creatively in new directions.

What is needed in the near future, in the 1990s, and into the twenty-first century, are creative approaches in community health programming and the provision of health care. It will mean development of new skills with new technology. By the year 2000, it is possible that organ transplants will be taking place with the use of connecting tubes. It will probably be possible to replace virtually every body organ. Today there is research in process attempting to develop artificial ear implants, red blood cells, and blood vessels. Work is also ongoing in the hopes of developing an implantable artificial lung and an artificial eye that are stimulated by electrodes implanted in the brain.

In the future, laser surgery will replace the need to cut open a person to perform surgery. Gene therapy, a procedure of replacing defective genes with nondefective ones, could reduce most genetics-related problems. It is likely that there will be as much technological development in the next decade as in all of the past century.

Computers will increasingly be used to operate various defective body parts. The role of computer technology in the field of community health has only begun to be explored. As the young generation becomes proficient with computers and other technological advances, it will mean drastic revamping of programming in community health.

It can be assumed that neither a national health program nor total reliance on the private sector will be effective in solving community health problems in the future. Nations having national health insurance or health care programs have not been able to solve the same problems faced by the United States nor have they been able to control the rising costs of health care. Cost containment is every bit as much of a concern in other developed, industrial nations as it is in our country. These nations have not solved the problems of maldistribution of health care services and facilities. The poor and disadvantaged, as well as those living in rural localities, often are as poorly served there as they are in the United States.

Just as one cannot expect national health programs to be totally successful, neither can it be expected that the private sector will be able to totally solve community health problems. Much of the private sector operates on the economic principle of profit and loss. It is impossible economically, and wrong morally, to suggest that the community health problems should be looked at from a profit point of view. The health, or lack thereof, of an individual, or a group of persons, should not be directly affected by an individual or an organization trying to make a profit.

Another component of the private sector, the volunteer movement, cannot be expected to totally solve the nation's community health problems. Though the volunteer movement has been very effective in the health fields, it is not possible to depend on volunteers to accomplish a task so complex as the provision of health for all.

New, different, and creative models of health care provision, community health services, and programming must be at the forefront in the years ahead. Whether traditional approaches found in community health will be effective remains doubtful. It seems likely that whatever model or models become the norm, they must be based upon sociological, economical, and political dynamics.

Only as "bridges" are built will the chasm be crossed, or narrowed, between medical technology and the state of well-being.[1] No single force is going to bridge the gap between existing health knowledge, skills, and technology on one hand, and the availability of adequate health care for all on the other. As has been indicated, economic and political concerns and attention to social and cultural values must be considered.

---

[1]Concept of the Great Chasm discussed in chapter 1.

A higher degree of wellness must be the ultimate goal for all people. Community health will need to present a model or several models to achieve that goal. The chasm can be bridged or filled. It will take creative thinking, new models of community health programming, and concern for the fellow man and woman in our communities and on our planet. Only as each of us moves and interacts within our various communities, developing an understanding and concern for the well-being of others, will effective community health be achieved. This is the future challenge for you . . . and community health.

Appendix: References

Corporate Organizations

Abbott Laboratories
Professional Relations D-383
Abbott Park, Ill. 60064

Aetna Life and Casualty
151 Farmington Ave.
Hartford, Conn. 06156

American Automobile Association
8111 Gatehouse Road
Falls Church, Va. 22047

Cereal Institute
1111 Plaza Drive
Schaumberg, Ill. 60195

Consumers Union
256 Washington Street
Mount Vernon, N.Y. 10550

Eli Lilly and Company
Public Relations Service Dept.
307 E. McCarty Street
Indianapolis, Ind. 46285

FMS Productions, Inc.
1777 North Vine St.
Los Angeles, Calif. 90028

Metropolitan Life Insurance Company
Health and Safety Education Division
One Madison Avenue
New York, N.Y. 10010

Sunburst Communications
Room G1414
39 Washington Avenue
Pleasantville, N.Y. 10570

National Dairy Council
6300 North River Road
Rosemont, Ill. 60018-4233

Governmental

Environmental Protection Agency
Washington, D.C. 20460

Food and Drug Administration
Washington, D.C.

National Center for Health Education
30 East 29th St.
New York, N.Y. 10016

National Clearinghouse for Alcohol Information
P.O. Box 2345
Rockville, Md. 20852

National Clearinghouse for Drug Abuse Information
P.O. Box 416, Dept. DQ
Kensington, Md. 20795

National Council on the Aging
600 Maryland Avenue, SW
West Wing 100
Washington, D.C. 20024

National Health Information Clearinghouse
P.O. Box 1133
Washington, D.C. 20013

Professional Organizations

American Academy of Dermatology
8120 Davis
Evanston, Ill. 60201

American Academy of Pediatrics
141 Northwest Point Boulevard
Elk Grove Village, Ill. 60007

American Dental Association
211 East Chicago Avenue
Chicago, Ill. 60611

American Dietetic Association
430 No. Michigan Ave.
Chicago, Ill. 60611

American Hospital Association
840 North Lake Shore Drive
Chicago, Ill. 60611

American Medical Association
Department of Health Education
535 N. Dearborn Street
Chicago, Ill. 60610

American Optometric Association
243 Lindberg Blvd.
St. Louis, Mo. 63141

American Pharmaceutical Association
2215 Constitution Avenue, NW
Washington, D.C. 20036

American Podiatry Association
20 Chevy Chase Circle, NW
Washington, D.C. 20015

American Psychiatric Association
1400 K Street NW
Washington, D.C. 20005

American Public Health Association
1015 15th Street NW
Washington, D.C. 20005

American School Health Association
P.O. Box 708
Kent, Oh. 44240

National League of Nursing, Inc.
Ten Columbus Circle
New York, N.Y. 10019

Voluntary Health Organizations

Alcoholics Anonymous
468 Park Avenue South
New York, N.Y. 10016

American Association for Maternal and Child Health,
Inc.
233 Prospect P. 209
LaJolla, Calif. 92037

American Association for Suicidology
2459 So. Ash
Denver, Colo. 80222

American Cancer Society
(contact state and/or local chapter)

American Cleft Palate Association
331 Salk Hall
University of Pittsburgh
Pittsburgh, Pa. 15261

American Diabetes Association
2 Park Avenue
New York, N.Y. 10016

American Heart Association
7320 Greenville Avenue
Dallas, Tex. 75231

American Lung Association
(contact state and/or local chapter)

American Social Health Association
260 Sheridan Avenue, Suite 307
Palo Alto, Calif. 94306

Association for Voluntary Sterilization
122 East 42nd St.
New York, N.Y. 10168

Cystic Fibrosis Foundation
6000 Executive Blvd.
Suite 510
Rockville, Md. 20852

March of Dimes, Birth Defects Foundation
Public Health Education Department
1275 Mamaroneck Avenue
White Plains, N.Y. 10605

National Hemophilia Foundation
19 West 34th St., Suite 1204
New York, N.Y. 10001

National Kidney Foundation
2 Park Avenue
New York, N.Y. 10016

National Mental Health Association
1021 Prince Street
Alexandria, Va. 22314

National Multiple Sclerosis Society
205 East 42nd St.
New York, N.Y. 10017

Planned Parenthood Federation of America
810 Seventh Avenue
New York, N.Y. 10019

Sex Information and Education Council of the United
States
80 Fifth Avenue
Suite 801–802
New York, N.Y. 10011

Sierra Club
530 Bush Street
San Francisco, Calif. 94108

United Cerebral Palsy Association, Inc.
66 East 34th St.
New York, N.Y. 10016

Glossary

A

Abortion Spontaneous or induced termination of a pregnancy before the fetus can survive by itself outside the womb

Acid rain Polluted rainfall resulting when the oxides of sulfur and nitrogen react with water vapor in the atmosphere and form acids

Acquired Immune Deficiency Syndrome (AIDS) Virus-caused illness characterized by a specific defect in the human body's natural immunity against disease

AIDS related complex (ARC) The presence of the HIV virus in an individual without the signs and symptoms associated with AIDS

Al-Anon A voluntary organization for relatives of alcoholic patients

Alcoholics Anonymous (AA) A voluntary fellowship of recovering alcoholics who come together to help each other stay away from the use of alcohol

Almshouses Facilities, such as jails or poorhouses, in which the mentally ill were kept in the early years of American and European history

Alzheimer's Disease Disorder of the elderly that produces memory loss and disorientation

AHEC Area Health Education Centers; program designed to encourage health care providers to work in medically underserved localities

Anorexia nervosa Eating disorder characterized by abnormal loss of weight and poor personal image of one's physical appearance

APHA American Public Health Association; professional organization of individuals employed in the various fields of community health

Asbestos A mineral used in various construction activities; ie. soundproofing and as a fireproofing agent

B

Bacteria Small, single-cell microorganisms, some of which cause diseases in humans

Barbiturates Drugs that depress the central nervous system to produce sleep or a quieting effect

Barden-LaFollette Act 1943 Federal legislation that provided for vocational counseling and training for the mentally ill

Battered wife syndrome Term used to refer to spouse abuse

BCG vaccine Vaccine that provides protection against tuberculosis

Beers, Clifford Author, in 1906, of *A Mind That Found Itself,* a classic of the state of affairs in mental hospitals at that time

Benign Noncancerous or nonmalignant

Bhopal City in India where a toxic gas accident killed hundreds in 1984

Black lung disease See pneumoconiosis

Brown lung disease See byssinosis

BSN (Bachelors of Nursing Degree) The bachelors of nursing degree earned upon completion of a four-year nursing degree program

Bubonic plague Disease transmitted to humans by fleas from infected rats; called "black death"

Bulimia Eating disorder characterized by binging, then purging by vomiting

Byssinosis Respiratory disease prevalent among textile workers; known as "brown lung disease"

C

Calorie Unit used to express the energy content of food; the amount of heat required to raise the temperature of a kilogram of water (2.2 pounds) one degree centigrade

Cannabis sativa   The Indian hemp plant from which marijuana is derived

Carbohydrate   Group of foods, such as sugars and starches, that contain only carbon, hydrogen, and oxygen; a major source of calories in an average diet

Carbon monoxide   A colorless, odorless gas that may cause death by asphyxiation

Cardiopulmonary resuscitation (CPR)   Basic emergency life support technique involving mouth-to-mouth breathing, or other ventilation technique and chest compression

Cataracts   A cloudiness or opacity of the lens of the eye that interferes with vision

Certificate-of-need (CON)   State laws that require state planning agency reviews and approval to spend capital expenditure monies

Cesarean section   Method of childbirth in which surgical incision is made in the abdominal and uterine walls to allow delivery of the fetus

Chlamydia   A sexually transmitted disease caused by the bacterium, *Chlamydia trachomatis*

Chernobyl   Location in the Soviet Union of a dangerous nuclear accident in 1986

Child sexual victimization   Term used to refer to sexual abuse of children and adolescents

Chloroquine   An antimalarial drug

Cholesterol   Substance found in the fatty parts of animal tissue and in egg yolks that contributes to atherosclerosis

Chronic disease   Disease that is long-term and permanent

Cirrhosis   Degenerative disease of the liver characterized by the destruction of liver cells and the formation of fibrous connective tissue; often associated with alcohol consumption

Clean Air Act   The principal federal legislation directed toward improving the air quality in the United States

Cocaine   Central nervous system stimulant extracted from the leaves of the coca plant

Cohort   The grouping of individuals who are free of the disease or problem being investigated in an epidemiological study

Communicable disease   Infection that is transmitted from human to human or from animal to human

Community Mental Health Services Act (1963)   Federal legislation that resulted in the establishment of community mental health centers throughout the country

Conception   Point in time when the sperm from a male is implanted into the egg of the female

Control group   The population in an experimental study that does not receive the specific treatment under examination

"Crack"   Smokable form of cocaine

Cross-sectional study   A type of retrospective study often used in epidemiological research

Crude birth rate   The standard statistical datum used for stating birth rates

Crude death rate   The standard statistical datum used for stating death rates

Curandero   Traditional healer using herbs and other modalities to cure various ailments; usually found in the Spanish-speaking countries of Central and South America

D

D.A.T.   Drugs, Alcohol, and Tobacco

Decibels (dbs)   Unit of measurement used to indicate the loudness (intensity) of sound

Decommission   Procedure of shutting down a nuclear power plant and closing its operation

Deinstitutionalization   Removal of the mentally ill from mental hospital institutions to community care facilities

Dental caries   Tooth decay

Depression   Abnormal state of sadness or feeling of dejection

Desertification   Process of land deterioration and encroachment of the desert into previously useful and productive lands

Detoxification   Process whereby a person who is physically dependent upon a drug is gradually withdrawn from the drug

Diagnostic related groups (DRGs)   A prospective system of reimbursement to health providers for Medicare patients

Diabetes   Disease in which the pancreas fails to produce sufficient insulin, causing an increase in blood-sugar level, or impairment of insulin activity

Dioxin   Toxic chemical associated with numerous health related problems in humans

Diphtheria   An infectious disease of the nose and throat

Doe v. Bolton   The case that the United States Supreme Court ruled on in 1973 that legalized abortion

Dracunuliasis   Parasitic disease transmitted by the guinea worm

Dram Shop Acts   Laws passed in some states which hold bartenders, servers of alcoholic beverages, and bar owners liable if they sell alcoholic beverages to an intoxicated person who later causes injury to a third person

E

Elisa test   Blood test to ascertain the presence of the HIV virus that causes AIDS

Emphysema   Chronic respiratory disease resulting from the loss of normal function of the lung tissue characterized by "wheezing" and difficult breathing

Environmental Protection Agency (EPA)   The principal governmental agency charged with maintaining environmental standards

Epidemiological model   The model used in epidemiological studies that includes the interrelationships between the host, the causative agent, and the environment

Epidemiology   Study of the occurrence of disease among people

Etiology   The cause of a specific disease

Experimental group   In an epidemiological study the group that receives the treatment being studied

Export cropping   Agricultural products are exported from Third World nations to developed nations rather than being used to feed the local population

F

Fee-for-service   Concept that an individual is obliged to pay for medical services rendered by a health care provider

Fetal Alcohol Syndrome   Condition in which babies are born with retardation and physical abnormalities resulting from alcohol consumption of the mother during pregnancy

Fetal death   A stillbirth

Fission   Splitting of the core of an atom when it is struck by a neutron

Fluoridation   Use of fluorides to provide protection against dental caries

Fomites   Inanimate objects or material on which disease-producing agents may be transmitted

Fungi   Parasitic, cellular organisms that lack chlorophyll

G

Galactosemia   Error of metabolism with inability to convert galactose to glucose

Gamma rays   One of the three kinds of radiation; has the ability to penetrate into the body

GMENAC   Graduate Medical Education National Advisory Committee; study of health manpower needs that was reported to the Secretary of Health and Human Services in 1980

Genital herpes   Infectious sexually transmitted diseases caused by a herpes simplex virus and characterized by painful blisters and lesions in the genital areas of both men and women

Gerontology   Study of the aging process

Glaucoma   Increased pressure of fluid within the eye that is a leading cause of blindness

Gonorrhea   Sexually transmitted disease that affects the genitourinary tract and is spread primarily through sexual intercourse

"Great Society" Program   Federal legislative program of the 1960s that resulted in establishment of federally funded and operated health and social service programs

Growing Healthy Curriculum Project   School health curriculum project combining the School Health Curriculum Project and the Primary Grades Curriculum Project

H

Health and Human Services, Department of   The federal cabinet level department responsible for health programming

Health Maintenance Organizations (HMOs)   An alternative system of health care where payment is made in advance on a fixed contract fee basis by a certain population

Health promotion   Term used to describe any combination of health education and related interventions designed to facilitate behavioral and environmental changes conducive to health

Hemoglobin   Substance in red blood cells that carries oxygen from the lungs to the tissues and gives blood its red color

Hepatitis   Inflammation of the liver caused by infection

Heroin   Narcotic synthesized from morphine

Hill-Burton Act   Legislation providing federal monies to construct and/or modernize health care facilities

Histoplasmosis   A fungal disease often marked by fever

Hispanic   Spanish-speaking population in the United States having come from Mexico, Puerto Rico, Cuba, and countries in Central and South America

HIV   The causative agent for Acquired Immune Deficiency Syndrome (AIDS)

Homeless   Individuals who find it necessary to live on the streets and in public shelters

Homicide   Taking the life of another person; the eleventh leading cause of death in the United States

Host   In an epidemiological study the group or individual affected by the causative agent

Hospital Survey and Construction Act   See Hill-Burton Act

Hydrocarbons   Compounds containing both hydrogen and carbon

Hypertension   High blood pressure

Hypothermia   An abnormally low body temperature

Hypothyroidism   Deficient secretion of hormones from the thyroid gland

I

Immunity   Resistance to disease and infection

Immunization   Process of providing protection against communicable diseases by use of killed or weakened strains of the causative agent to produce antibodies

Incest   Term used to refer to sexual abuse of children and adolescents; usually used when the abuser is a parent, guardian, or caretaker of the abused

Incubation period   Period of time from the invasion into the body of a causative agent until the first signs and symptoms of the disease appear

Indian Health Service   Principal federal agency providing health care for Native Americans

Individual Practice Association (IPA)   One of two types of health maintenance organizations; the HMO reimburses the physician on a fee-for-service basis

Industrial hygienist   Individual that deals with environmental factors in the workplace that may cause sickness and injury

Incidence rate   Numerical statistic used to express the number of cases that develop over a specific period of time

Infant mortality   Death that occurs in infants under one year of age

Influenza   A viral respiratory disease

Inpatient care   Medical care provided in the hospital

Intrauterine device   Small plastic or metal device inserted into the uterus to prevent pregnancy

J

"Joints"   Slang term used for marijuana cigarettes

K

Kwashiorkor   A protein deficiency disease often characterized by bloated stomachs among children

L

L.S.D.   Lysergic acid diethylamide, a potent hallucinogenic drug; sometimes referred to as "acid"

Lead   Chemical that causes various health problems

Leprosy   A communicable disease caused by mycobacterium leprae that affects the skin and peripheral nerves

Low infant birthweight   Weight at birth of less than 2,500 grams (5.5 pounds); popularly referred to as premature birth

M

MADD   Acronym for Mothers Against Drunk Driving, a voluntary group interested in solving the problem of drunken driving

Mainlining   The practice of injecting heroin directly into the vein

Malaria   Infectious disease caused by protozoan parasites within the red blood cells and transmitted by the bite of a mosquito

Malignant   Cancerous

Malnutrition   Poor nutrition resulting in the lack of essential nutrients

Marine Health Service   The forerunner of the Public Health Service

Maternal mortality   Death of a woman from causes associated with childbirth

Measles   Infectious disease causing eruption of small red spots on the skin, referred to as rubeola

Medical montris   Village health workers as they are referred to in Indonesia

Medicaid   Federal program of health insurance for certain low-income individuals

Medicare   Federal program of health insurance for the elderly

Mescaline   A hallucinogenic drug sometimes known as peyote

Metastasis   Transfer of cancerous cells through the bloodstream and lymphatic system to form a growth in another part of the body not directly connected to the original cancerous site

Metazoa   Animal organisms that can infect humans

Mumps   Contagious viral disease with inflammation and swelling of the parotid and other salivary glands, fever, and pain

N

Narcotics   Drugs that have a depressant effect on the central nervous system

National Health Service Corps   A federal program designed to encourage the placement of health manpower personnel in medically underserved areas

Neonatal death   Infant death that occurs within the first twenty-eight days after birth

New Federalism   Federal program of placing responsibility for planning, administration, and management of health and social service programs to the states; created the block-grant programs

Nicotine   A central nervous system stimulant that is present in the leaf of tobacco

Nitrogen oxides   Colorless, odorless gas making up most of the atmosphere and found in all living things

Norepinephrine   Neurotransmitter that is important in normal brain functioning that governs emotions

Nurse-midwives   Nurses with specialty training in the care and delivery of the pregnant woman

Nurse-practitioner   A health professional with specialty training beyond that of a registered nurse

Nursing home   The principal health care facility providing long-term care for the elderly

O

Occupational health nurse   A nurse who has specific training, experience, and skills unique to problems found in the industrial setting

Occupational physician   Medical doctor who services the medical needs in the occupational setting

Occupational Safety and Health Act   Federal legislation that established the Occupational Safety and Health Administration and the National Institute of Occupational Safety and Health

Official health organization   Health agency that receives a majority of its funding from tax sources

Omnibus Budget Reconciliation Act   Federal legislation that created the "block-grant" program

Onchocerciasis   A filarial disease caused by Onchocerca, a filarial parasitic worm; popularly known as "river blindness"

Oncology   The study of and treatment of cancer

Opiates   Drugs that are derived from opium, such as codeine, morphine, and heroin

Optometrist   A nonmedical doctor trained in the diagnosis of refractive errors of the eyes

Oral rehydration therapy (ORT)   An inexpensive, effective measure used to orally rehydrate patients. Procedure is particularly useful where children have suffered dehydration from diarrhea

OSHA   Term used to identify the Occupational Safety and Health Administration

Osteopathic medicine   The diagnosis and treatment of diseases with particular attention to impairments of the musculoskeletal system

Osteoporosis   Loss of bone or thinning of bones that can result in pain and disability

Otitis media   An inflammation of the middle ear

Outpatient care   Medical care provided in such a manner that the patient does not need to be hospitalized

Ozone   Photochemical oxidant formed when atomic oxygen combines with oxygen already in the atmosphere that irritates the lungs, eyes, and throat, damages plants, and causes rubber to crack and decompose

P

Particulate matter   Airborne particles of solid or liquid substances; soot, dirt, dust, fly ash

Pellagra   Dietary deficiency disease

Pelvic inflammatory disease (PID)   Severe inflammation of the upper part of the female reproductive system and the abdominal cavity

Pertussis   Whooping cough

Peyote   See mescaline

Phenylketonuria   Metabolic disorder caused by the absence of the enzyme phenylalanine hydroxylase

Philanthropic foundations   Nonprofit funding foundations that support a broad range of social, education, and health services

Physician's assistant   An individual with one to two years of specialty training who can provide primary health care under the supervision of a physician

Pneumoconiosis   Respiratory disease that results from exposure to various dusts, principally found among coal miners; known as "black lung disease"

Pneumonia   Inflammation of the lungs caused by bacteria, viruses, chemical irritants, and allergens

Podiatrist   An allied health professional who provides care and treatment of problems of the feet

Polychlorinated biphenyls (PCB)   Chemical compounds found in industrial products and wastes that may accumulate in animal tissue and cause birth defects and liver damage

Postpartum   That which occurs after childbirth; after the delivery

Prevalence rate   Statistical data that indicates the number of persons with a given problem at a particular point in time

Pro-Choice   Term used to describe those who favor abortion

Prohibition   Period of time in the 1920s when it was illegal to manufacture and market alcoholic beverages

Pro-Life   Term used by those who are opposed to abortion

Promotores del salud   Village health workers as they are referred to in Latin America

Prospective study   A type of epidemiological study that examines a given factor over a long-term period of time

Psychiatrist   A medical doctor whose specialty includes the diagnosis and treatment of emotional disturbances and mental disorders

Psychologist   An individual who studies the nonmedical science of human behavior

Public Health Service   Governmental agency that is part of the Department of Health and Human Services; principally responsible for maintaining and protecting the health of the American public

PVOs   Term used in international health work to designate those organizations in the private sector; private voluntary organizations, nongovernment agencies

R

Radioactivity   The release of radiation

Radon   An odorless, colorless, tasteless, natural radioactive gas that is produced naturally in the ground; the product of underground uranium decay

Rape   An act of violence involving sex or attempted sex without the consent of the victim

Recommended Dietary Allowances (RDAs)   Standards of adequate nutritional intake published by the Food and Nutrition Board of the National Research Council

"Reefers"   Slang term used for marijuana cigarettes

Respite care   Type of care for the elderly that provides periodic relief for the family; adult day-care centers

Retrospective study   In epidemiological study an observational technique in which the specific population group is examined for a particular factor under investigation

Roe v. Wade   The legal case upon which the United States Supreme Court ruled that abortion was legal

Roentgens   Basic unit of measurement of radiation

Rubella   Infectious disease causing eruption of small red spots on the skin; referred to as German measles; of shorter duration than rubeola

Rubeola   See measles

S

Saccharin   Artificial sweetening substance used as a substitute for sugar

SADD   Acronym for Students Against Drunk Driving, a voluntary group of adolescents interested in assuring that they will not drive intoxicated or ride with others who have been drinking

Safety engineer   Worker involved in dealing with potential hazards in the workplace

Salmonella   Most common cause of foodborne disease in the United States

Sanitarian   An individual employed by health departments to conduct environmental inspections and carry out sanitation measures as required by rules and regulations of the local and state health department

Sanitary landfill   Site where solid wastes are buried in layers under dirt as a means of waste disposal and land reclamation

Scurvy   A dietary deficiency disease resulting from inadequate ascorbic acid

Sedative   A drug that produces a calming effect, relaxes muscles, and relieves feelings of tension, anxiety, and irritability

Senile dementia   Results from narrowing of blood vessels that supply brain with oxygen

Schistosomiasis   Parasitic disease carried by snails that reside in slow-moving or stagnant water

Sickle-cell anemia   An inherited disorder of the red blood cells in which the normal flow of blood is blocked; this condition is found principally among the black population and those individuals from the Mediterranean region

Sidestream smoke   That smoke that affects the person in proximity to the individual who is smoking

Silicosis   Respiratory disease prevalent among workers exposed to silica

Smallpox   Acute, contagious disease (caused by a virus) that is characterized by fever, headache, abdominal pain, and lesions of the skin; has been eradicated since the early 1980s

Smokeless tobacco   Use of tobacco as snuff or chewing tobacco

Social Security   Social retirement insurance program for the elderly established by the federal government in 1935

Sodium   Salt

Stimulant   Drug that increases central nervous system function

Sudden Infant Death Syndrome (SIDS)   Condition in which a child dies unexpectedly from unknown causes, usually while asleep in bed

Suicide   The taking of one's own life

Superfund   Federally authorized fund to provide support for cleaning up toxic waste sources

Synanon   First therapeutic community program for drug addicts founded in 1959

Syphilis   Sexually transmitted disease that is spread by sexual contact

T

Temperance movement   A movement that started in the early 1800s that called for total abstinence from the use of alcohol; a leading organization in the movement to bring about Prohibition in the 1920s.

Temperature inversion   Meteorological condition in which cooler air becomes trapped under a warmer layer of air and the cooler layer becomes heavily polluted

Tetanus   Acute infectious disease caused by the toxin of *Clostridium tetani:* lockjaw

Tetrahydrocannabinol (THC)   Active ingredient in marijuana that causes the euphoric effects

Thalidomide   Tranquilizing drug taken by many pregnant women during the late 1950s that caused severe birth defects

Therapeutic community   Residential programs providing drug abuse treatment

Toxemia   Condition in which toxic substances are in the blood cells; caused by bacteria

Tuberculosis   Respiratory disease caused by the tubercle bacillus

Tumor   Abnormal, nonfunctional cell mass that grows independent of surrounding structures

Typhus   Acute infectious disease usually prevalent in unsanitary localities

V

Vaccine   Preparations of weakened or killed pathogens that stimulate antibody formation without causing observable signs of the disease

Vector   An organism that transmits a disease-producing microorganism

Veterans Administration   Operates a network of medical centers and clinics for former members of the military

Vinyl chloride   Toxic chemical that can cause respiratory distress in humans

Virus   Microscopic infectious organism that is parasitic and depends on nutrients inside cells for metabolic and reproductive survival

Voluntary health organizations   Nonprofit organizations whose programming involves much use of voluntary time and financial support from nongovernmental sources

W

W.I.C. A federally funded nutritional program for women, infants, and children

World Health Assembly The governing body of the World Health Organization

World Health Organization International health organization with headquarters in Geneva, Switzerland

Y

Yellow fever An acute viral disease that affects the liver and is transmitted by certain mosquitoes

Z

Zoonosis Animal diseases that can be transmitted to humans

Credits

Unless otherwise indicated all photographs are © Dean Miller.

Chapter 1
Page 7 left: UPI-Bettmann News Photos, **right:** © Rich Rosenkoetter; **page 9:** © Dean Miller photographed by James L. Shaffer; **page 13 top:** © Rick Smolan, **lower left:** White Coyote Enterprises, **lower right:** © James L. Shaffer.

Chapter 2
Pages 26, 27 all: Centers for Disease Control, Atlanta; **page 32 both lower:** National Institute of Health; **pages 35, 36, 39, 40:** National Institute of Health.

Chapter 3
Pages 58 all, 59, 60 all: Erie County General Health District; **pages 61, 62 both:** photograph provided by Health Commissioner, Fulton/Henry County Health Department, Ohio; **page 63:** Erie County General Health District; **page 64:** Photograph provided by Health Commissioner, Fulton/Henry County Health Department, Ohio.

Chapter 4
Pages 70, 78 both: WHO; **page 85 both:** WHO/Photo by Mr. Steve Pavik; **page 86:** WHO/UNICEF/ Photo by H. Cerni; **page 87:** WHO/FAO/F. Botts.

Chapter 5
Page 100: National Institute of Health; **page 102:** Kimberly-Clark Corporation; **page 105:** Veterans Administration.

Chapter 7
Page 142: Courtesy Veterans Administration; **page 144:** © James L. Shaffer; **pages 154, 155 both, 157:** Kaiser-Permanente Medical Care.

Chapter 8
Pages 168, 169: American Cancer Society; **page 170:** American Heart Association; **pages 171, 172:** American Cancer Society; **pages 173, 174:** Ohio Department of Education; **pages 179 both, 182:** provided by the W. K. Kellogg Foundation, Battle Creek, Michigan.

Chapter 9
Page 199: courtesy of HEW; **page 204:** courtesy of WHO.

Chapter 10
Page 215: © Michael DeSpezio; **page 219:** © EKM-Nepenthe; **page 224 both:** photographs provided by the Ohio Environmental Protection Agency, Northwest District Office.

Chapter 11
Page 237: American Heart Association; **pages 240, 241:** Erie County General Health District.

Chapter 12
Page 257: National Library of Medicine; **page 266 all:** National Institute of Mental Health; **page 267:** © David M. Grossman; **page 269:** © Cathy Cheney/EKM-Nepenthe.

Chapter 13
Page 279: W. K. Kellogg Foundation; **page 280:** Ohio Department of Education; **page 283:** © James L. Shaffer; **page 290:** Erie County General Health District; **page 291:** photograph provided by the Ohio Environmental Protection Agency, Northwest District Office.

Chapter 14

Page 303: W. K. Kellogg Foundation; **page 309 top:** American Heart Association, **bottom both:** W. K. Kellogg Foundation; **page 312:** Ohio Department of Education.

Chapter 15

Page 321: The National Council on Aging; **pages 325, 326:** © Donna Jernigan; **page 329:** © Bob Combs/ Free Vision; **page 332:** W. K. Kellogg Foundation.

Chapter 16

Page 340: © Ron Byers; **page 347:** © James L. Ballard; **page 351:** © Jean-Claude Lejeune.

Chapter 17

Page 358: National Institute of Health; **page 366:** Erie County General Health District; **page 368:** Veterans Administration; **page 369:** W. K. Kellogg Foundation; **page 370:** © Julie O'Neil.

Chapter 18

Page 378: © Chuck Isaacs; **page 385:** © Donna Jernigan.

Chapter 19

Page 407: UPI-Bettmann News Photos; **page 410:** Kimberly-Clark Corporation; **page 413:** American Red Cross.

Chapter 20

Pages 424–432: Courtesy of Julie Coyle.

Index